Headache

Blue Books of Practical Neurology
(Volumes 1–14 published as BIMR Neurology)

Headache

Edited by

Peter J. Goadsby MD, PhD, DSc, FRACP
Wellcome Senior Research Fellow and Reader in Clinical Neurology, University Department of Clinical Neurology, and Consultant Neurologist, Institute of Neurology, The National Hospital for Neurology and Neurosurgery, London

and

Stephen D. Silberstein MD, FACP
Clinical Professor of Neurology, Temple University School of Medicine, Philadelphia; Chief, Section of Neurology, and Co-Director, Comprehensive Headache Center, Germantown Hospital and Medical Center, Philadelphia

Butterworth-Heinemann
Boston   Oxford   Johannesburg   Melbourne   New Delhi   Singapore

Library of Congress Cataloging-in-Publication Data

Headache / edited by Peter J. Goadsby, Stephen D. Silberstein.
      p.   cm. -- (Blue books of practical neurology ; 17)
    Includes bibliographical references and index.
    ISBN 0-7506-9871-3
    1. Headache.   I. Goadsby, Peter J.   II. Silberstein, Stephen D.
   III. Series.
    [DNLM: 1. Headache. WI BU9749 v.17 1997 / WL 342 H43155 1997]
   RC392.H412   1997
   616.8'491--dc21
   DNLM/DLC
   for Library of Congress   96-50464
                                           CIP

British Library Cataloguing-in-Publication Data
A catalogue record for this book is available from the British Library.

The publisher offers special discounts on bulk orders of this book.
For more information, please contact:
Manager of Special Sales
Butterworth–Heinemann
313 Washington Street
Newton, MA 02158–1626
Tel: 617-928-2500
Fax: 617-928-2620

For information on all Butterworth-Heinemann medical publications available, contact our World Wide Web home page at: http://www.bh.com/med

10 9 8 7 6 5 4 3 2

Printed in the United States of America

Contents

Contributing Authors

Lea Averbuch-Heller MD
Assistant Professor of Neurology, Case Western Reserve University School of Medicine and University Hospitals of Cleveland, Cleveland

Nikolai Bogduk MD, PhD
Professor of Anatomy, Faculty of Medicine and Health Sciences, University of Newcastle, Newcastle, New South Wales, Australia; Visiting Medical Officer in Pain Management, Master Misericordiae Hospital, Newcastle

J. Keith Campbell MD
Emeritus Professor of Neurology, Mayo Medical School, Rochester, Minnesota

Richard J. Caselli MD
Associate Professor of Neurology, Mayo Medical School, Rochester, Minnesota; Consultant Neurologist, Mayo Clinic, Scottsdale, Arizona

James J. Corbett MD
McCarty Professor and Chairman of Neurology and Professor of Ophthalmology, University of Mississippi Medical Center, Jackson

F. Michael Cutrer MD
Instructor of Neurology, Harvard Medical School, Boston; Assistant in Neurology, Massachusetts General Hospital, Boston

Robert B. Daroff MD
Professor of Neurology and Associate Dean, Case Western Reserve University School of Medicine, Cleveland; Chief of Staff and Senior Vice President for Medical Affairs, University Hospitals of Cleveland

John Edmeads MD
Professor of Medicine (Neurology), University of Toronto Faculty of Medicine, Toronto, Ontario, Canada; Physician-in-Chief, Department of Medicine, Sunnybrook Health Science Center, University of Toronto

Michel D. Ferrari MD, PhD
Associate Professor of Neurology and Consultant Neurologist, Leiden University Hospital, Leiden, The Netherlands

Howard L. Fields MD, PhD
Professor of Neurology and Physiology, University of California, San Francisco, School of Medicine; Attending Neurologist, University of California, San Francisco, Hospitals and Clinics

Peter J. Goadsby MD, PhD, DSc, FRACP
Wellcome Senior Research Fellow and Reader in Clinical Neurology, University Department of Clinical Neurology, and Consultant Neurologist, Institute of Neurology, The National Hospital for Neurology and Neurosurgery, London

Steven B. Graff-Radford DDS
Adjunct Associate Professor of Orofacial Pain, UCLA School of Dentistry, Los Angeles; Director, The Pain Center, Cedars-Sinai Medical Center, Los Angeles

Joost Haan MD, PhD
Senior Researcher in Neurology, University Hospital, Leiden, The Netherlands; Neurologist, Rijnland Hospital, Leiderdorp, The Netherlands

Gene G. Hunder MD
Professor of Medicine, Division of Rheumatology, Mayo Medical School, Rochester, Minnesota; Consultant in Rheumatology and Internal Medicine, Mayo Clinic, Rochester

Lee Kudrow MD
Co-Director, California Medical Clinic for Headache, Encino, California

James W. Lance MD, FRCP, FRACP
Professor Emeritus of Neurology, University of New South Wales, Sydney, New South Wales, Australia; Consultant Neurologist, Institute of Neurological Sciences, Prince of Wales Hospital, Sydney

Christine L. Lay MClSc, MD
Department of Neurology, Mayo Clinic, Rochester, Minnesota

Volker Limmroth
Research Fellow, Department of Neurosurgery, Harvard Medical School and Massachusetts General Hospital, Boston

Richard B. Lipton MD
Professor of Neurology, Epidemiology, and Social Medicine, Albert Einstein College of Medicine, Bronx, New York; Co-Director, Headache Unit, Montefiore Medical Center, Bronx

Graeme R. Martin PhD
Head of Molecular Pharmacology Department, Institute of Pharmacology, Roche Bioscience, Palo Alto, California

George R. Merriam MD
Professor of Medicine, Obstetrics, and Gynecology, Division of Metabolism, Endocrinology, and Nutrition, University of Washington School of Medicine, Seattle

Bahram Mokri MD
Professor of Neurology, Mayo Medical School, Rochester, Minnesota; Consultant Neurologist, Mayo Clinic, Rochester

Michael A. Moskowitz MD
Professor of Neurology, Harvard Medical School, Boston; Director, Stroke and Neurovascular Regulation, Neuroscience Center, Massachusetts General Hospital, Boston

Lawrence C. Newman MD
Assistant Professor of Neurology, Albert Einstein College of Medicine, Bronx, New York; Director, Montefiore Headache Unit, Montefiore Medical Center, Bronx

Jes Olesen MD, DrMedSci
Professor of Neurology, University of Copenhagen, Copenhagen, Denmark; Chairman of Department of Neurology, Glostrup Hospital, Copenhagen

Russell C. Packard MD, FACP
Adjunct Professor of Psychology, University of West Florida, Pensacola; Director, Headache Management and Neurology, Pensacola

Stephen J. Peroutka MD, PhD
President and CEO, Spectra Biomedical, Inc., Menlo Park, California

Birthe Krogh Rasmussen MD, DrMedSci
University of Copenhagen, Copenhagen, Denmark; Neurologist, Hilleroed Hospital, Hilleroed, Denmark

Jean Schoenen MD, PhD
Clinical Professor of Neurology and Research Director, NFSR, University of Liège, Belgium; Clinical Professor of Neurology, CHR Citadelle, Liège

Stephen D. Silberstein MD, FACP
Clinical Professor of Neurology, Temple University School of Medicine, Philadelphia; Chief, Section of Neurology, and Co-Director, Comprehensive Headache Center, Germantown Hospital and Medical Center, Philadelphia

Walter F. Stewart PhD, MPH
Associate Professor of Epidemiology, Johns Hopkins University School of Medicine, Baltimore

Christian Waeber
Research Fellow, Department of Neurosurgery, Harvard Medical School and Massachusetts General Hospital, Boston

Wei Wang BMed, DSc
Department of Neurology, Anhui Provincial Hospital, Hefei, Anhui, China

William B. Young MD
Clinical Instructor of Neurology, Temple University School of Medicine, Philadelphia; Active Staff Neurologist and Co-Director, Comprehensive Headache Center, The Germantown Hospital and Medical Center, Philadelphia

Xian Yu
Research Fellow, Department of Neurosurgery, Harvard Medical School and Massachusetts General Hospital, Boston

Series Preface

The *Blue Books of Practical Neurology* series is the new name for the *BIMR Neurology* series, which was itself the successor to the *Modern Trends in Neurology* series. As before, the volumes are intended for use by physicians who grapple with the problems of neurologic disorders on a daily basis, be they neurologists, neurologists in training, or those in related fields such as neurosurgery, internal medicine, psychiatry, and rehabilitation medicine.

Our purpose is to produce monographs on topics in clinical neurology in which progress through research has brought about new concepts of patient management. The subject of each monograph is selected by the Series Editors using two criteria: first, that there has been significant advance in knowledge in that area and, second, that such advances have been incorporated into new ways of managing patients with the disorders in question. This has been the guiding spirit behind each volume, and we expect it to continue. In effect we emphasize research, both in the clinic and in the experimental laboratory, but principally to the extent that it changes our collective attitudes and practices in caring for those who are neurologically afflicted.

C. David Marsden
Arthur K. Asbury
Series Editors

Preface

As we approach the next millennium, neurologic practice will see the fruits of the developments in the basic neurosciences that have taken place in the last quarter of this century. Perhaps no single area of neurologic practice will have been so utterly transformed as that for the most common of the neurologic problems—headache. Headache is the last common neurologic problem to be added to the *Blue Books* series, a fact that reflects in some considerable measure the efforts of many who were asked to contribute to the volume.

Not so very long ago, diagnosis in headache was literally by ad hoc arrangements that, while stating some very clear truths, had little hope of underpinning careful clinical neuroscience. The impact of the disease was underestimated and ill-understood because it had never been subject to careful study, and to some extent because headache was the last of the "Cinderella" neurologic subspecialties. In the recent past, to speak of the anatomy and physiology of head pain might have seemed a delusion requiring psychiatric referral, much less to have an understanding at the molecular level of drug actions as we now have for the treatments of the acute attack migraine. Our authors now speak of genetics and pharmacology, but we have been careful not to abandon our clinical roots with the inclusion of the clinical manifestations of both primary and secondary headaches that confront many medical practitioners daily.

As we wrote this preface, the field evolved before us with the exciting and thought-provoking description of voltage-gated calcium channel abnormalities in patients with familial hemiplegic migraine (*Cell* 1996;87:543). At any point, a book can only reflect what was already known. We hope by covering a broad range of headache-related topics to provide a knowledge base to the reader and that this will be supplemented by the reader's ongoing interest and experience.

We have tried to recruit authors with particular interests to exercise their expertise. We are grateful that they did so with clarity and care. We thank them for their cooperation, particularly in response to our editorial suggestions, which we hope have given the volume the overall thrust that good patient care is based on knowledge of a condition and its treatments and that in the application of science to clinical practice, we should always remain focused on our patients.

Peter J. Goadsby
Stephen D. Silberstein

Headache

ONE

MIGRAINE

I
ISSUES IN BASIC NEUROSCIENCE

1
Pathophysiology of Migraine: A Disease of the Brain

Peter J. Goadsby

INTRODUCTION

An understanding of the pathophysiology of headache must be based on the anatomy and physiology of the pain-sensitive structures within the cranium. Such an approach may at first seem daunting; however, headache is by far the most common neurologic problem and as such merits some detailed attention. Time devoted to understanding migraine is particularly well spent when one attempts to match the patient's symptoms and signs to safe and effective therapeutic intervention.[1] In this chapter the pathophysiology is discussed against a clinical background so that the reader may see where new knowledge can be integrated into clinical practice.

WHAT CAUSES MIGRAINE: THE GENETICS OF HEADACHE

Migraine is predominantly an affliction of young people who are otherwise well, although it can be seen at virtually any age. The genetics of the disorder will be dealt with in detail elsewhere in this volume (Chapter 7). From a pathophysiologic viewpoint the genetic developments provide a substrate upon which one can integrate the available clinical data. The prevalence of a family history and early onset of the disorder suggest that there is a strong genetic component. Indeed the first description of a genetic locus for a migrainous disease, that of the location on chromosome 19p13 of the gene for familial hemiplegic migraine,[2] announced the beginning of a large effort to unravel the fundamental defect, or defects, that lead to migraine. Recent data have shown that not all patients with familial hemiplegic migraine map to this locus.[3] Regarding migraine with and without aura, some researchers suggest that migraine in certain families may also be linked to chromosome 19,[4] whereas others have found linkage to other regions (Chapter 7). Equally interesting is the description of a possible genetic contribution[5] to cluster headache (Chapter 13). Taken together, the clinical features suggest a subtle structural or functional defect that is not usually life-threatening. A useful clinical comparison may be with the so-called channelopathies, such as hyperkalemic periodic paralysis, paramyotonia congenita, hypokalemic periodic paralysis, myotonia congenita, and episodic ataxia with myokymia,[6] particularly because the gene for episodic ataxia with cerebellar vermal atrophy[7] is located on chromosome 19p.[8] In these disorders, patients have no abnormal symptoms between attacks yet have profound clinical problems during attacks. It is thus of great interest that it has been anecdotally reported that acetazolamide, which can be useful in some paroxysmal ataxias, is also useful in familial hemiplegic migraine. A patient thus inherits a diathesis or constitution that is liable to headache. This susceptibility is the basic neurobiology of migraine. The female predominance (Chapter 5) and the association with menstruation (Chapter 10) do not help to differentiate the site of the problem, since the hormonal changes described[9] could affect either neural or vascular structures.

PREMONITORY FEATURES

Approximately 25% of patients report symptoms of elation, irritability, depression, hunger, thirst, or drowsiness during the 24 hours preceding headache. Most of those manifestations can arise in the hypothalamus,[10] and this suggests a central site for their evolution. In addition, the suprachiasmatic nucleus of the hypothalamus[11] has been suggested as one of two primary oscillators in the generation of circadian rhythms[12] and thus could easily be implicated in the periodicity of migraine that is such an important clinical feature. The recent description of bilateral oligemia in a patient with migraine without aura, who complained only of visual blurring, may have significance to understanding the complex biology of the initiation of migraine attacks that goes beyond its contribution of information about aura since the patient did not have typical aura.[13] Much experimental work remains to be done in this area to understand the fundamental triggering process involved in migraine.

PRODROME OF MIGRAINE WITH AURA

Cerebral Blood Flow and the Aura

Numerous studies over some years have confirmed that the aura phase of migraine is associated with a reduction in cerebral blood flow.[14–27] Visual disturbances such as the scintillating scotoma (flashing lights that move across the visual field), paresthesias, or other focal neurologic signs are associated with this reduction in cerebral blood flow.[28] The flow change moves across the cortex as a "spreading oligemia" at 2–3 mm per minute,[28] corresponding to the rate that Lashley estimated from plotting the progression of his own visual aura[29] and the phenomenon of spreading cortical depression of Leão.[30,31] The patterns of blood flow changes that have been observed share some common threads.[32] First, there is a focal reduction in flow that usually occurs in the posterior cortex near Brodman area 7 and the superior part of area 19, although focal frontal oligemia without visual aura has been rarely reported.[33] Second, this reduction enlarges and may involve the whole hemisphere. The changes noted previously, first reported by Olesen and his colleagues, were produced by carotid angiography,[23] but similar changes have been seen in spontaneous attacks with single-photon emission computed tomography (SPECT).[34] The progression of the oligemia across the cortex does not respect vascular territories and is thus unlikely to be primarily vasospastic. Furthermore, there are reports that the oligemia is preceded by a phase of focal hyperemia.[28] Such a change is again exactly what would be expected if a phenomenon similar to cortical spreading depression was involved.[35] Following the passage of the oligemia, the cerebrovascular response to hypercapnia is blunted while autoregulation is intact.[36] Again this pattern is repeated in spreading depression.[35] Recently, the description of a patient with migraine without aura who had an attack during a positron-emission tomographic (PET) study[13] placed beyond doubt the phenomenon of spreading oligemia. Given these clear PET data and the observation of a patient without hypoxia, again using PET,[37] the earlier arguments that the spreading oligemia is due to Compton scatter and ischemia[27,38–40] can be consigned to the dustbin of scientific history. The new PET data did, however, raise a more interesting question. The patient studied did not have aura in any traditional sense; in fact, she had only some transient visual blurring. These data open up the exciting possibility that blood flow changes may occur in migraine both with and without aura. Indeed it is remarkable that a spreading oligemia can traverse cortex usually considered clinically eloquent and have few clinical sequelae. However, the flow–headache relationship is complex. Flow changes reported during aura are often accompanied by a contralateral aura, and the unilateral headache is then homolateral with respect to the oligemia; but patients have been reported to have unilateral headache with a homolateral aura, suggesting a mismatch of the aura with the subsequent headache.[28] Headache may begin while cortical blood flow is still reduced[28] and while bilateral flow changes can be seen, thus the suggestion that the pain arises from a primary vascular abnormality is untenable.

How Can Aura Data Be Reconciled in Humans?

The neurologic changes during aura parallel what is seen when the brain is directly stimulated[41,42] and resemble what might be predicted if ocular dominance columns[43] were serially activated. Direct attempts at measuring spreading depression in humans, either using electrophysiologic techniques[44] or laser Doppler flowmetry,[45] have been unsuccessful. Indirect measurements in humans—indirect because spreading depression is essentially defined by electrical events—give conflicting results. Welch and his colleagues, using magnetoencephalography, have shown that changes similar to those seen in rabbits undergoing spreading depression can be seen in humans, although the relative novelty of the method requires that further such observations be made.[46] Observations of a low intracellular magnesium in the occipital cortex of migraine patients have been seen in the clinical phenomenon of the migraine aura. A low intracellular magnesium would render the cortex more easily excitable via glutamate-activated N-methyl-

D-aspartate–mediated (NMDA-mediated) receptor mechanisms. Taken together, these factors suggest that spreading depression or a human homologue of spreading depression is the neurobiologic basis for aura in migraine. Spreading depression in humans, however, must be different in some yet-to-be-understood way from what is seen in animals, to account for the difficulty of observing it in vivo in humans. Integration of the cerebral blood flow and clinical aura data also leads to the inescapable conclusion that aura is not the initiator of a migraine attack but a parallel and not always present part of a larger syndrome. Moreover, it is most likely that the syndrome and the bulk of its manifestations are driven from within the central nervous system.

HEADACHE

Trigeminal Innervation of Pain-Sensitive Intracranial Structures

Surrounding the large cerebral vessels, pial vessels, large venous sinuses, and dura mater is a plexus of largely unmyelinated fibers that arise from the trigeminal ganglion[47] and, in the posterior fossa, from the upper cervical dorsal roots.[48,49] This plexus is seen in the monkey[50] and cat.[51] Tracing studies have shown that fibers innervating cerebral vessels arise from within the trigeminal ganglion from neurons that contain substance P and calcitonin gene-related peptide (CGRP),[52] both of which can be released when the trigeminal ganglion is stimulated either in humans or in cats.[53] Moreover, the cell bodies in the trigeminal ganglion are bipolar neurons that innervate the large cerebral arteries and dura mater and arise from the first, or ophthalmic, division of the trigeminal nerve. Stimulation of the cranial vessels, such as the superior sagittal sinus, is certainly painful in humans.[54] Human dural nerves that innervate the cranial vessels consist largely of small-diameter myelinated and unmyelinated fibers that subserve a nociceptive function.[55,56]

What Is the Source of Pain in Migraine?

There are few studies of humans that directly answer the question of the source of migraine pain. Certainly, two-thirds of migraineurs experience relief if the carotid artery is occluded ipsilateral to the side of headache, although this does not account for the remaining one-third at all.[57] Moreover, distension of major cerebral vessels by balloon dilatation leads to pain referred to the ophthalmic division of the trigeminal nerve.[58,59] Moskowitz and Cutrer have provided an elegant series of experiments whose results suggest that the pain of migraine may be a form of sterile neurogenic inflammation.[60] These studies are considered briefly here as they affect the interpretation of the clinical question of pain, and the phenomenon is dealt with in detail by Cutrer and colleagues elsewhere in this volume (Chapter 4). Neurogenic plasma extravasation can be seen during electrical stimulation of the trigeminal ganglion in the rat.[61] Plasma extravasation can be blocked by ergot alkaloids,[62] indomethacin, acetylsalicylic acid,[63] the serotonin (5-HT)$_{1B/D}$–like agonist sumatriptan,[64] gamma-aminobutyric acid

Table 1.1   Ability of migraine models to predict response to treatment

	Model				
	AVA	*PPE*	*CGRP*	*Vn*	*Migraine*
DHE	+++	+++	+++	+++	+++
Sumatriptan	+++	+++	+++	+/x[a]	+++
Zolmitriptan[b]	+++	+++	+++	+++	+++
Alniditan	+++	+++	?	?	+++
Rizatriptan	+++	+++	?	++	++
Avitriptan	+++	?	?	?	++
CP-122,288	++	+++++	?	?	?
Substance P antagonist[c]	x	+++	?	?	x
Bosentan	x	+++	x	x	x

AVA = arteriovenous anastomosis model[151]; PPE = plasma protein extravasation model[60]; CGRP = release of calcitonin gene-related peptide with trigeminal activation[159]; Vn = inhibits activity in the trigeminal nucleus caudalis[92]; + = effective; x = ineffective; ? = not known or not studied; DHE = dihydroergotamine.
[a]Effective after blood–brain barrier disruption.[92]
[b]Zolmitriptan: 311C90.
[c]Largely peripherally acting RPR100893.

(GABA) agonists such as valproate and benzodiazepines,[65] neurosteroids,[66] substance-P antagonists,[67,68] and the endothelin antagonist bosentan.[69,70] The pharmacology of the newer abortive antimigraine drugs is dealt with in more detail in Chapter 2.

What will become clearer in the next few years is the extent to which experimental models of migraine can predict the effects of drug therapy.[71] Bosentan's lack of effect in migraine—seen in the unequivocal outcome of a double-blind, placebo-controlled study of its intravenous use[72]—contrasts with data from the neurogenic inflammation model[71] but is in line with our observations.[73] Furthermore, the demonstration of a lack of clinical effect in acute migraine attacks of the orally administered substance-P antagonist RPR 100893, in a double-blind, placebo-controlled study,[74] casts into doubt the importance of peripherally released substance P in migraine. Moreover, these substance-P data are in line with clinical observations of a lack of release of substance P in migraineurs during headache.[75] The comparative ability of various models of the migraine process to predict response to treatment (Table 1.1) will help to define more precisely the pathophysiology of the disease. There has certainly been some effort to move away from drugs with a vascular action, which all the 5-HT$_{1B/D}$–like agonist compounds possess, to compounds that are perhaps more neurally active, such as CP-122,288, substance-P antagonists, and endothelin antagonists. It has been suggested, based on initial molecular biological studies, that the trigeminal ganglion may preferentially contain 5-HT receptors of the ID class[76] and the blood vessels 5-HT$_{1B}$ receptors.[77] Extensive studies from Hamel's group suggest that, as a general rule, to some extent both receptors may be found in both tissues

Table 1.2   Location of 5-HT$_1$-like receptors in humans*

Site	5-HT$_{1D}$	5-HT$_{1B}$
Extracerebral vessels	+/–	+++
Cerebral microvessels	+	–
Trigeminal ganglion	+++	++
Coronary vessels	+/–	+++

*Plus and minus signs indicate relative strength of mRNA signal from tissue: not quantitative.

and even in the human coronary vessels (E. Hamel, personal communication, 1995; see Table 1.2), a target most clinicians would seek to avoid.

In addition to the physiologic responses seen with trigeminal ganglion stimulation, there are structural changes seen in the dura mater. These include mast cell degranulation[78] and changes in postcapillary venules including platelet aggregation.[79] The latter is not surprising given the very close anatomic relationship between nerves and mast cells in the dura mater.[80] Such changes would account for the changes in serotonin, and indeed in platelet serotonin, reported in migraine.[81] Although it is generally accepted that such changes, and particularly the initiation of a sterile inflammatory response, would cause pain, it is not clear whether these changes are sufficient of themselves or whether other stimulators or promoters are required. It is my view that the changes are secondarily driven from the brain stem as part of the migrainous process.

Brain Stem Processing of Trigeminovascular Pain

The sites within the brain stem that are responsible for craniovascular pain have now begun to be mapped. Using c-*fos* immunocytochemistry, a method for looking at activated cells, after meningeal irritation with blood, expression is reported in the trigeminal nucleus caudalis,[82] whereas after stimulation of the superior sagittal sinus, *fos*-like immunoreactivity is seen in the trigeminal nucleus caudalis and in the dorsal horn at the C-1 and C-2 levels in cat[83] and rat.[84] These latter findings are in accord with two similar results using 2-deoxyglucose measurements with superior sagittal sinus stimulation[85] and with our most recent studies demonstrating a similar organization in the monkey.[86] These data contribute to our view that the trigeminal nucleus extends beyond the traditional nucleus caudalis to the dorsal horn of the high cervical region in a functional continuum that includes a cervical extension that could be regarded as a *trigeminal nucleus cervicalis*. These data clearly demonstrate that a substantial portion of the trigeminovascular nociceptive information comes by way of the most caudal cells. The rather diffuse activation of neurons in the trigeminal nucleus in visceral-type pain, such as that arising from intracranial vessels, contrasts with what is seen when pain stimuli are applied to discrete facial structures. In the latter case, neuronal activation is more restricted,[87,88] in line with the relatively good spatial localization of more superficial pain. This concept provides an anatomic explanation for

Table 1.3　Processing of craniovascular pain

Order	Structures	Comments
First	Trigeminal ganglion	Located in middle cranial fossa
Second	Trigeminal nucleus	Trigeminal nucleus caudalis C-1/C-2 dorsal horn (processing in laminae I/II$_o$)
	(Quintothalamic tract)	Afferents to thalamus
Third	Thalamus	Ventrobasal complex
		Medial nucleus of posterior group
		Intralaminar complex
Final	Cortex	Site unknown

the referral of pain to the back of the head in migraine. Moreover, experimental pharmacologic evidence suggests that some abortive antimigraine drugs, such as ergots,[89,90] acetylsalicylic acid,[91] sumatriptan (after blood–brain barrier disruption),[92,93] and zolmitriptan (311C90)[94] can have actions at these second-order neurons to reduce cell activity, suggesting a further possible site for therapeutic intervention in migraine.

Following transmission in the caudal brain stem and high cervical spinal cord, information is relayed in a group of fibers (the quintothalamic tract) to the thalamus. Processing of vascular pain in the thalamus occurs in the ventroposteromedial thalamus, medial nucleus of the posterior complex, and intralaminar thalamus.[95] Zagami and Lambert have shown by application of capsaicin to the superior sagittal sinus that trigeminal projections with a high degree of nociceptive input are processed in neurons, particularly in the ventroposteromedial thalamus and in its ventral periphery.[96] The properties and further higher center connections of these neurons are the subject of ongoing studies that will allow us to build a more complete picture of the trigeminovascular pain pathways (Table 1.3).

Experimental Cerebral Blood Flow Studies

Experimental evidence suggests that the trigeminovascular system promotes vasodilatation. Nerves that innervate the cerebral vessels through the trigeminovascular system contain almost exclusively vasodilator transmitters, such as CGRP and substance P. Available data suggest that lesions of the trigeminal ganglion do not affect resting cerebral blood flow or glucose use in the cat.[97] They do, however, affect vasodilator protector mechanisms such as those seen during hyperemia following ischemia or epilepsy,[98] and vasodilator mechanisms usually entrained when cerebral vessels are constricted by such substances as noradrenaline.[99] In addition, it has recently been shown that in subarachnoid hemorrhage, with threatened cerebrovascular compromise from vasospasm, venous calcitonin gene-related peptide levels are elevated in humans.[100] Electrical stimulation of the trigeminal ganglion in both humans and cats leads to increases in extracerebral blood flow and to local release of both CGRP and substance P.[53] In the cat trigeminal ganglion, stimulation also increases cerebral blood flow by a pathway traversing the greater superficial petrosal branch of the facial nerve,[101] again releasing a powerful vasodilator peptide, vasoactive intestinal polypeptide (VIP).[102] Interestingly, the VIP-ergic innervation of the cerebral vessels is predominantly anterior rather than posterior[103]; this may contribute to the region's vulnerability to spreading depression and in part explain why the aura is so often seen to commence posteriorly. Stimulation of the more specifically vascular and pain-sensitive superior sagittal sinus increases cerebral blood flow and jugular vein CGRP levels.[104] Human evidence that CGRP is elevated in the headache phase of migraine[75,105] and cluster headache[106,107] supports the view that the trigeminovascular system may be activated in a protective role in these conditions. Taken together, the data suggest that the trigeminovascular system is unlikely to be the source of the generation of the aura, but rather is either activated by it or is activated in parallel by the same process that activates the aura. What is yet to be determined is whether other neuropeptides besides CGRP and VIP are involved, such as a pituitary adenylate cyclase–activating peptide[108] or helodermin-related peptides.[109] These latter peptides are also vasodilators and are found widely in the cerebral and extracerebral circulation.

Central Modulation of Trigeminovascular Pain

It has been shown in experimental animals that stimulation of a discrete nucleus in the brain stem, nucleus locus coeruleus (the main central noradrenergic nucleus), reduces cerebral blood flow in a frequency-dependent manner[110] through an α-adrenoceptor–linked mechanism.[111] This reduction is maximal in the occipital cortex.[112] Although a 25% overall reduction in cerebral blood flow is seen, extracerebral vasodilatation occurs in parallel.[113] In addition, the main serotonin-containing nucleus in the brain stem, the midbrain dorsal raphe nucleus, can increase cerebral blood flow when activated.[114–116] These animal studies have been the subject of renewed interest since the description in humans of activation of the periaqueductal gray in the region of the dorsal raphe nucleus and in the dorsal pons near the locus coeruleus in PET studies during migraine without aura.[117] Moreover, these areas are active immediately after successful treatment of the headache but are not active interictally. From the clinical standpoint, aura can exist in isolation from the pain as "migraine equivalent"; it is thus possible that the aura originates in the central nervous system and that the vascular changes are a secondary feature (Figure 1.1).

With respect to the idea of aminergic modulation of trigeminovascular processing, some further clinical work should be considered. First, placement of an electrode into the region of the periaqueductal gray matter can evoke a migraine-like headache.[118] Second, it has been shown that the contingent negative variation (CNV), which is an event-related slow cerebral potential, is increased in amplitude and its habituation lacking in patients with migraine without aura.[119] Furthermore, the CNV normalizes after treatment with β-blockers.[120] More recently, the same group has shown that the visual evoked potential is potentiated, rather than habituated, in migraine patients when studied between attacks.[121] The CNV is under aminergic control,[122] and these data fit nicely with both the animal data and the human PET data. Moreover, returning to recent animal stud-

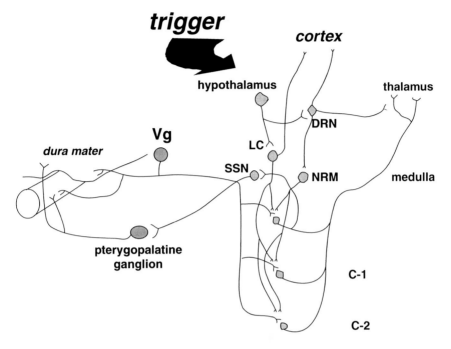

Figure 1.1 Schematic summary of the neural elements required for a proposed unified central neural hypothesis for migraine. The peripheral input from the trigeminovascular system that arises in the dura mater and blood vessels passes through the ophthalmic division of the trigeminal nerve and has its cell body in the trigeminal ganglion (Vg). The second-order neurons lie in the most caudal trigeminal nucleus caudalis and in the dorsal horn of the upper cervical spinal cord at the C-1 and C-2 levels. These cells project via the quintothalamic tract, which decussates before synapsing on third-order neurons in the thalamus. There is a reflex connection with the parasympathetic outflow from the seventh cranial nerve, which arises in the superior salivatory nucleus (SSN). This pathway synapses in cranial autonomic ganglion, pterygopalatine, and otic ganglion (the latter not shown) projecting to cerebral vessels and dura mater. To account for the many central nervous system manifestations of migraine, including the recent positron-emission tomographic data,[117] the aminergic cells in the locus coeruleus (LC; noradrenergic) and dorsal raphe nucleus (DRN; serotonergic) are illustrated. The LC projects both to cortex and to the trigeminal nucleus, which gates incoming pain. DRN projections are to be found to cerebral blood vessels, to thalamus, and to the nucleus raphe magnus (NRM), which in turn gates trigeminal nucleus input. Well-established connections between the LC and DRN and the hypothalamus may account for manifestations of migraine seen in the premonitory phase, such as hunger or thirst.

ies, we have seen activation of cells in the ventrolateral periaqueductal gray using c-*fos* immunocytochemistry after superior sagittal sinus stimulation.[123] Migraine is thus most likely to be primarily a disorder of the central nervous system, and with advances in PET and other imaging technologies the central dysfunction should soon be better understood.

Clinical Observations of the Trigeminovascular System

Drummond and Lance have shown that in at least one-third of patients there is a significant extracerebral vascular component to the headache.[57] The level of CGRP is elevated in the external jugular vein blood of migraineurs during headache,[75] clearly demonstrating some activation of trigeminovascular neurons during migraine with or without aura. These data have been confirmed in adolescent migraineurs.[105] Whether the activity is peripherally generated is again uncertain, although it is clear that such changes can in part be seen in both humans and cats with direct stimulation of the trigeminal ganglion.[53] The release of peptides, such as CGRP or neurokinin A, offers the prospect of a marker for migraine that could be readily determined from a venous blood sample.

Migraine and the Blood–Brain Barrier

Some compelling data from a clinical study of aura raise the possibility that the blood–brain barrier may not be normal in migraine. This is not a new suggestion,[124] although there has been little direct evidence for an altered barrier apart from a case report based on computed tomography.[125] The era of more modern therapeutics, which has arguably started with sumatriptan, has provided more and interesting data. The effect of sumatriptan on the aura was examined in a well-conducted study of patients with migraine with aura. In a placebo, double-blinded, parallel groups study, the drug was administered at the onset of aura as a 6-mg subcutaneous injection, thus assuring absorption. In this setting, sumatriptan neither shortened nor lengthened the aura when compared with placebo. The most fascinating aspect of the study was that the incidence of headache in the placebo group and the treated group was the same: Despite having good delivery and a suitable drug level, with a 20-minute mean length of aura, headache still occurred. What is perhaps even more remarkable is that the developed headache responded to a further sumatriptan injection.[126] Ferrari, in analyzing his extensive clinical experience with sumatriptan, has also noted that treatment failure is particularly associated with early use of the subcutaneous formulation, again suggesting that some process must take hold that facilitates the action of sumatriptan (Chapter 8). These data suggest that sumatriptan does not have access to a crucial receptor site during aura and that the interaction of the drug concentration and rate of absorption, along with access to the appropriate site, are the elements of the equation required to terminate the attack.

To what site in the body does sumatriptan not have ready access? The obvious suggestion is a site behind the blood–brain barrier, which reopens the exciting possibility that the blood–brain barrier may not be normal in the headache phase of migraine. Indeed, better access to sites within the central nervous system may be advantageous for drug development, rather than a drawback. Results of phase II clinical studies with zolmitriptan (311C90), a 5-HT–like agonist with access to central nervous system 5-HT$_{1D}$ sites, confirm that such an advantage may have a clinical correlate.[127] A recent report of a study of zolmitriptan in treatment of aura[128] was inconclusive, attempting to analyze the outcome at 24 hours rather than at the time when the headache would be expected after the aura. We can only await further analysis of the data and further studies with suitable compounds and clinical endpoints to evaluate this concept.

Perhaps a link in the overall chain of events that occurs in migraine may again be found in the brain stem and, given the recent human PET data,[117] in the aminergic nuclei. It was shown many years ago that the locus coeruleus, the main noradrenaline-containing cell group in the central nervous system, could alter brain–blood flow and blood–brain barrier permeability.[129–131] Modulation of central noradrenergic systems using tricyclic antidepressants can alter blood–brain barrier permeability in experimental animals[132]; and it has been shown that the noradrenergic innervation arising in the locus coeruleus is essential for maintaining blood–brain barrier integrity during some pathophysiologic states.[133] One interesting differentiating feature between the central aminergic nuclei is the presence of nicotinamide-adenine dinucleotide phosphate (NADPH) diaphorase activity in the dorsal raphe nucleus but its absence from the locus coeruleus.[134] This marker correlates with nitric oxide synthase activity, and given recent interest in nitric oxide–induced models of headache, provides a curious overlap from the laboratory, through the clinical PET studies, to the clinical manifestations of a disease, and finally to therapeutic uses of drugs and their relationship to the integrity of the blood–brain barrier.

THERAPY AND PATHOPHYSIOLOGY

The current era of antimigraine compounds began in 1973 with attempts to synthesize a more cranially selective serotonin agonist. More detail about the serotonin receptor system is found in Chapter 2. The project was commenced because it had been shown that (1) urinary excretion of 5-hydroxyindoleacetic acid, the main metabolite of serotonin, was increased in association with migraine attacks[81,135]; (2) platelet 5-HT also dropped rapidly during the onset of the migraine attack[136]; and (3) intravenous injection of 5-HT could abort either reserpine-induced or spontaneous headache.[136,137]

At that time it was thought that there were two serotonin receptors: D (dibenzyline phenoxybenzamine–sensitive) and M (morphine-sensitive). By the mid-1980s it had become obvious that there was at least a further, atypical class that could be found, among other places, in the dog carotid circulation. Characterization of the biology of such serotonergic responses led in part to a reclassification of serotonin receptors in 1986[138] and then to the current system as defined in detail[139] and reviewed in Chapter 2. Class 1 has been subdivided; this subdivision is presented in an abbreviated form (Table 1.4) to elucidate the action of some of the antimigraine drugs. Sumatriptan,[140] zolmitriptan (311C90),[141] alniditan,[142,143] MK-462 (rizatriptan),[144] and BMS180048 (avitriptan)[145] belong to class 1 at the 1B and 1D subclasses. The concept that the 5-HT$_{1B/D}$–like receptor is the pivotal antimigraine site has recently been called into question. Sumatriptan, zolmitriptan, and a number of other agonists have actions on protein plasma extravasation and have been shown to be agonists at both 5-HT$_{1B}$ and 5-HT$_{1D}$ receptors. However, a recently tested compound that is a conformationally restricted analogue of sumatriptan, CP-122,288,[146] is at least 1,000 times more potent in the protein plasma extravasation model than suma-

Table 1.4   Classification of serotonin (5-HT) subclass 1 receptors

Subtype	Agonist	Antagonist	Function
1A	8-OH-DPAT[a]	WAY 100135	Hypotension Behavioral (satiety) (Rat)
1B	CP-93, 129[a]		Craniovascular receptor
	Sumatriptan		(human)
	Dihydroergotamine		
	Zolmitriptan		—
	Alniditan		—
	Rizatriptan (MK-462)		—
	Avitriptan (BMS-180048)		—
	Naratriptan		—
	Eletriptan (UK116044)		—
	CP-122,228	GR127935[a]	—
1D	Sumatriptan		Trigeminal neuronal
	Dihydroergotamine		receptor
	Zolmitriptan		—
	Alniditan		—
	Rizatriptan		—
	Avitriptan		—
	Naratriptan		—
	Eletriptan		—
	CP-122,288	GR127935[a]	—
1E	Rizatriptan[b]	—	?
1F	Sumatriptan	—	?
	Zolmitriptan		
	CP-122,228		
1?	CP-122,228	—	Is the effect due to an undescribed receptor?

[a]8-OH-DPAT (8-hydroxy-2-(di-n-propylamino)tetralin), WAY 100135, CP-93,129, and GR127935 are all compounds used in the laboratory for pharmacologic purposes and have no current clinical indications.
[b]Drug agonist actions are relative and the inclusion of rizatriptan (MK-462) as an agonist at 5-HT$_{1E}$ sites is based on a published comparison with sumatriptan.[144]
Source: Modified from GR Martin, PPA Humphrey. Receptors for 5-hydroxytryptamine: current perspectives on classification and nomenclature. Neuropharmacology 1994;33:261. Revisions based on PR Hartig, D Hoyer, PPA Humphrey, et al. Alignment of receptor nomenclature with the human genome: classification of 5HT$_{1B}$ and 5HT$_{1D}$ receptor subtypes. Trends Pharmacol Sci 1996;17:103.

triptan yet equipotent at the 5-HT$_{1D}$–like receptors (Table 1.5). This observation brings into focus what might usefully be labeled as the 5-HT$_1$–like conundrum: Whereas the vasoconstrictor effect is blocked by methiothepin,[147] a potent but not specific 5-HT$_{1D}$ antagonist,[148,149] the response is not antagonized by metergoline either in vivo[150,151] *or* in vitro,[150,152,153] although metergoline is more potent than methiothepin at the 5-HT$_{1D}$ receptor.[154,155] It is also noted that metergoline may exhibit noncompetitive antagonism[147] or in some situations have intrinsic efficacy.[154,156] The development of a potent 5-HT$_{1D}$ antagonist, GR127935,[157] might then allow this problem to be resolved, although the fact that GR127935 has ago-

Table 1.5   What is the 5-HT antimigraine site?

Model	Compound			
	Sumatriptan	*Zolmitriptan[a]*	*Rizatriptan*	*CP-122,288*
PPE ED$_{50}$ μg/kg	31.0[b]	15.0	30.0	0.001
pKi 1D	7.9	9.2	7.9	8.1
pKi 1B	7.9	8.2	7.9	7.9
pKi 1F	7.5	7.1		7.6

PPE = plasma protein extravasation; ED$_{50}$ = median effective dose.
[a]Zolmitriptan, 311C90.
[b]These values represent published values for the 5-HT$_{1B/D}$ receptor without subclassification.[144]

nist action at the 5-HT$_{1D}$ receptor[158] may serve to complicate any analysis. All of these data point to the existence of a further receptor site of interest, which may be the crucial site for the action of these drugs. Only clinical studies with the new class of compounds will determine the direction for further pharmacologic research.

What can be gleaned from the actions of the antimigraine drugs? Recent developments have certainly identified pathophysiologic mechanisms that may be active during the migraine attack. The common theme has been activation and nociceptive transmission through the pain-sensitive intracranial innervation, the trigeminovascular system. The trigeminovascular system, perhaps not surprisingly, is the common focus of activity for vascular headache.[159,160] Consequently, modulation of activity in the trigeminovascular system, be it in the vessels, at the level of the peripheral innervation, or in processing within the trigeminal nucleus, can probably exert a favorable influence on headache. It does not, however, follow that the modulated structures are the primary site of the abnormality. Rather, it is more likely that they represent a final common nociceptive pathway activated or acted on by central nervous system processing or by triggering events.

SUMMARY

An understanding of the basic anatomy and physiology of the cranial circulation facilitates the assessment and management of patients with headache, particularly vascular-type headache such as migraine. Migraine should be viewed as an episodic syndrome of pain, probably involving intracranial structures, and certainly associated with other neurologic disturbances. It is the syndromic nature of migraine that is its core characteristic, and this attribute is conferred by the brain and the connections that process and control head pain. The aminergic nuclei, whose usual role is to gate afferent nociceptive information, modulate cerebral blood flow and blood–brain barrier permeability, and control the signal-to-noise aspect of sensory inputs, are the crucial sites in migraine. Indeed they are strong candidates for the lesion in the classical neurologic sense. When these modulatory controls are triggered or timed to dysfunction, the migrainous process is driven by the brain, releasing sensory inputs to create Liveing's "nerve storm." At once, vessels pulsing normally can be felt to throb; fluid in an otherwise satisfied stomach is perceived as nausea; normal lights, sounds, or smells are perceived as pungent or unpleasant; and normal movement is perceived to jar and disturb the head. The trigeminovascular system provides a therapeutic target for attack treatment. Treatment arrests the final common pathway for expression of vascular head pain; the brain, however, provides the essential key to the disorder, its genesis, and its ultimate understanding and control.

Acknowledgments

The work of the author reported herein has been supported by the Wellcome Trust and the Migraine Trust. P.J.G. is a Wellcome Senior Research Fellow.

REFERENCES

1. Goadsby PJ. The challenge of headache for the nineties. Curr Opin Neurol 1994;7:255.
2. Joutel A, Bousser MG, Biousse V, et al. A gene for familial hemiplegic migraine maps to chromosome 19. Nat Genet 1993;5:40.
3. Ducros A, Joutel A, Vahedi K, et al. Towards the identification of a second locus for familial hemiplegic migraine. Cephalalgia 1995;15(Suppl 14):9.
4. Terwindt GM, Ophoff RA, May A, et al. Familial hemiplegic migraine locus on 19P13 is involved in the common forms of migraine with and without aura. Cephalalgia 1995;15(Suppl 14):8.
5. Russell MB, Andersson PG, Thomsen LL, Iselius L. Cluster headache is an autosomal dominantly inherited disorder in some families: A complex segregation analysis. J Med Genet 1995;32:954.
6. Griggs RC, Nutt JG. Episodic ataxias as channelopathies. Ann Neurol 1995;37:285.
7. Goadsby PJ, Boyce G. Paroxysmal cerebellar ataxia. Aust N Z J Med 1990;20:103.
8. Vahedi K, Joutel A, van Bogaert P, et al. A gene for hereditary paroxysmal cerebellar ataxia maps to chromosome 19p. Ann Neurol 1995;37:289.
9. Somerville BW. The role of estradiol withdrawal in the etiology of menstrual migraine. Neurology 1972;22:355.
10. Kupfermann I. Hypothalamus and Limbic System. II: Motivation. In ER Kandel, JH Schwartz (eds), Principles of Neural Science. Amsterdam: Elsevier, 1985;626.
11. Swaab DF, Hofman MA, Lucassen PJ, Purba JS, et al. Functional neuroanatomy and neuropathology of the hypothalamus. Anat Embryol 1993;187:317.
12. Moore-Ede MC. The circadian timing system in mammals: Two pacemakers preside over many secondary oscillators. Fed Proc 1983;42:2802.
13. Woods RP, Iacoboni M, Mazziotta JC. Bilateral spreading cerebral hypoperfusion during spontaneous migraine headache. N Engl J Med 1994;331:1689.
14. Skinhoj E, Paulson OB. Regional cerebral blood flow in the internal carotid artery distribution during migraine. BMJ 1969;3:569.
15. O'Brien MD. Cerebral blood flow changes in migraine. Headache 1971;10:139.
16. Skinhoj E. Hemodynamic studies within the brain during migraine. Arch Neurol 1973;29:95.
17. Simard D, Paulson OB. Cerebral vasomotor paralysis during migraine attack. Arch Neurol 1973;29:207.
18. Norris JW, Hachinski VC, Cooper PW. Changes in cerebral blood flow during a migraine attack. BMJ 1975;3:676.
19. Mathew NT, Hrastnik F, Meyer JS. Regional cerebral blood flow in the diagnosis of vascular headache. Headache 1976;15:252.
20. Edmeads J. Cerebral blood flow in migraine. Headache 1977;17:148.

21. Hachinski VC, Olesen J, Norris JW, Larsen B, et al. Cerebral hemodynamics in migraine. Can J Neurol Sci 1977;4:245.
22. Sakai F, Meyer JS. Regional cerebral hemodynamics during migraine and cluster headaches measured by the 133-Xe inhalation method. Headache 1978;18:122.
23. Olesen J, Larsen B, Lauritzen M. Focal hyperemia followed by spreading oligemia and impaired activation of rCBF in classic migraine. Ann Neurol 1981;9:344.
24. Staehelin-Jensen T, Voldby B, Olivarius BF, Jensen FT. Cerebral hemodynamics in familial hemiplegic migraine. Cephalalgia 1981;1:121.
25. Lauritzen M, Skyhoj-Olsen T, Lassen NA, Paulson OB. The changes of regional cerebral blood flow during the course of classical migraine attacks. Ann Neurol 1983;13:633.
26. Lauritzen M, Olesen J. Regional cerebral blood flow during migraine attacks by Xenon-133 inhalation and emission tomography. Brain 1984;107:447.
27. Skyhoj-Olsen T, Friberg L, Lassen NA. Ischemia may be the primary cause of the neurological deficits in classic migraine. Arch Neurol 1987;44:156.
28. Olesen J, Friberg L, Skyhoj-Olsen T, et al. Timing and topography of cerebral blood flow, aura, and headache during migraine attacks. Ann Neurol 1990;28:791.
29. Lashley KS. Patterns of cerebral integration indicated by the scotomas of migraine. Arch Neurol Psychiatry 1941;46:331.
30. Leão AAP. Pial circulation and spreading activity in the cerebral cortex. J Neurophysiol 1944;7:391.
31. Leão AAP. Spreading depression of activity in cerebral cortex. J Neurophysiol 1944;7:359.
32. Lauritzen M. Pathophysiology of the migraine aura: The spreading depression theory. Brain 1994;117:199.
33. Olesen J. Cerebral and extracranial circulatory disturbances in migraine: Pathophysiological implications. Cerebrovasc Brain Metab Rev 1991;3:1.
34. Andersen AR, Friberg L, Skyhoj-Olsen T, Olesen J. SPECT demonstration of delayed hyperemia following hypoperfusion in classic migraine. Arch Neurol 1988;45:154.
35. Lauritzen M. Long-lasting reduction of cortical blood flow of the rat brain after spreading depression with preserved autoregulation and impaired CO_2 response. J Cereb Blood Flow Metab 1984;4:546.
36. Lauritzen M, Skyhoj-Olsen T, Lassen NA, Paulson OB. Regulation of regional cerebral blood flow during and between migraine attacks. Ann Neurol 1983;14:569.
37. Herold S, Gibbs JM, Jones AKP, Brooks DJ, et al. Oxygen metabolism in migraine. J Cereb Blood Flow Metab 1985;5(Suppl):S445.
38. Friberg L, Skyhoj-Olsen T, Roland PE, Lassen NA. Focal ischemia caused by instability of cerebrovascular tone during attacks of hemiplegic migraine. Brain 1987;110:917.
39. Skyhoj-Olsen T. Migraine with and without aura: The same disease due to cerebral vasospasm of different intensity. A hypothesis based on CBF studies during migraine. Headache 1990;30:269.
40. Skyhoj-Olsen T, Lassen NA. Blood flow and vascular reactivity during attacks of classic migraine: Limitations of the Xe-133 intra-arterial technique. Headache 1989;29:15.
41. Brindley GS, Lewin WS. The sensations produced by electrical stimulation of the visual cortex. J Physiol 1968;196:479.
42. Penfield W, Perot P. The brain's record of auditory and visual experience. Brain 1963;86:595.
43. Hubel DH, Weisel TN. Receptive fields and functional architecture of monkey striate cortex. J Physiol 1968;195:215.
44. McLachlan RS, Girvin JP. Spreading depression of Leão in rodent and human cortex. Brain Res 1994;666:133.
45. Piper RD, Matheson JM, Hellier M, et al. Cortical spreading depression is not seen intraoperatively during temporal lobectomy in humans. Cephalalgia 1991;11(Suppl 11):1.
46. Welch KMA, D'andrea G, Tepley N, Barkeley GL, et al. The concept of migraine as a state of central neuronal hyperexcitability. Headache 1990;8:817.
47. Liu-Chen L-Y, Gillespie SA, Norregaard TV, Moskowitz MA. Co-localization of retrogradely transported wheat germ agglutinin and the putative neurotransmitter substance P within trigeminal ganglion cells projecting to cat middle cerebral. J Comp Neurol 1984;225:187.
48. Saito K, Moskowitz MA. Contributions from the upper cervical dorsal roots and trigeminal ganglia to the feline circle of Willis. Stroke 1989;20:524.
49. Arbab MA-R, Wiklund L, Svendgaard NA. Origin and distribution of cerebral vascular innervation from superior cervical, trigeminal, and spinal ganglia investigated with retrograde and anterograde WGA-HRP tracing in the rat. Neuroscience 1986;19:695.
50. Ruskell GL, Simons T. Trigeminal nerve pathways to the cerebral arteries in monkeys. J Anat 1987;155:23.

51. Liu-Chen LY, Mayberg MR, Moskowitz MA. Immunohistochemical evidence for a substance P–containing trigeminovascular pathway to pial arteries in cats. Brain Res 1983;268:162.
52. Uddman R, Edvinsson L, Ekman R, Kingman T, et al. Innervation of the feline cerebral vasculature by nerve fibers containing calcitonin gene-related peptide: Trigeminal origin and co-existence with substance P. Neurosci Lett 1985;62:131.
53. Goadsby PJ, Edvinsson L, Ekman R. Release of vasoactive peptides in the extracerebral circulation of man and the cat during activation of the trigeminovascular system. Ann Neurol 1988;23:193.
54. Feindel W, Penfield W, McNaughton F. The tentorial nerves and localisation of intracranial pain in man. Neurology 1960;10:555.
55. Penfield W, McNaughton FL. Dural headache and the innervation of the dura mater. Arch Neurol Psychiatry 1940;44:43.
56. Kimmel DL. The nerves of the cranial dura mater and their significance in dural headache and referred pain. Clin Med Sch Quart 1961;22:16.
57. Drummond PD, Lance JW. Extracranial vascular changes and the source of pain in migraine headache. Ann Neurol 1983;13:32.
58. Nichols FT, Mawad M, Mohr JP, Hilal S, et al. Focal headache during balloon inflation in the vertebral and basilar arteries. Headache 1993;33:87.
59. Martins IP, Baeta E, Paiva T, Campo T, et al. Headaches during intracranial endovascular procedures: A possible model of vascular headache. Headache 1993;33:227.
60. Moskowitz MA, Cutrer FM. Sumatriptan: A receptor-targeted treatment for migraine. Annu Rev Med 1993;44:145.
61. Markowitz S, Saito K, Moskowitz MA. Neurogenically mediated leakage of plasma proteins occurs from blood vessels in dura mater but not brain. J Neurosci 1987;7:4129.
62. Markowitz S, Saito K, Moskowitz MA. Neurogenically mediated plasma extravasation in dura mater: Effect of ergot alkaloids. A possible mechanism of action in vascular headache. Cephalalgia 1988;8:83.
63. Buzzi MG, Sakas DE, Moskowitz MA. Indomethacin and acetylsalicylic acid block neurogenic plasma protein extravasation in rat dura mater. Eur J Pharmacol 1989;165:251.
64. Buzzi MG, Moskowitz MA. The antimigraine drug sumatriptan (GR43175) selectively blocks neurogenic plasma extravasation from blood vessels in dura mater. Br J Pharmacol 1990;99:202.
65. Cutrer FM, Limmroth V, Ayata G, Moskowitz MA. Valproate reduces c-*fos* expression in the trigeminal nucleus caudalis (TNC) after noxious meningeal stimulation. Cephalalgia 1995;15(Suppl 14):96.
66. Limmroth V, Lee WS, Cutrer FM, Waeber C, et al. Progesterone and its ring-A–reduced metabolites suppress dural plasma protein extravasation by activation of peripheral $GABA_A$ receptors. Cephalalgia 1995;15(Suppl 14):98.
67. Lee WS, Moussaoui SM, Moskowitz MA. Blockade by oral or parenteral RPR100893 (a non-peptide NK1 receptor antagonist) of neurogenic plasma protein extravasation in guinea-pig dura mater and conjunctiva. Br J Pharmacol 1994;112:920.
68. Cutrer FM, Garret C, Moussaoui SM, Moskowitz MA. The non-peptide neurokinin-1 antagonist, RPR100893, decreases c-*fos* expression in trigeminal nucleus caudalis following noxious chemical meningeal stimulation. Neuroscience 1995;64:741.
69. Clozel M, Breu V, Gray AG, et al. Pharmacological characterisation of bosentan, a new potent orally active nonpeptide endothelin receptor antagonist. J Pharmacol Exp Ther 1994;270:228.
70. Brandli P, Loffler B-M, Breu V, Osterwalder R, et al. Role of endothelin in mediating neurogenic plasma extravasation in rat dura mater. Pain; in press.
71. Goadsby PJ. Animal Models of Migraine: Which One and for What? In FC Rose (ed), Migraine: New Concepts. Amsterdam: Elsevier, in press.
72. Gijsman HJ, May A, Wallnofer A, Jones CR, Deiner HC, Ferrari MD. The endothelin antagonist bosentan is not effective in the acute treatment of migraine. Cephalalgia 1995;15(Suppl 14):267.
73. Goadsby PJ, Adner M, Edvinsson L. Characterisation of endothelin ETA receptors in the cerebral vasculature and their lack of effect upon spreading depression. J Cereb Blood Flow Metab 1996;16, in press.
74. Diener HC. Substance-P Antagonist RPR100893-201 Is Not Effective in Human Migraine Attacks. In J Olesen, P Tfelt-Hansen (eds), Trial Methodology and New Drugs. New York: Raven, in press.
75. Goadsby PJ, Edvinsson L, Ekman R. Vasoactive peptide release in the extracerebral circulation of humans during migraine headache. Ann Neurol 1990;28:183.
76. Rebeck GW, Maynard KI, Hyman BT, Moskowitz MA. Selective 5-HT_{1D} alpha serotonin receptor gene expression in trigeminal ganglion: Implications for antimigraine drug development. Proc Natl Acad Sci U S A 1994;91:3666.

77. Hamel E, Fan E, Linville D, Ting V, et al. Expression of mRNA for the serotonin 5-hydroxytrypta-mine$_{1DB}$ receptor subtype in human bovine and cerebral arteries. Mol Pharmacol 1993;44:242.
78. Dimitriadou V, Buzzi MG, Moskowitz MA, Theoharides TC. Trigeminal sensory fiber stimulation induces morphological changes reflecting secretion in rat dura mater mast cells. Neuroscience 1991;44:97.
79. Dimitriadou V, Buzzi MG, Theoharides TC, Moskowitz MA. Ultrastructural evidence for neuro-genically mediated changes in blood vessels of the rat dura mater and tongue following antidromic trigeminal stimulation. Neuroscience 1992;48:187.
80. Dimitriadou V, Aubineau P, Taxi J, Seylaz J. Ultrastructural evidence for a functional unit between nerve fibers and type II cerebral mast cells in the cerebral vascular wall. Neuroscience 1987;22:621.
81. Curran DA, Hinterberger H, Lance JW. Total plasma serotonin, 5-hydroxyindoleacetic acid and p-hydroxy-methoxymandelic acid excretion in normal and migrainous subjects. Brain 1965;88:997.
82. Nozaki K, Boccalini P, Moskowitz MA. Expression of c-*fos*–like immunoreactivity in brain stem after meningeal irritation by blood in the subarachnoid space. Neuroscience 1992;49:669.
83. Kaube H, Keay K, Hoskin KL, Bandler R, et al. Expression of c-*fos*–like immunoreactivity in the trigeminal nucleus caudalis and high cervical cord following stimulation of the sagittal sinus in the cat. Brain Res 1993;629:95.
84. Strassman AM, Mineta Y, Vos BP. Distribution of *fos*-like immunoreactivity in the medullary and upper cervical dorsal horn produced by stimulation of dural blood vessels in the rat. J Neurosci 1994;14:3725.
85. Goadsby PJ, Zagami AS. Stimulation of the superior sagittal sinus increases metabolic activity and blood flow in certain regions of the brain stem and upper cervical spinal cord of the cat. Brain 1991;114:1001.
86. Goadsby PJ, Keay KA, Hoskin KL. Distribution of pain processing trigeminovascular neurons in the brain stem and high cervical spinal cord of the monkey. Cephalalgia 1995;15(Suppl 14):57.
87. Strassman AM, Vos BP. Somatotopic and laminar organization of *fos*-like immunoreactivity in the medullary and upper cervical dorsal horn induced by noxious facial stimulation in the rat. J Comp Neurol 1993;331:495.
88. Strassman AM, Vos BP, Mineta Y, Naderi S, et al. *Fos*-like immunoreactivity in the superficial medullary dorsal horn induced by noxious and innocuous thermal stimulation of the facial skin in the rat. J Neurophysiol 1993;70:1811.
89. Goadsby PJ, Gundlach AL. Localization of [H]- dihydroergotamine binding sites in the cat central nervous system: Relevance to migraine. Ann Neurol 1991;29:91.
90. Hoskin KL, Kaube H, Goadsby PJ. Central activation of the trigeminovascular pathway in the cat is inhibited by dihydroergotamine: A c-*fos* and electrophysiology study. Brain 1996;119; in press.
91. Kaube H, Hoskin KL, Goadsby PJ. Intravenous acetylsalicylic acid inhibits central trigeminal neu-rons in the dorsal horn of the upper cervical spinal cord in the cat. Headache 1993;33:541.
92. Kaube H, Hoskin KL, Goadsby PJ. Sumatriptan inhibits central trigeminal neurons only after blood-brain barrier disruption. Br J Pharmacol 1993;109:788.
93. Shepheard SL, Williamson DJ, Williams J, Hill RG, et al. Comparison of the effects of sumatriptan and the NK1 antagonist CP-99,994 on plasma extravasation in the dura mater and c-*fos* mRNA expression in the trigeminal nucleus caudalis of rats. Neuropharmacology 1995;34:255.
94. Goadsby PJ, Edvinsson L. Peripheral and central trigeminovascular activation in cat is blocked by the serotonin (5-HT)-1D receptor agonist 311C90. Headache 1994;34:394.
95. Zagami AS, Lambert GA. Stimulation of cranial vessels excites nociceptive neurones in several thal-amic nuclei of the cat. Exp Brain Res 1990;81:552.
96. Zagami AS, Lambert GA. Craniovascular application of capsaicin activates nociceptive thalamic neu-rons in the cat. Neurosci Lett 1991;121:187.
97. Edvinsson L, McCulloch J, Kingman TA, Uddman R. On the Functional Role of the Trigemino-Cerebrovascular System in the Regulation of Cerebral Circulation. In CH Owman, JE Hardebo (eds), Neural Regulation of the Cerebral Circulation. Stockholm: Elsevier, 1986;407.
98. Sakas DE, Moskowitz MA, Wei EP, Kontos HA, et al. Trigeminovascular fibers increase blood flow in cortical gray matter by axon-dependent mechanisms during severe hypertension or seizures. Proc Natl Acad Sci U S A 1989;86:1401.
99. Edvinsson L, Olesen I, Kingman TA, McCulloch J, et al. Modification of vasoconstrictor respons-es in cerebral blood vessels by lesioning of the trigeminal nerve: Possible involvement of CGRP. Cephalalgia 1995;15:373.
100. Edvinsson L, Juul R, Uddman R. Peptidergic innervation of the cerebral circulation: Role in sub-arachnoid hemorrhage in man. Neurosurg Rev 1990;13:265.
101. Goadsby PJ, Duckworth JW. Effect of stimulation of trigeminal ganglion on regional cerebral blood flow in cats. Am J Physiol 1987;253:R270.
102. Goadsby PJ, Shelley S. High frequency stimulation of the facial nerve results in local cortical release of vasoactive intestinal polypeptide in the anesthaetised cat. Neurosci Lett 1990;112:282.

103. Matsuyama T, Shiosaka S, Matsumoto M, et al. Overall distribution of vasoactive intestinal polypeptide containing nerves on the wall of the cerebral arteries: An immunohistochemical study using whole-mounts. Neuroscience 1983;10:89.
104. Zagami AS, Goadsby PJ, Edvinsson L. Stimulation of the superior sagittal sinus in the cat causes release of vasoactive peptides. Neuropeptides 1990;16:69.
105. Gallai V, Sarchielli P, Floridi A, et al. Vasoactive peptides levels in the plasma of young migraine patients with and without aura assessed both interictally and ictally. Cephalalgia 1995;15:384.
106. Goadsby PJ, Edvinsson L. Human in vivo evidence for trigeminovascular activation in cluster headache. Brain 1994;117:427.
107. Fanciullacci M, Alessandri M, Figini M, Geppetti P, et al. Increases in plasma calcitonin gene-related peptide from extracerebral circulation during nitroglycerin-induced cluster headache attack. Pain 1995;60:119.
108. Uddman R, Goadsby PJ, Jansen I, Edvinsson L. PACAP, a VIP-like peptide: Immunohistochemical localization and effect upon cat pial arteries and cerebral blood flow. J Cereb Blood Flow Metab 1993;13:291.
109. Uddman R, Goadsby PJ, Jansen I, Edvinsson L. Helospectin-like peptides: Immunohistochemical localization and effects on cat pial arteries and on cerebral blood flow. J Cereb Blood Flow Metab 1993;13(Suppl 1):S206.
110. Goadsby PJ, Lambert GA, Lance JW. Differential effects on the internal and external carotid circulation of the monkey evoked by locus coeruleus stimulation. Brain Res 1982;249:247.
111. Goadsby PJ, Lambert GA, Lance JW. The mechanism of cerebrovascular vasoconstriction in response to locus coeruleus stimulation. Brain Res 1985;326:213.
112. Goadsby PJ, Duckworth JW. Low frequency stimulation of the locus coeruleus reduces regional cerebral blood flow in the spinalized cat. Brain Res 1989;476:71.
113. Goadsby PJ, Lambert GA, Lance JW. Effects of locus coeruleus stimulation on carotid vascular resistance in the cat. Brain Res 1983;278:175.
114. Goadsby PJ, Piper RD, Lambert GA, Lance JW. The effect of activation of the nucleus raphe dorsalis (DRN) on carotid blood flow. I: The monkey. Am J Physiol 1985;248:R257.
115. Goadsby PJ, Piper RD, Lambert GA, Lance JW. The effect of activation of the nucleus raphe dorsalis (DRN) on carotid blood flow. II: The cat. Am J Physiol 1985;248:R263.
116. Underwood MD, Bakalian MJ, Arango V, Smith RW, et al. Regulation of cortical blood flow by the dorsal raphe nucleus: Topographic organization of cerebrovascular regulatory regions. J Cereb Blood Flow Metab 1992;12:664.
117. Weiller C, May A, Limmroth V, et al. Brainstem activation in spontaneous human migraine attacks. Nature Med 1995;1:658.
118. Raskin NH, Hosobuchi Y, Lamb S. Headache may arise from perturbation of brain. Headache 1987;27:416.
119. Maertens de Noordhout A, Timsit-Berthier M, Timsit M, Schoenen J. Contingent negative variation and headache. Ann Neurol 1986;19:78.
120. Bocker KB, Timsit-Berthier M, Schoenen J, Brunia CH. Contingent negative variation in migraine. Headache 1990;30:604.
121. Schoenen J, Wang W, Albert A, Delwaide PJ. Potentiation instead of habituation characterizes visual evoked potentials in migraine patients between attacks. Eur J Neurol 1995;2:115.
122. Schoenen J, Timsit-Berthier M. Contingent negative variation: Methods and potential interest in headache. Cephalalgia 1993;13:28.
123. Keay KA, Kaube H, Hoskin KL, Bandler R, et al. Fos expression in the midbrain periaqueductal gray of the cat evoked by electrical stimulation of the superior sagittal sinus. Proc Aust Neuro Soc 1993;4:179.
124. Harper AM, MacKenzie ET, McCulloch J, Pickard JD. Migraine and the blood-brain barrier. Lancet 1977;1(8020):1034.
125. Alvarez-Cermeno J, Gobernado JM, Aimeno A. Transient blood-brain barrier (BBB) damage in migraine. Headache 1986;26:437.
126. Bates D, Ashford E, Dawson R, et al. Subcutaneous sumatriptan during the migraine aura. Neurology 1994;44:1587.
127. Dahlof C, Diener HC, Goadsby PJ, et al. A multicentre, double-blind, placebo-controlled, dose-range finding study to investigate the efficacy and safety of oral doses of 311C90 in the acute treatment of migraine. Headache 1995;35:292.
128. Dowson A, Ramphul-Gokulsing S, Klein K, Cox R, et al. Can oral 311C90, a novel 5-HT$_{1D}$ agonist, prevent migraine headache when taken during an aura? Cephalalgia 1995;15(Suppl 14):173.
129. Raichle ME, Hartman BK, Eichling JO, Sharpe LG. Central noradrenergic regulation of cerebral blood flow and vascular permeability. Proc Natl Acad Sci U S A 1975;72:3726.

130. Raichle ME, Eichling JO, Grubb RL, Hartman BK. Central Noradrenergic Regulation of Brain Micro-Circulation. In HM Pappius, W Feindel (eds), Dynamics of Brain Edema. New York: Springer, 1976;11.
131. Hartman BK, Swanson LW, Raichle ME, Preskorn SH, et al. Central adrenergic regulation of cerebral microvascular permeability and blood flow: Anatomic and physiologic evidence. The cerebral microvasculature. Adv Exp Med Biol 1980;131:113.
132. Preskorn SH, Hartman BK, Raichle ME, Clark HB. The effect of dibenzazepine (tricyclic antidepressants) on cerebral capillary permeability in the rat in vivo. J Pharmacol Exp Ther 1980;213:313.
133. Harik SI, McGunigal T. The protective influence of the locus ceruleus on the blood-brain barrier. Ann Neurol 1984;15:568.
134. Johnson MD, Ma PM. Localization of NADPH diaphorase activity in monoaminergic neurons of the rat brain. J Comp Neurol 1993;332:391.
135. Sicuteri F, Testi A, Anselmi B. Biochemical investigations in headache: Increases in hydroxyindoleacetic acid excretion during migraine attacks. Int Arch Allergy 1961;19:55.
136. Anthony M, Hinterberger H, Lance JW. Plasma serotonin in migraine and stress. Arch Neurol 1967;16:544.
137. Kimball RW, Friedman AP, Vallejo E. Effect of serotonin in migraine patients. Neurology (Minneapolis) 1960;10:107.
138. Bradley PB, Engel G, Feniuk W, et al. Proposals for the classification and nomenclature of functional receptors for 5-hydroxytryptamine. Neuropharmacology 1986;25:563.
139. Hoyer D, Clarke DE, Fozard JR, et al. International Union of Pharmacology classification of receptors for 5-hydroxytryptamine (serotonin). Pharmacol Rev 1994;46:157.
140. Humphrey PPA, Feniuk W, Marriott AS, et al. Preclinical studies on the antimigraine drug sumatriptan. Eur Neurol 1991;31:282.
141. Martin GR. Preclinical Profile of the Novel 5-HT$_{1D}$ Receptor Agonist 311C90. In FC Rose (ed), New Advances in Headache Research, Vol. 4. London: Smith-Gordon, 1994;3.
142. Leysen JE, Gommeren W, Luyten WHML, Van Hoenacker P, et al. [3H]-Alniditan, a new high-affinity ligand for human 5-HT$_{1D\alpha}$ and human 5-HT$_{1D\beta}$ receptors. Proceedings of the Society for Neuroscience (USA) 1995;21:1854.
143. Goldstein J, Schellens R, Diener HC, et al. Alniditan, a Novel Non-Indole 5-HT$_{1D}$–Receptor Agonist: A sc Dose-Finding Trial. In J Olesen, P Tfelt-Hansen (eds), Trial Methodology and New Drugs. New York: Raven, 1996.
144. Beer M, Middlemiss D, Stanton J, et al. In vitro pharmacological profile of the novel 5-HT$_{1D}$–receptor agonist MK-462. Cephalalgia 1995;15(Suppl 14):203.
145. Yocca FD, Buchanan I, Gylys IA, et al. The preclinical pharmacological profile of the putative antimigraine agent BMS-180048, a structurally novel 5-HT$_{1D}$ agonist. Cephalalgia 1995;15(Suppl 14):174.
146. Lee WS, Moskowitz MA. Conformationally restricted sumatriptan analogs, CP-122,288 and CP-122,638, exhibit enhanced potency against neurogenic inflammation in dura mater. Brain Res 1993;626:303.
147. Hamel E, Bouchard D. Contractile 5-HT$_1$ receptors in human isolated pial arterioles: Correlation with 5-HT$_{1D}$ binding sites. Br J Pharmacol 1991;102:227.
148. Peroutka SJ, McCarthy BG. Sumatriptan (GR43175) interacts selectively with 5-HT$_{1B}$ and 5-HT$_{1D}$ binding sites. Eur J Pharmacol 1989;163:133.
149. Schoeffter P, Hoyer D. How selective is GR43175? Interactions with functional 5-HT$_{1A}$, 5-HT$_{1B}$, 5-HT$_{1C}$, and 5-HT$_{1D}$ receptors. Naunyn Schmiedebergs Arch Pharmacol 1989;340:135.
150. Perren MJ, Feniuk W, Humphrey PPA. Vascular 5-HT$_1$–like receptors that mediate contraction of the dog isolated saphenous vein and carotid arterial vasoconstriction in anaesthetised dogs are not of the 5-HT$_{1A}$ or 5-HT$_{1D}$ subtype. Br J Pharmacol 1991;102:191.
151. Villalon CM, Bom AH, Den Boer MO, Heiligers JP, et al. Effects of S9977 and dihydroergotamine in an animal experimental model for migraine. Pharmacol Res 1992;25:125.
152. Bax WA, Van Heuven-Nolsen D, Simoons ML, Saxena PR. 5-Hydroxytryptamine-induced contractions of the human isolated saphenous vein: Involvement of 5-HT$_2$ and 5-HT$_{1D}$–like receptors, and a comparison with grafted veins. Naunyn Schmiedebergs Arch Pharmacol 1992;345:500.
153. Deckert V, Pruneau D, Elghozi J-L. Mediation by the 5-HT$_{1D}$ receptors of 5-hydroxytryptamine-induced contractions of rabbit middle and posterior cerebral arteries. Br J Pharmacol 1994;112:939.
154. Schoeffter P, Waeber C, Palacios JM, Hoyer D. The 5-hydroxytryptamine 5-HT$_{1D}$ receptor subtype is negatively coupled to adenylate cyclase in calf substantia nigra. Naunyn Schmiedebergs Arch Pharmacol 1988;337:602.
155. Waeber C, Schoeffter P, Palacios JM, Hoyer D. Molecular pharmacology of 5-HT$_{1D}$ recognition sites: Radioligand binding studies in human, pig and calf brain membranes. Naunyn Schmiedebergs Arch Pharmacol 1988;337:595.

156. Miller KJ, King A, Demchyshyn L, Niznik H, et al. Agonist activity of sumatriptan and metergoline at the human 5-HT$_{1D\beta}$ receptor: Further evidence for a role of the 5-HT$_{1D}$ receptor in the action of sumatriptan. Eur J Pharmacol 1992;227:99.
157. Clitherow JW, Scopes DI, Skingle M, et al. Evolution of a novel series of [(N,N-dimethylamino) propyl]- and peperazinylbenzanilides as the first selective 5-HT$_{1D}$ antagonists. J Med Chem 1994;37:2253.
158. Pauwels PJ, Colpaert FC. The 5-HT$_{1D}$ receptor antagonist GR127935 is an agonist at cloned human 5-HT$_{1D\alpha}$ receptor sites. Neuropharmacology 1995;34:235.
159. Goadsby PJ, Edvinsson L. The trigeminovascular system and migraine: Studies characterising cerebrovascular and neuropeptide changes seen in man and cat. Ann Neurol 1993;33:48.
160. Martin GR, Humphrey PPA. Receptors for 5-hydroxytryptamine: Current perspectives on classification and nomenclature. Neuropharmacology 1994;33:261.

2
Serotonin Receptor Involvement in the Pathogenesis and Treatment of Migraine

Graeme R. Martin

INTRODUCTION

Speculation concerning the possible roles for serotonin (5-hydroxytryptamine; 5-HT) receptors in migraine holds an intriguing ambivalence. On the one hand, there is a long-standing implied role for serotonin mobilization and depletion during a migraine attack, suggesting that a tonic activation of serotonin receptors is in some way crucial to the normal modulation of cranial nociception. On the other hand, drugs that activate specific serotonin receptor subtypes are clearly effective in the symptomatic treatment of an attack. Perhaps such a dichotomy is not unreasonable given that as many as 14 distinct 5-HT receptors have now been identified.

The possibility that serotonin might be an important endogenous factor responsible for the pain of migraine was first proposed by Wolff and colleagues in the late 1950s.[1,2] It is therefore remarkable that even though definitive proof for its involvement remains elusive, the concept remains in vogue more than 40 years later. Following a limited clinical study by Ostfeld[3] showing that intravenous injection of serotonin provoked a migraine attack in four of 13 migraineurs, Sicuteri et al.[4] reported that the urinary concentration of 5-hydroxyindoleacetic acid, the primary metabolite of serotonin, was elevated during an attack. These observations led to the idea that migraine might be triggered by a mobilization of the transmitter, a notion that was subsequently reinforced by Lance and coworkers[5] with the demonstration that blood concentrations of serotonin decreased at the onset of migraine as a consequence of its liberation from platelets.[6,7] In subsequent years, additional evidence favoring a "serotonin mobilization" theory came from clinical studies showing that drugs that either release endogenous serotonin (reserpine, fenfluramine) or mimic its actions at specific serotonin receptors (m-chlorophenylpiperazine; m-CPP) reliably provoke an attack in susceptible individuals (see Fozard[8] for a review). Although undeniably circumstantial, this body of accumulated information continues to encourage the view that serotonin and serotonin receptors are somehow implicated in migraine pathogenesis; this view is strengthened by the fact that many of the current prophylactic drugs are powerful serotonin receptor antagonists.

Whether the action of these drugs can be explained in terms of antagonism at a common serotonin receptor site remains, however, an open question.

In an apparent contradiction of Ostfeld's early finding that migraine could be induced by intravenous serotonin, two subsequent independent studies reported that serotonin injection aborted an ongoing attack, whether spontaneous[9] or induced by prior administration of reserpine.[10] Both noradrenaline[11] and ergotamine[12] were likewise shown to be effective in providing relief of acute symptoms. By contrast, interventions resulting in dilation[13,14] or stretch[15] of cerebral blood vessels cause head pain, which can evolve to migraine in migraineurs (see also Chapter 1). These observations led to the development of sumatriptan, a serotonin mimetic that has selective cranial vasoconstrictor actions by virtue of its specificity for vascular "5-HT$_{1D}$–like" receptors.[16,17] Extensive clinical experience with this drug has confirmed its excellent efficacy in migraine with or without aura, as well as in cluster headache,[18] and stimulated the development of several newer so-called 5-HT$_{1D}$ agonist drugs (Figure 2.1; see also Chapter 8). However, the recent rapid evolution of molecular approaches to receptor characterization has revealed that the drugs in this class act at more than one serotonin receptor type, raising new questions about the precise molecular mechanisms responsible for their efficacy against migraine. This chapter deals with the current classification of serotonin receptors and draws on available direct and indirect evidence that implicates a role for specific receptor subtypes in the symptomatic and prophylactic treatment of migraine.

CLASSIFICATION OF SEROTONIN RECEPTORS

Historical Classification

Until the beginning of the 1990s, receptor and ion channel classification was based principally on functional pharmacologic, biochemical, and electrophysiologic experiments in isolated intact tissues, cells, and cell membranes. Gaddum and Picarrelli[19] first provided evidence that serotonin effects are mediated by more than one receptor and proposed the first subclassification of receptors into neurotropic morphine-sensitive (M) and musculotropic dibenzyline-sensitive (D) types. The subsequent development of better discriminatory ligands, coupled with the emergence of radioligand binding assays as a means of identifying receptors, confirmed this early subclassification and quickly revealed the presence of many more serotonin binding sites. This progress culminated in the first attempt to rigorously classify serotonin receptors using well-defined pharmacologic and biochemical criteria and resulted in a nomenclature that recognized three main receptor classes: 5-HT$_1$, 5-HT$_2$, and 5-HT$_3$.[20] In this scheme, the 5-HT$_2$ and 5-HT$_3$ receptors corresponded to D and M receptors, respectively, whereas the 5-HT$_1$ class accommodated a number of receptor subtypes denominated 5-HT$_{1A}$, 5-HT$_{1B}$, 5-HT$_{1C}$, and, later, 5-HT$_{1D}$. Although additional putative receptors and recognition sites for serotonin continued to be identified using these largely operational criteria, the advent of gene-cloning techniques paved the way to a more fundamental basis for classifying receptors, namely the receptor protein primary structure.

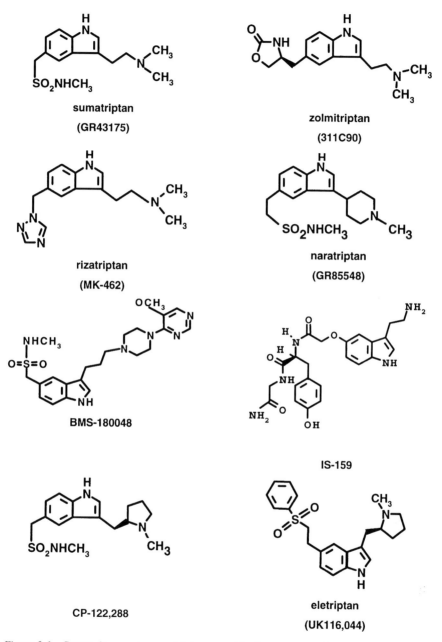

Figure 2.1 Serotonin receptor agonist drugs used in the treatment of acute migraine.

Table 2.1   1996 IUPHAR classification of serotonin receptors based on operational and

Receptor name	$5\text{-}HT_{1A}$	$5\text{-}HT_{1B}$
Previous name(s)	—	$5\text{-}HT_{1D\beta}$
Selective agonists	8-OH-DPAT	Sumatriptan
Selective antagonists	(±)WAY 100165	GR55562
Radioligands	[^{3}H]8-OH-DPAT	[^{125}I]GTI
Effector pathway	Gi / Go	Gi / Go
Structural data	421 aa 7TM	390 aa 7TM

Receptor name	$5\text{-}HT_{2A}$	$5\text{-}HT_{2B}{}^a$
Previous name(s)	D / $5\text{-}HT_2$	$5\text{-}HT_{2F}$
Selective agonists	α-me-5-HT	α-me-5-HT
		BW723C86
Selective antagonists	Ketanserin	SB204741
Radioligands	[^{3}H]ketanserin	[^{3}H]5-HT
Effector pathway	Gq / G_{11}	Gq / G_{11}
Structural data	471 aa 7TM	479 aa 7TM

Receptor name	$5\text{-}ht_{5A}$	$5\text{-}ht_{5B}$
Previous name(s)	$5\text{-}HT_{5\alpha}$	$5\text{-}HT_{5\beta}$
Selective agonists	—	—
Selective antagonists	—	—
Radioligands	[^{3}H]5-CT	[^{3}H]5-CT
Effector pathway	—	—
Structural data	357 aa 7TM	r $5\text{-}ht_{5A}$: 371 aa 7TM^b

IUPHAR = International Union of Pharmacology.
^{a}Rodent $5\text{-}HT_{1B}$ receptor displays unique pharmacology.
^{b}No human structural data are available.

Modern Classification

During the last 6 years, gene products encoding 14 different serotonin receptors have been cloned and sequenced from a variety of species, including
humans. Many of these have been shown to encode already well-defined receptors, but a number still lack clear physiologic correlates. Nevertheless, it is clear
that the combination of primary structural information with precise operational data offers a powerful basis for the differential classification of receptors,
and these attributes now form the basis of the current, NC-IUPHAR–sanc-
tioned* scheme for naming and classifying receptors.[21] This scheme, summarized in Table 2.1, has recently been further modified to more closely align
receptor nomenclature with the human genome.[22] Hence, the $5\text{-}HT_{1D\alpha}$ and

---

*NC-IUPHAR is the receptor nomenclature committee of the International Union of
Pharmacology.

structural criteria in which the human species assumes primacy

$5\text{-}HT_{1D}$	$5\text{-}ht_{1E}$	$5\text{-}ht_{1F}$
$5\text{-}HT_{1D\alpha}$	—	$5\text{-}HT_{1E\beta}$ $5\text{-}HT_6$
Sumatriptan	—	—
—	—	—
$[^{125}I]$GTI	$[^3H]$5-HT	$[^{125}I]$LSD
Gi / Go	Gi / Go	Gi / Go
377 aa 7TM	365 aa 7TM	366 aa 7TM
$5\text{-}HT_{2C}$	**$5\text{-}HT_3$**	**$5\text{-}HT_4$**
$5\text{-}HT_{1C}$	M	—
α-me-5-HT	2-me-5-HT	RS39604
	m-chlorophenyl-biguanide	BIMU-8
SB200646	Granisetron	GR113808
	Ondansetron	SB204070
$[^3H]$mesulergine	$[^3H]$zacopride	$[^3H]$GR113808
		$[^{125}I]$SB204070
Gq / G_{11}	Intrinsic ion channel	Gs
458 aa 7TM	m $5\text{-}HT^3$: 487 aa 4TM[b]	421 aa 7TM
$5\text{-}HT_6$	**$5\text{-}HT_7$**	
—	—	
—	—	
—	—	
$[^3H]$5-CT	$[^3H]$5-CT	
Gs	Gs	
436 aa 7TM	445 aa 7TM	

$5\text{-}HT_{1D\beta}$ receptor subtypes have been renamed $5\text{-}HT_{1D}$ and $5\text{-}HT_{1B}$, respectively, reflecting more accurately the fact that they are distinct gene products. In accommodating this change, which, for nomenclature purposes, establishes primacy for the human genome, the well-characterized rodent $5\text{-}HT_{1B}$ receptor is subsumed within the human $5\text{-}HT_{1B}$ class, with the appellation r $5\text{-}HT_{1B}$ (denoting rat $5\text{-}HT_{1B}$ receptor). However, it is important to remember that the pharmacology of the human and rodent $5\text{-}HT_{1B}$ receptors is completely different as a consequence of a single amino acid difference in the seventh transmembrane domain.[23,24]

Thus, the combination of structural and operational characteristics that define serotonin receptors presently enables seven distinct classes or families to be delineated: $5\text{-}HT_1$ to $5\text{-}HT_7$. As illustrated in Table 2.1, all but one of these receptor classes are members of the 7-TM G-protein-coupled superfamily, the sole exception being the $5\text{-}HT_3$ class, which belongs to the ligand-gated ion-channel superfamily. This multiplicity of receptor types is magnified by the existence of receptor subtypes, allelic variants, or both, within each class. In this respect the 5-HT_1 class exhibits a marked heterogeneity.

Although diverse in their pharmacology, the subtypes within each class appear to share the same transduction system, presumably reflecting a common ancestry in terms of the evolution and differentiation of the serotonin receptor family.[25] Indeed, analysis of the evolution of serotonin receptors suggests that yet more serotonin receptor families remain to be discovered, although these receptors are likely to exhibit poor homology ($< 25\%$) with those currently identified.[25] Obviously, the possibility that as yet undiscovered serotonin receptors might contribute further to an understanding of migraine mechanism and therapeutics is tantalizing, especially in light of the recent demonstration that indole derivatives such as CP-122,288 (see the section titled "CP-122,288–Sensitive" Receptor) potently inhibit neurogenic inflammation in the dura by a mechanism that does not involve any of the currently recognized serotonin receptors.[26]

RECEPTORS IMPLICATED IN THE SYMPTOMATIC TREATMENT OF MIGRAINE

5-Hydroxytryptamine $_{1B}$ and 5-Hydroxytryptamine $_{1D}$ Receptors

The advent of sumatriptan has been a fundamental advance not just in the treatment of migraine, but also in accelerating the understanding of the disease's pathophysiology. Although the drug was developed as a selective agonist at "5-HT_{1D}–like" receptors mediating vascular contraction,[16,17] it is now clear that, like the newer 5-HT_{1D} agonist drugs, its profile is more accurately regarded as that of a $5\text{-HT}_{1B}/5\text{-HT}_{1D}$ agonist. This class of drugs, together with the ergots, block or reverse the consequences of trigeminovascular activation by constricting cranial blood vessels and inhibiting the release of sensory neuropeptides from perivascular trigeminal afferents.[27,28] Elegant studies by Goadsby and colleagues have shown that activation of $5\text{-HT}_{1B}/5\text{-HT}_{1D}$ receptors can also attenuate the excitability of cells in the trigeminal nucleus caudalis that receive a primary input from the trigeminal nerve.[29,30] Hence, $5\text{-HT}_{1B}/5\text{-HT}_{1D}$ agonists such as zolmitriptan, which access central as well as peripheral components of the trigeminovascular system, interrupt cranial nociceptive input at three sites. However, whether or not the 5-HT_{1B} and 5-HT_{1D} receptor subtypes exhibit distinct distributions within the trigeminovascular system remains unknown. The extremely close pharmacologic identity between these receptors in nonrodents has hampered attempts to differentiate them in terms of functional effects. Nevertheless, a consensus based on available data favors the view that cerebral vessel constriction is mediated predominantly by the 5-HT_{1B} subtype.[31–33] This is supported by studies in the rat,[34] a species in which the unique pharmacology of the 5-HT_{1B} receptor enables its unambiguous functional differentiation from the 5-HT_{1D} receptor. Subsequent speculation that a 5-HT_{1D} subtype–selective agonist might therefore produce inhibition of the trigeminal nerve without causing vasoconstriction was initially encouraged by a report indicating that messenger RNA for 5-HT_{1D} receptors, but not 5-HT_{1B} receptors, could be found in postmortem human trigeminal ganglia.[35] Although unpublished preliminary data with a novel agonist reported to be highly selective for 5-HT$_{1D}$ over 5-HT$_{1B}$ receptors has been presented in support of this concept,[36] there is increasing evidence to question its validity across species. First, in mice lacking the 5-HT$_{1B}$ receptor gene, sumatriptan and the selective 5-HT$_{1B}$ agonist CP-93,129 lose the ability to inhibit neurogenic inflammation evoked by trigeminal ganglion stimulation,[37] implying that 5-HT$_{1D}$ receptors do not mediate trigeminal neuroinhibition in this species. Second, a number of studies using tissue from humans and other species have now shown that message for both 5-HT$_{1B}$ and 5-HT$_{1D}$ receptors can be detected not only in the trigeminal ganglion but also in the cerebrovascular smooth muscle.[38–40] If this mRNA signals the presence of functional 5-HT$_{1D}$ as well as 5-HT$_{1B}$ receptors in cerebral vessels, it may not be possible to achieve subtype-selective, nonconstrictor antimigraine agents from the 5-HT$_{1B}$/5-HT$_{1D}$ drug class.

Autoradiographic studies using [³H]-dihydroergotamine (DHE),[41] [³H]-sumatriptan,[42] or [³H]-zolmitriptan[43,44] have shown that in addition to their presence in the blood vessels and the perivascular sensory nerves innervating them, 5-HT$_{1B}$/5-HT$_{1D}$ receptors are localized in the trigeminal nucleus caudalis (TNC), the nucleus tractus solitarius (NTS), and, in higher regions, in the area postrema and subnucleus gelatinosus. Attempts to determine whether this binding corresponds to a predominance of 5-HT$_{1B}$ or 5-HT$_{1D}$ receptors have been inconclusive, possibly because both subtypes coexist in these regions.[43] Nevertheless, specific binding to the TNC is consistent with the ability of 5-HT$_{1B}$/5-HT$_{1D}$ agonists to attenuate the excitability of these cells during sensory nerve activation,[29,30] while binding to the NTS and area postrema raises the intriguing possibility that these drugs might also exert a direct effect to prevent the nausea and vomiting associated with migraine. Also of possible therapeutic relevance is that both [³H]-DHE and [³H]-zolmitriptan access the TNC and NTS following systemic administration,[41,45] indicating that these drugs can act centrally as well as peripherally to inhibit trigeminovascular activation. This is not the case for sumatriptan, which inhibits cell excitability in the TNC only after disruption of the blood–brain barrier.[30]

5-Hydroxytryptamine$_{1A}$ Receptors

One unsubstantiated report has suggested that the 5-HT$_{1A}$-receptor–selective agonist buspirone can alleviate migraine,[46] but formal placebo-controlled clinical studies have not been conducted. Although it is clear from Table 2.2 that, like the ergots, sumatriptan and many of the 5-HT$_{1D}$–agonist drugs in development display affinity at the 5-HT$_{1A}$ receptor, it is unlikely that an action at this receptor subtype accounts for their cranial analgesic effects. Whether agonist action at this receptor might nevertheless contribute to other facets of these drugs' therapeutic profile, for example, their ability to reduce nausea and vomiting or the sensory disturbances that accompany the headache, remains an intriguing but unanswered question.

5-ht$_{1F}$ Receptors

Speculation that 5-ht$_{1F}$ receptors might be target sites of action for sumatriptan, zolmitriptan, and the ergot alkaloids arose shortly after the human receptor had

Table 2.2   Affinities ($-\log K_i$ or $-\log [IC_{50}]$) at human recombinant 5-HT$_1$ receptors of antimigraine drugs known to be or putatively effective in the treatment of acute migraine

Drug	5-HT$_{IA}$	5-HT$_{IB}$	5-HT$_{ID}$	5-ht$_{IE}$	5-ht$_{IF}$
Sumatriptan	7.0	7.9	7.9	5.6	7.6
Zolmitriptan	6.5	8.2	9.2	<5.0	7.1
Rizatriptan	6.3	7.3	7.7	6.5	—
IS 159	6.0	8.5	8.8*	<5.0	<5.0
Naratriptan	7.1	8.7	8.3	—	—
BMS-180,048	6.7	7.7	8.3	<6.0	—
CP-122,288	—	7.5	8.1	—	—
Ergotamine	9.5	8.3	9.4	8.0	6.8
Dihydroergotamine	9.1	8.2	9.3	8.1	—

IC_{50} = concentration of ligand producing 50% displacement of radiolabel.
*Total 5-HT$_{1D}$ binding.

been cloned and expressed in mammalian cells.[47] Radioligand binding experiments showed that in addition to their high affinity at 5-HT$_{1B}$ and 5-HT$_{1D}$ receptors, these drugs also had high affinity for the 5-ht$_{1F}$ subtype (Table 2.2) and behaved as agonists when effects on cAMP formation were measured.[48] However, a significant role for 5-ht$_{1F}$ receptors in the therapeutic actions of antimigraine drugs can probably be eliminated. Although 5-ht$_{1F}$ mRNA has recently been detected in the human trigeminal ganglion and cerebral vessels,[40] receptor message has not been found in other anatomic regions associated with the processing of head pain.[39] Second, and more pertinent, one of the newer 5-HT$_{1D}$ agonist drugs in development, IS 159, exhibits low affinity ($pK_i < 5.0$; see Table 2.2) at the 5-ht$_{1F}$ subtype, yet shares with sumatriptan and zolmitriptan a high affinity at 5-HT$_{1B}$ and 5-HT$_{1D}$ receptors and a high therapeutic efficacy in aborting migraine (Chauveau J. Immunotech; personal communication, 1995).

5-Hydroxytryptamine$_3$ Receptors

The rationale for developing and evaluating 5-HT$_3$ receptor antagonists as antimigraine drugs arose from knowledge of the potent dermal algesic properties of 5-HT[49] and the realization that neuroexcitatory 5-HT$_3$ receptors mediated this effect.[50] Subsequently, it has been shown that these receptors are also discretely concentrated in brain stem nuclei that receive sensory input from the trigeminal nerve (trigeminal nucleus caudalis) and are present in a high density in the nucleus tractus solitarius and area postrema.[44,51] Within the brain stem, the distribution of 5-HT$_3$ receptors is similar to that reported for 5-HT$_{1D}$ receptors, but with an even higher density of sites.[44] Clearly, this anatomic distribution is attractive in terms of a potential role for both receptor types in the modulation of cranial nociception, and in this regard 5-HT$_3$ receptor antagonists have been shown to inhibit potassium-evoked release of sensory neuropeptides from dorsal spinal cord, implying inhibition of C-fiber activation.[52] Although an early clinical trial with the first drug designed specifically to test this hypothesis, MDL 72222, appeared to show moderate efficacy in migraine patients,[53] subsequent studies with more potent and selective 5-HT$_3$ antagonists have failed to confirm therapeutic benefit with these drugs in migraine, either as prophylactics or in the treatment of acute symptoms.[54] However, the drugs *are* effective against the nausea and vomiting of migraine, consistent with their ability to inhibit radiation- and chemotherapy-induced vomiting in animals and humans.[54]

"CP-122,288–Sensitive" Receptor

CP-122,288 is an indole analogue of sumatriptan, conformationally restricted in the 3 position by substitution of an N-methylpyrrolidine (see Table 2.1). Like the ergots and the more selective 5-HT$_{1D}$ agonist drugs, this compound also blocks neurogenic plasma protein extravasation, but at an intravenous dose at least 1,000 to 40,000 times lower than the inhibitory dose of sumatriptan.[26,55,56] A similar low dose of the drug also attenuates the expression of c-*fos*–like immunoreactivity in the trigeminal nucleus caudalis provoked by intracisternal capsaicin,[55] and again the effective dose is much lower than that at which sumatriptan or DHE is effective.[57]

The pattern of c-*fos* inhibition with CP-122,288 mimics that described with sumatriptan, DHE, and the selective 5-HT$_{1B}$ agonist CP-93,129, but the nature of the receptor involved remains unclear. The drug displays similar agonist potency to sumatriptan at 5-HT$_{1D}$–like receptors mediating vasoconstriction and also has a similar affinity at recombinant human 5-HT$_{1B}$ and 5-HT$_{1D}$ receptors.[56] The more than 1,000 to 1 potency ratio observed for CP-122,288 and sumatriptan in both the extravasation and c-*fos* assays therefore makes it highly unlikely that these drugs mediate their effects through the same receptor type or types. Indeed, confirmation that this is so was recently obtained using 5-HT$_{1B}$ receptor knockout mice, in which the ability of sumatriptan to inhibit plasma protein extravasation into the dura was lost, whereas the potency of CP-122,288 in the same assay was unaffected.[37] Evidently CP-122,288 recognizes a novel receptor type. To date, limited pharmacologic studies have shown that CP-122,288 effects are insensitive to the 5-HT$_{1B}$/5-HT$_{1D}$ antagonist GR127935[58] and are only partially reversed by the nonselective 5-HT$_{1D}$ antagonist metergoline.[26] Furthermore, increasing evidence indicates that 5-CT exhibits a similar profile to CP-122,288 in terms of extravasation responses, suggesting that both agents inhibit neurogenic inflammation via the same CP-122,288–sensitive receptor type.[58] That drugs of this type could provide migraine relief in the absence of any direct vascular actions is a truly exciting possibility. Whether or not this turns out to be the case, they clearly offer a means to more thoroughly understand the relation between existing animal models and the disease itself.

RECEPTORS INVOLVED IN THE PREVENTATIVE TREATMENT OF MIGRAINE

5-Hydroxytryptamine$_{2B}$/5-Hydroxytryptamine$_{2C}$ Receptors

The first rational approach to the prevention of migraine was aimed at blocking the actions of serotonin by using lysergic acid derivatives.[59] This led to the

Table 2.3   Drugs used in migraine prophylaxis: daily doses and their potencies (pK_B/pKi) at the 5-HT_2 receptor subtypes

Drug	Dose (mg/day)	5-HT_{2A}	5-HT_{2B}	5-HT_{2C}
Methysergide	2–6	8.3	(9.5)	8.7
Pizotifen	4.5–9.0	9.4	(8.5)	7.8
Cyproheptadine	12–24	8.9	(7.5)	7.4
Mianserin	30–60	8.1	7.7	7.9
Amitriptyline	30–75	—	6.6	7.5
DL-Propranolol	80–320	6.2	6.2	4.0
Ketanserin (inactive)	—	8.6	<5.0	5.1
m-CPP[a]	—	—	7.1/0.5	6.9/0.65[b]

[a]Denotes agonist.
[b]Result from pig choroid plexus.[71]
Source: Drug dose data are from MG Buzzi, DE Sakas, MA Moskowitz. Indomethacin and acetylsalicylic acid block neurogenic plasma protein extravasation in rat dura mater. Eur J Pharmacol 1989;165:251. Potency data are unpublished results obtained within species (rabbit) by R Martin, Wellcome Research Laboratories, Beckenham, Kent, UK.

introduction of methysergide and a number of other drugs that, in retrospect, clearly share a common property of 5-HT_2 receptor antagonism (Table 2.3). Available evidence, carefully reviewed in recent years by Fozard and colleagues,[60–62] shows that prophylactic drugs from various chemical classes display an affinity at both 5-HT_{2B} and 5-HT_{2C} receptors that corresponds closely with the effective daily dose of these drugs (Table 2.3). Although most of these agents are also powerful D (5-HT_{2A}) receptor antagonists, the inability of the highly selective antagonist ketanserin to prevent migraine suggests that the 5-HT_{2A} subtype is not involved.[63] Of particular interest in this regard, Brewerton et al. have shown that m-CPP, a metabolite of the antidepressant trazodone and an agonist at both 5-HT_{2B} and 5-HT_{2C} receptors, reliably provokes migraine about 3–4 hours after administration to migraineurs.[64] The possibility that mobilization of endogenous serotonin culminates in 5-HT_{2B}, 5-HT_{2C}, or both receptor activation to precipitate a migraine accords with long-standing theories of migraine pathogenesis, but the locus of drug action is unclear. 5-HT_{2C} receptors are widespread throughout the central nervous system; there is no obvious concentration in regions involved in pain processing and no convincing evidence for their presence in peripheral tissues. However, the epithelium of the choroid plexus is especially enriched in these receptors, implying a role in the modulation of cerebrospinal fluid production. Moreover, recent studies have shown that 5-HT_{2C} receptors also activate lipoxygenase and cyclo-oxygenase pathways, an action that might conceivably promote a local inflammatory response.[65] Perhaps a more plausible possibility is that prophylactic drugs act at 5-HT_{2B} receptors on the endothelium of cerebral blood vessels. The endothelial 5-HT_{2B} receptor couples to nitric oxide synthase, promoting the local release of nitric oxide ($NO^{\bullet}$).[66] In cerebral vessels, $NO^{\bullet}$ liberated in this way might be expected to excite and sensitize perivascular trigeminal afferents because NO• donors activate trigeminovascular fibers to cause release of sensory neuropeptides.[67] Moreover, there is evidence for the involvement of NO• in the initiation of migraine. First, the NO• donor nitroglycerin provokes migraine in migraineurs.[13] Second, histamine acting at endothelial H_1 receptors likewise liberates NO• and can also induce migraine in susceptible individuals.[14] Interestingly, after nitroglycerine infusion, migraine appeared with a similar latency to that reported after the administration of m-CPP. It is therefore conceivable that NO• serves as an important intermediary in the initiation, and possibly in the propagation, of a neurogenic cranial vessel inflammatory response that ultimately results in headache. Because a role for endogenous serotonin is clearly implicit in such a scenario, it bears emphasis that the transmitter exhibits an affinity for the endothelial 5-HT_{2B} receptor that is higher than its affinity for any other native, functional serotonin receptor.[68]

SUMMARY

The therapy for migraine has long relied on the use of drugs suspected to mimic or block the actions of serotonin, but the recent introduction of selective $5\text{-HT}_{1B}/5\text{-HT}_{1D}$ receptor agonists has established beyond doubt that serotonin receptors can be exploited in symptomatic treatment. A major current question is whether actions at both of these receptor subtypes is necessary for therapeutic benefit, or whether development of drugs with an improved therapeutic index might be achieved by targeting just one subtype. Early evidence suggesting that a 5-HT_{1D} subtype–selective agonist might maintain the antimigraine efficacy of sumatriptan while reducing the potential for unwanted vascular side effects (which are presumed to be 5-HT_{1B}–receptor mediated) now seems less tenable, since mRNA for both subtypes appears to be present in smooth muscle and neuronal elements of the trigeminovascular system. However, a new class of agent, exemplified by CP-122,288, blocks trigeminal-evoked plasma protein extravasation into the dura without producing vasoconstriction. Although the drug is chemically related to sumatriptan, the receptor mediating this neuroinhibitory effect does not correspond with any of the known serotonin receptor types. Nevertheless, it is clear that, regardless of its pharmacology, clinical evaluation of CP-122,288 will provide valuable insights on the relevance of available preclinical models of migraine to the disease itself.

   In terms of migraine pathogenesis, the evidence regarding involvement of serotonin receptors remains ambiguous. Many of the most effective prophylactic drugs, including propranolol, block 5-HT_{2B} receptors with a potency that matches the drug dose. Furthermore, the functional affinity of serotonin for this receptor subtype is high, so that activation can be anticipated at serotonin concentrations as low as 1 nmol per liter.[68,69] Because clinical studies have shown that agents that evoke NO• release can precipitate a migraine attack, the demonstration that vascular endothelial 5-HT_{2B} receptors likewise promote local NO• release makes them an attractive candidate target for the prophylactics. However, until selective antagonist drugs are made available to test and challenge this hypothesis, the evidence for a modulatory role of serotonin in migraine will remain circumstantial.

REFERENCES

1. Ostfeld AM, Chapman LF, Goodell H, Wolff HG. Studies in headache: Summary of evidence concerning a noxious agent active locally during migraine headache. Psychosom Med 1957;19:199.
2. Wolff HG. Headache and Other Pain. New York: Oxford University Press, 1963.
3. Ostfeld AM. Some aspects of cardiovascular regulation in man. Angiology 1959;10:34.
4. Sicuteri F, Testi A, Anselmi B. Biochemical investigations in headache: Increase in the hydroxyindoleacetic acid excretion during migraine attacks. Int Arch Allergy Appl Immunol 1961;19:55.
5. Lance JW, Anthony M, Gonski A. Serotonin, the carotid body, and cranial vessels in migraine. Arch Neurol 1967;16:553.
6. Anthony M, Hinterberger H, Lance JW. The possible relationship of serotonin to the migraine syndrome. Res Clin Stud Headache 1969;2:29.
7. Dalsgaard-Nielsen T, Genefke IK. Serotonin (5-hydroxytryptamine) release and uptake in platelets from healthy persons and migrainous patients in attack-free intervals. Headache 1974;14:26.
8. Fozard JR. Serotonin, migraine, and platelets. In PA van Zwieten, E Schönbaum (eds), Drugs and Platelets (Vol 4). Stuttgart: Gustaf Fisher Verlag, 1982;135.
9. Kimball RW, Friedman AP, Vallejo E. Effects of serotonin in migraine patients. Neurology 1960;10:107.
10. Anthony M, Hinterberger H, Lance JW. Plasma serotonin in migraine and stress. Arch Neurol 1967;16:544.
11. Ostfeld AM, Wolff HG. Studies on headache: Arterenol (norepinephrine) and vascular headache of the migraine type. Arch Neurol Psychiatry 1955;74:131.
12. Lance JW. The Mechanism and Management of Headache (2nd ed). London: Butterworth Publishers, 1973.
13. Olesen J, Iversen HK, Thomsen LL. Nitric oxide supersensitivity: A possible molecular mechanism of migraine pain. Neuroreport 1993;4:1027.
14. Krabbe AA, Olesen J. Headache provocation by continuous infusion of histamine: Clinical results and receptor mechanisms. Pain 1990;8:253.
15. Nichols FT, Mawad M, Mohr JP, Stein B, et al. Focal headache during balloon inflation in the internal carotid and middle cerebral arteries. Stroke 1990;21:555.
16. Humphrey PPA, Apperley E, Feniuk W, Perren MJ. A Rational Approach to Identifying a Fundamentally New Drug for the Treatment of Migraine. In PR Saxena, DI Wallis, W Wouters, P Bevan (eds), Cardiovascular Pharmacology of 5-Hydroxytryptamine. Dordrecht, The Netherlands: Kluwer, 1990;417.
17. Humphrey PPA, Feniuk W, Perren MJ, Connor HE, et al. The pharmacology of the novel 5-HT$_1$–like receptor agonist GR43175. Cephalalgia 1989;9(Suppl 9):23.
18. The Sumatriptan Cluster Headache Study Group. N Engl J Med 1991;325:322.
19. Gaddum JH, Picarrelli ZP. Two kinds of tryptamine receptor. Br J Pharmacol 1957;12:323.
20. Bradley PB, Engel G, Feniuk W, et al. Proposals for the classification and nomenclature of functional receptors for 5-hydroxytryptamine. Neuropharmacology 1986;25:563.
21. Hoyer D, Clarke DE, Fozard JR, et al. International Union of Pharmacology classification of receptors for 5-hydroxytryptamine (serotonin). Pharmacol Rev 1994;46:157.
22. Hartig PR, Hoyer D, Humphrey PPA, Martin GR. Alignment of receptor nomenclature with the human genome: Classification of 5-HT$_{1B}$ and 5-HT$_{1D}$ receptor subtypes. Trends Pharmacol Sci 1996;17:103.
23. Oksenberg D, Masters SA, O'Dowd BF, et al. A single amino-acid difference confers major pharmacological variation between human and rodent 5-HT$_{1B}$ receptors. Nature 1992;360:161.
24. Parker EM, Grisel DA, Iben LG, Shapiro RA. A single amino-acid difference accounts for the pharmacological distinctions between the rat and human 5-hydroxytryptamine$_{1B}$ receptors. J Neurochem 1993;60:380.
25. Peroutka SJ. Serotonin receptor subtypes: Their evolution and clinical relevance. CNS Drugs 1995;4(Suppl 1):18.
26. Lee WS, Moskowitz MA. Conformationally restricted sumatriptan analogues, CP-122,288 and CP-122,638, exhibit enhanced potency against neurogenic inflammation in dura mater. Brain Res 1993;626:303.
27. Moskowitz MA. Neurogenic versus vascular mechanisms of sumatriptan and ergot alkaloids in migraine. Trends Pharmacol Sci 1992;13:307.
28. Humphrey PPA, Feniuk W. Mode of action of the antimigraine drug sumatriptan. Trends Pharmacol Sci 1991;12:444.
29. Goadsby PJ, Edvinsson L. Peripheral and central trigeminovascular activation in cat is blocked by the serotonin (5-HT)-1D receptor agonist 311C90. Headache 1994;34:394.

30. Kaube H, Hoskin KL, Goadsby PJ. Sumatriptan inhibits central trigeminal neurones only after blood-brain barrier disruption. Br J Pharmacol 1993;109:788.
31. Kauman AJ, Parsons AA, Brown AM. Human arterial constrictor serotonin receptors. Cardiovasc Res 1993;27:2094.
32. Hamel E, Fan E, Linville D, et al. Expression of mRNA for the serotonin 5-hydroxytryptamine$_{1D}$ receptor subtype in human and bovine cerebral arteries. Mol Pharmacol 1993;44:242.
33. Connor HE, Beattie DT, Feniuk W, et al. Use of GR55562, a selective 5-HT$_{1D}$ antagonist, to investigate 5-HT$_{1D}$ receptor subtypes mediating cerebral vasoconstriction. Cephalalgia 1995;15(Suppl 14):99.
34. Craig DA, Martin GR. 5-HT$_{1B}$ receptors mediate potent contractile responses to 5-HT in rat caudal artery. Br J Pharmacol 1993;109:609.
35. Rebeck GW, Maynard KI, Hyman BT, Moskowitz MA. Selective 5-HT$_{1D}$ alpha serotonin receptor gene expression in trigeminal ganglia: Implications for antimigraine drug development. Proc Natl Acad Sci U S A 1994;91:3666.
36. Moskowitz MA. Paper presented at the International Headache Congress, Toronto, 1995.
37. Yu X-J, Waeber C, Castanon N, et al. Knock-out mice lacking 5-HT$_{1B}$ receptors: 5-CT and CP-122,288, but not sumatriptan or CP-93,129, block dural plasma protein extravasation. Cephalalgia 1995;15(Suppl 14):59.
38. Bruinvels AT, Landwehrmeyer B, Palacios JM, et al. Localisation of 5-HT$_{1D\alpha}$ and 5-HT$_{1B}$ receptor messenger RNA in rat brain and trigeminal ganglia. Br J Pharmacol 1993;108:95P.
39. Bruinvels AT, Landwehrmeyer B, Gustafson EL, et al. Localisation of 5-HT$_{1B}$, 5-HT$_{1D\alpha}$, 5-HT$_{1E}$ and 5-HT$_{1F}$ receptor messenger RNA in rodent and primate brain. Neuropharmacology 1994;33:367.
40. Bouchelet I, Cohen Z, Seguela P, Hamel E. Differential Expression of Sumatriptan-Sensitive 5-HT$_1$ Receptors in Human Neuronal and Vascular Tissues. In M Sandler, M Ferrari (eds), Migraine Research: Towards the Third Millennium. London: Chapman and Hall, 1996;55.
41. Goadsby PJ, Gundlach AL. Localisation of [³H]-dihydroergotamine binding sites in the cat central nervous system: Relevance to migraine. Ann Neurol 1991;29:91.
42. Mills A, Martin GR. Autoradiographic mapping of [³H]-sumatriptan binding in cat brain stem and spinal cord. Eur J Pharmacol 1995;280:175.
43. Mills A, Rhodes P, Martin GR. [³H]-311C90 binding sites in cat brain stem: Implications for migraine treatment. Cephalalgia 1995;15(Suppl 14):116.
44. Mills A, Martin GR. Labelling of cat brainstem sections with the novel antimigraine drug [³H]-311C90 and the 5-HT$_3$ receptor ligand [³H]-BRL43694. Cephalalgia 1995;15(Suppl 14):213.
45. Knight YE, Goadsby PJ. Direct evidence for central sites of action of 311C90: An autoradiographic study in the cat. Cephalalgia 1995;15(Suppl 14):214.
46. Pascual J, Berciano J. An open trial of buspirone in migraine prophylaxis: Preliminary report. Clin Neuropharmacol 1991;14:245.
47. Adham N, Kao H-T, Schechter LE, et al. Cloning of another human serotonin receptor (5-HT$_{1F}$): A fifth 5-HT$_1$ receptor subtype coupled to the inhibition of adenylate cyclase. Proc Natl Acad Sci U S A 1993;90:408.
48. Adham N, Borden LA, Schechter LE, et al. Cell-specific coupling of the cloned human 5-HT$_{1F}$ receptor to multiple signal transduction pathways. Naunyn Schmiedebergs Arch Pharmacol 1993;348:566.
49. Keele CA, Armstrong D. Substances Producing Pain and Itch. Baltimore: Williams & Wilkins, 1964.
50. Richardson BP, Engel G, Donatsch P, Sadler PA. Identification of 5-hydroxytryptamine M-receptor subtypes and their specific blockade by a new class of drugs. Nature 1985;316:126.
51. Pratt GD, Bowery N, Kilpatrick GJ, et al. Consensus meeting agrees distribution of 5-HT$_3$ receptors in mammalian hindbrain. Trends Pharmacol Sci 1990;11:135.
52. Saria A, Javorsky F, Humpel C, et al. 5-HT$_3$ receptor antagonists inhibit sensory neuropeptide release from the rat spinal cord. Neuroreport 1990;1:104.
53. Fozard JR. 5-HT in Migraine: Evidence from 5-HT Receptor Antagonists for a Neuronal Aetiology. In M Sandler, G Collins (eds), Migraine: A Spectrum of Ideas. Oxford: Oxford University Press, 1990;128.
54. Ferrari MD. 5-HT$_3$ receptor antagonists and migraine. J Neurol 1991;238(Suppl 1):S53.
55. Cutrer FM, Schoenfeld D, Limmroth V, et al. Suppression by the sumatriptan analogue CP-122,288 of c-*fos* immunoreactivity in trigeminal nucleus caudalis induced by intracisternal capsaicin. Br J Pharmacol 1995;114:987.
56. Beattie DT, Connor HE. The pre- and postjunctional activity of CP-122,288, a conformationally restricted analogue of sumatriptan. Eur J Pharmacol 1995;276:271.
57. Nozaki K, Moskowitz MA, Boccalini P. CP-93,129, sumatriptan, dihydroergotamine block c-*fos* expression in rat trigeminal nucleus caudalis caused by chemical stimulation of the meninges. Br J Pharmacol 1992;106:409.

58. Yu X-J, Waeber C, Moskowitz MA. Additional 5-HT receptor subtypes (besides 5-HT$_{1D}$) inhibit neurogenic plasma extravasation within guinea-pig dura mater. Cephalalgia 1995;15(Suppl 14):117.
59. Sicuteri F. Prophylactic and therapeutic properties of 1-Methyl-lysergic acid Butanolamide in migraine. Int Arch Allergy 1959;15:300.
60. Fozard JR, Gray JA. 5-HT$_{1C}$ receptor activation: A key step in the initiation of migraine? Trends Pharmacol Sci 1989;10:307.
61. Fozard JR. 5-HT$_{1C}$ Receptor Agonism as an Initiating Event in Migraine. In J Olesen, PR Saxena (eds), 5-Hydroxytryptamine Mechanisms in Primary Headache. New York: Raven, 1992;200.
62. Kalkman HO. Is migraine prophylactic activity caused by 5-HT$_{2B}$ or 5-HT$_{2C}$ receptor blockade? Life Sci 1994;54:641.
63. Winther K. Ketanserin: A selective serotonin antagonist, in relation to platelet aggregation and migraine attack rate. Cephalalgia 1985;5(Suppl 3):402.
64. Brewerton TD, Murphy DL, Mueller EA, et al. Induction of migraine-like headaches by the serotonin agonist m-chlorophenylpiperazine. Clin Pharmacol Ther 1988;43:605.
65. Kaufman MJ, Hartig P, Hoffman BJ. Serotonin 5-HT$_{2C}$ receptor stimulates cyclic GMP formation in choroid plexus. J Neurochem 1995;64:199.
66. Martin GR, Bolofo ML, Giles H. Inhibition of endothelium-dependent vasorelaxation by arginine analogues: A pharmacological analysis of agonist- and tissue-dependence. Br J Pharmacol 1992; 105:643.
67. Wei EP, Moskowitz MA, Boccalini P, et al. Calcitonin gene-related peptide mediates nitroglycerine and sodium nitroprusside vasodilation in feline cerebral arterioles. Circ Res 1992;70:1313.
68. Martin GR. Vascular receptors for 5-hydroxytryptamine: Distribution, function, and classification. Pharmacol Ther 1994;62:283.
69. Hoyer D, Schoeffter P. Are TFMPP, mCPP, and CGS 12066 selective for 5-hydrioxytryptamine 5-HT$_{1B}$ receptors? Br J Pharmacol 1989;96:9P.

GLOSSARY

MK-462 (rizatriptan): N,N-dimethyl-[5-(1H-1,2,4-triazol-1yl-methyl)-1*H*-indole-3yl]ethanamine

311C90 (zolmitriptan): (*S*)-4[[3-[2-(dimethylamino)ethyl]-1*H*-indol-5yl]methyl]-2-oxazolidinone

GR85548 (naratriptan): N-methyl-3-(1-methyl-4-piperidinyl)-1H-indole-5-ethanesulphonamide

BMS-180048: 3-(2-aminoethyl)-5-(acetamidyl-3-(4-hydroxyphenyl)-propionamidyl-acetamidyloxy)-indole

IS 159: 3-(aminoethyl-5-(acetamidyl-3-(4-hydroxyphenyl)-propionamidyl-acetamidyloxy)-1*H*-indole

UK116,044 (eletriptan): (*R*)-3-[(1-methyl-2-pyrrolidinyl)methyl]5-[2(phenyl-sulphonyl)ethyl-1H-indole

CP-122,288: 5-methylaminosulphonylmethyl-3{N-methylpyrrolidin-2R-yl-methyl}-1H-indole

CP-93,169: 5-hydroxy-3-(4-1,2,5,6-tetrahydropyridyl)-4-azaindole

GR127,935: 3-[3-(dimethylamino)propyl]-4-hydroxy-N-[4-(4-pyridinyl)phenyl]benzamide

3
Pain Modulation and Headache

Howard L. Fields

Our current level of understanding of the neural mechanisms underlying idiopathic recurrent head pain is primitive. We have yet to identify the source of the pain signal, much less the initial triggering events. Most hypotheses of headache generation stress peripheral mechanisms, either extracranial (muscle contraction, vascular dilatation) or intracranial (dural vascular innervation).[1] The strength of such proposals is that they are clearly applicable to head pains with an identifiable pathology such as meningitis, vasculitis, myofascial syndromes, intracranial masses, or head trauma. According to these "peripheralist" ideas, the critical initiating event for head pain occurs in the vicinity of the peripheral terminals of primary afferent nociceptors. Some process at that site leads to depolarization of the nociceptor terminal and to the generation of action potentials in its axon. These action potentials propagate to synapses on second-order neurons in the trigeminal complex. From there, the encoded message is relayed via well-known trigeminothalamic pathways to the cortex, resulting in the perception of head pain.

Such straightforward theories of head pain have the advantage of simplicity and they have been of heuristic value, leading to extensive and valuable studies of the properties of the sensory pathways that innervate and represent cranial structures (see Chapters 1 and 4). However, idiopathic headaches such as migraine have features that are difficult to explain if only nociceptors and pain transmission pathways are considered. For example, it is well established that headache frequency and intensity can be influenced, and perhaps even attacks triggered, by psychological factors such as emotional stress, attention, expectation, relaxation-based therapies, and suggestion (Chapter 9). Furthermore, exposure to bright lights and noise can worsen and sleep onset can abort severe headaches. Finally, despite the early suggestion that dilated blood vessels, plasma serotonin, or cortical spreading depression precedes or accompanies certain headache types, the great majority of idiopathic headaches (migraine without aura and tension type) are not associated with demonstrated objective changes in peripheral tissues.[2]

Even if some chemical change in or near peripheral nociceptors is ultimately shown to be crucial to their initiation, the powerful effects of psychological factors will have to be explained before we reach any profound understanding of idiopathic headaches. How are we to understand the contribution of psychological factors such as arousal, attention, expectation, and affect in headache? In this chapter, this issue is approached by first reviewing the evidence that psychological factors modify pain perception. The better-known central nervous system (CNS) pain-modulating circuits are described and evidence is presented that they are activated by psychological factors and exert powerful and selective bidirectional control over pain transmission pathways.

VARIABILITY OF PAIN

Cognitive Interventions That Reduce Pain

It is now accepted that, except under highly constrained experimental conditions, there is no simple relationship of tissue damage to the subjective experience of pain. This point was appreciated and extensively explored by the Harvard anesthesiologist Henry Beecher, who marveled at World War II soldiers who sustained serious injuries but complained little compared with civilians in hospitals with comparable injuries.[3,4] He also reported on the apparently high incidence and degree of placebo-induced relief, even in those with severely painful conditions.[3] His extensive though anecdotal experience has been amply confirmed in controlled studies of clinically significant and experimentally induced pain.[5] It is now established that dummy tablets and suggestion can relieve pain. Evidence is also accumulating that cognitive-behavioral methods such as hypnosis, biofeedback, guided imagery, and insight-based psychotherapy can relieve pain, including headache pain.[6]

Explanations for the relief provided by such psychologically based interventions are of three general classes. One, which may be thought of as an essentially peripheralist view, proposes that the relief produced by cognitive and behavioral treatments results from a reduction of anxiety (fear, stress) or of muscle contraction. Reduction of anxiety would reduce sympathetic outflow and blood pressure, which in turn would reduce nociceptor activation. This model derives from the "vicious circle" concept proposed by Livingston[7] to explain reflex sympathetic dystrophy. According to this idea, both pain and the anxiety it produces increase sympathetic outflow and muscle contraction, which in turn produce more pain, and so on. Although such a mechanism may contribute to pain in some chronic conditions, there is little evidence that it plays a major role in the most common headache syndromes.

A second class of explanation depends on the proposal that there are several separate components to the pain experience: sensation (i.e., quality and intensity), affect (fear, anxiety, depression), and evaluation (meaning). According to this "centralist" view, cognitive interventions reduce the affect or change the meaning of the pain so that the patient, with no change in the afferent pain signal, perceives less threat, has greater tolerance, and suffers less.

A third class of explanation, and the one that is emphasized in this chapter, is that the pain signal, when it arrives at its first synaptic relay in the spinal cord dorsal horn or medullary nucleus caudalis, becomes subject to modulating signals arising from the CNS. In other words, the pain message is altered in transit by modulating circuits that are activated by psychological factors.

Attention and Expectation Can Generate or Worsen Pain

Attention and affect are influenced by and can powerfully modulate subjective responses to noxious stimuli. The effect of attention on pain is widely appreciated by the lay public, and many people use distraction to cope with pain. Formal psychophysical studies have confirmed that drawing attention away from a noxious stimulus raises its perceptual threshold.[8] Conversely, pain intensity ratings are increased when a subject's attention is focused on a pain assessment task.[9]

One important study indicating that attention and expectation or suggestion may induce headache was carried out by Bayer et al.[10] They observed that placing dummy electrodes on the heads of normal volunteers can induce head pain if the subjects believe they will be electrically stimulated. In their study, head pain was not correlated with increases in heart rate or electrodermal responses, a correlation that might be expected if stress or anxiety alone were responsible for the pain.

Emotional Stress, Anxiety, and Negative Affect Are Correlated with Increased Pain

The most common and most commonly studied affective variable is depressive symptomatology. Patients with chronic pain, including those with frequent moderate-to-severe migraine or tension-type headaches are likely to have depressive symptoms.[11–13] Breslau and colleagues[14] have reported that persons with depression are at increased risk for developing migraine. A high percentage of depressed patients report somatic pain.[15] More relevant to the current discussion is the limited evidence that depression can cause or worsen pain. For example, inducing sadness in normal volunteers reduces pain tolerance.[16] Furthermore, in patients undergoing surgery, postoperative pain ratings are positively correlated with preoperative Beck Depression Inventory scores.[17]

In addition to the correlation of sad mood and depressive symptoms with pain, there is a strong correlation of anxiety with pain states. Anxiety is an integral part of the subjective experience of pain, and anxiety can induce or worsen pain. For example, several population-based studies demonstrate a positive correlation of migraine with anxiety disorders.[12,14,18] Significantly, there is evidence that perceived stressful life events increase prior to the onset of migraine or chronic tension-type headache.[19]

Although the positive correlation of emotional stress with headache is such a common experience that it is virtually a cliché, only a few rigorous studies have addressed the question of whether clinically significant pains can be produced by emotional stress. In an important prospective study, Gannon and colleagues[20] confirmed the widespread anecdotal experience that a stressful situation can reliably induce headache. They exposed subjects to the experimental stress of performing rapid mental arithmetic for an hour. Subjects were grouped according to three categories: those with frequent migraine, those with frequent tension-type headaches, and those with infrequent headaches. Eleven of 16 frequent headache subjects but only two of eight infrequent headache subjects developed a headache during the 1-hour stress session. Increases in heart rate, cephalic blood volume pulse, and neck muscle electromyography were observed in all subject groups and were correlated with headache severity.

The idea that affect, attention, and expectation have powerful and clinically relevant effects on pain is reinforced by the report that, compared with subjects with infrequent headaches, patients with frequent severe tension-type headaches show high scores on a questionnaire that measures fear of pain.[21] In that study, scores on the questionnaire were positively correlated with measures of both anxiety and depression but not with headache characteristics such as frequency, severity, or duration.

In summary, psychological variables have powerful modulating actions that can either increase or decrease pain. Headache in particular appears to be highly susceptible to the influence of psychological factors. More complete understanding of headache at the level of neural mechanisms therefore requires us to address the question of how psychological variables can modulate pain. One possibility is that they do so through the action of pain-modulating circuitry.

The past two decades have brought enormous advances in our knowledge of pain-modulating systems. We know that these systems exert bidirectional control over pain transmission, that they can be engaged by environmental stimuli that influence the psychological state of the individual, and that their component neurons release both opioid and biogenic amine neurotransmitters. Our knowledge of these systems is reviewed in the following sections.

PAIN-MODULATING CIRCUITS: A NEURAL SUBSTRATE FOR PSYCHOLOGICAL INFLUENCES ON PAIN?

As briefly noted previously, under conditions of strong emotion (e.g., anger, fear, elation), major injuries may be essentially painless. Conversely, in situations associated with dysphoria or when pain is anticipated, subjects often report the occurrence or worsening of pain without an imposed noxious stimulus. The point is that whether a noxious stimulus produces no pain or severe pain depends as much on the state of the subject as on the qualities of the stimulus. Our understanding of this stimulus-independent variability of pain has increased greatly with the discovery and elucidation of CNS circuits that selectively modulate pain transmission.[22–24]

Psychological Factors Influence the Firing of Dorsal Horn Pain Transmission Neurons

The clearest evidence that pain transmission neurons can be modulated by learning and attentional factors comes from studies of neurons in the nucleus caudalis, which receive direct input from primary afferent nociceptors that innervate cranial structures. Despite the technical challenges, it has been possible to record from trigeminothalamic pain transmission neurons in awake primates.[25] In a set of elegant experiments, monkeys were trained to detect small noxious heat pulses to their upper lip. The paradigm involved training the monkey to press and hold a lever in response to a light cue signaling the task to be performed. To obtain a reward, the monkey was required to hold the lever down until the occurrence of a small noxious heat pulse. All neurons showed increasing firing frequency when noxious stimuli of increasing intensity were applied within their receptive fields, thus identifying them as pain transmission neurons. What was striking, however, was that many of these cells increased or decreased their firing rates in response to either the signal light *or* the act of pushing the lever. These changes in firing rate occurred *prior to any noxious stimulus being applied to the monkey.* The cells had apparently acquired the property of changing their activity in anticipation of a noxious stimulus. These experiments show that in the primate nervous system there are pathways that mediate the modulatory actions of attention and learning on pain transmission neurons. What are those pathways?

Stimulation-Produced Analgesia and the Discovery of Brain Stem Pain-Modulating Nuclei

Rapid progress in understanding the CNS mechanisms of pain modulation began with the serendipitous discovery of stimulation-produced analgesia in rats and its confirmation in humans with chronic pain.[22,24,26] In rats, electrical stimulation in the midbrain periaqueductal gray (PAG) suppresses responses to noxious stimulation whereas responses to innocuous stimuli are preserved. In humans, stimulation of the PAG produces a gradual fading of ongoing pain without any other consistent sensory or motor effects. The combination of these two apparently similar observations is very powerful, because one cannot determine whether the rats actually are analgesic or simply not responding, and in humans the possibility of a placebo effect is difficult to rule out. By drawing attention to the PAG, these observations opened up a fruitful line of research.

Subsequent work has established that the PAG is part of a circuit that controls nociceptive neurons in the dorsal horn (Figure 3.1). Its major outflow is caudally to the rostral ventromedial medulla (RVM). The RVM in turn projects massively and selectively to pain-transmitting neurons in the dorsal horn of the spinal cord and the trigeminal nucleus caudalis. Electrical stimulation in the PAG or the RVM produces behavioral analgesia and inhibition of spinal and trigeminal pain transmission neurons. Another brain stem region involved in pain modulation is the dorsolateral pontine tegmentum (DLPT). The DLPT is directly linked to both the PAG and the RVM and projects directly to the spinal cord dorsal horn (Figure 3.2).

Neurotransmitters in Pain-Modulating Circuits

Endogenous Opioids

When opioid agonists such as morphine are microinjected into either the PAG or the RVM, a powerful analgesic effect is produced. Furthermore, when opioid

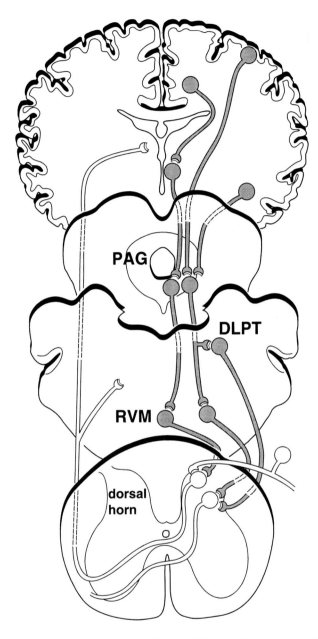

Figure 3.1   The major pain-modulating pathways of the central nervous system. Projections arising in the cortex, primarily limbic system–related, and the hypothalamus connect to the midbrain periaqueductal gray (PAG). The PAG projects to both the dorsolateral pontine tegmentum (DLPT) and the rostral ventromedial medulla (RVM). The RVM and DLPT in turn project to nociceptive neurons in the trigeminal nucleus caudalis and spinal cord dorsal horn. Thus, pain transmission is controlled at the first central synapse of primary afferent nociceptors.

analgesics are given systemically, microinjection of opioid antagonists into these sites blocks the analgesic effect. This indicates that opioid analgesics work in part by activating these brain stem pain-modulating sites.[23]

The RVM, PAG, and DLPT contain opioid receptors and dense concentrations of endogenous opioid peptides. There are three types of opioid receptors (μ, δ, and κ). Although all three types contribute to pain modulation, the μ-receptor produces the most profound and consistent analgesia both in animal models and in human clinical situations. All three opioid receptors belong to the G-protein–coupled family of neurotransmitter receptors.[27] When coupled to a ligand (the endogenous opioid peptide or an exogenous opioid analgesic), opioid receptors produce two well-described actions: either they reduce transmitter release by closing a Ca^{++} channel[28] or they inhibit neurons postsynaptically by opening a K^+ channel, which causes hyperpolarization.[29,30]

There are also three families of endogenous opioid peptides: the enkephalins, which are derived from the precursor preproenkephalin; the endorphin group, which includes β-endorphin and is derived from prepro-opioimelanocortin; and the dynorphin family, which is derived from preprodynorphin. The PAG, DLPT, and RVM each contain high concentrations of one or more of the endogenous opioid peptides. Furthermore, these brain stem sites are linked to each other by opioid synapses. For example, when μ-opioids are injected into the PAG, an endogenous opioid—probably enkephalin—is released in the RVM.[31–33] Thus, opioid analgesics not only mimic the action of endogenous opioid peptides, they induce the release of endogenous opioids at pain-modulating sites.

Biogenic Amines

About 30% of the neurons in the RVM contain serotonin. In fact, the RVM is the major, perhaps the exclusive, location of serotonin neurons that project to the spinal cord dorsal horn and the trigeminal nucleus caudalis (Figure 3.2). This serotonergic projection to the dorsal horn contributes to the modulation of nociceptive dorsal horn neurons.[34] Note that the RVM itself receives a major projection from midbrain serotonergic neurons.[35]

The DLPT is the major source of noradrenergic projections to the dorsal horn.[36] These noradrenergic projections are activated by analgesia-producing electrical stimulation of the RVM.[37,38] Their analgesic effect in rodents is mediated by the alpha$_2$-adrenergic receptor. Alpha$_2$-agonists (e.g., clonidine) produce analgesia in humans and are particularly effective when applied directly to the spinal cord.[39]

Thus, spinally released serotonin and norepinephrine both contribute to the analgesia produced by electrical stimulation of the RVM. Both neurotransmitters inhibit nociceptive dorsal horn neurons.[23] It is of interest that the antidepressant medications that are most effective for treating pain, including headache, block the reuptake of both norepinephrine and serotonin, suggesting that these two transmitters act synergistically. The possibility that antidepressants relieve pain by acting on the biogenic amine–containing spinal terminals of brain stem pain-modulating neurons is supported by the observation that antidepressants applied directly to the spinal cord enhance the antinociceptive effect of systemically administered morphine.[40]

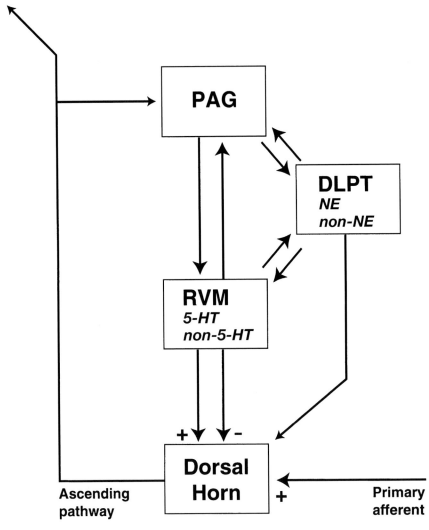

Figure 3.2   Interconnections of brain stem pain-modulating sites. The periaqueductal gray (PAG), rostral ventromedial medulla (RVM), and dorsolateral pontine tegmentum (DLPT) are reciprocally connected, and there is evidence that RVM exerts both excitatory and inhibitory control over pain transmission neurons. (5-HT = 5-hydroxytryptamine; NE = norepinephrine.)

On- and Off-Cells in the Rostral Ventromedial Medulla: Bidirectional Control of Pain

Electrophysiologic recordings in the RVM have revealed unexpected and interesting properties of neurons.[23,41] One class of RVM neuron, the on-cell, shows a burst of activity beginning just prior to withdrawal from a noxious stimulus. The other major class, the off-cell, has the opposite firing pattern (Figure 3.3), pausing during withdrawal from noxious heat. On-cells, which facilitate pain transmission, receive an enkephalinergic input,[42] are inhibited by opioids through an action at the μ-receptor, and project to the spinal cord dorsal horn. Off-cells, which also project to the spinal cord dorsal horn, are inhibited by on-cells and thus are activated indirectly (disinhibited) by opioids (Figure 3.3) and inhibit pain transmission.[43] Important support for the hypothesis that on-cell activity facilitates pain is that on-cells show rebound hyperactivity following withdrawal of opioid administration. Rats given morphine followed within minutes by the opioid antagonist naloxone develop hyperalgesia that is directly related to the preceding dose of morphine.[44] The hyperalgesia is correlated with an increased discharge rate of RVM on-cells and is abolished by inactivation of the RVM.[45,46] This result shows that opioid analgesics induce two opposing processes in pain-modulating circuits: analgesia (inhibition of on-cells) and a longer-lasting "compensatory" hyperalgesia (rebound excitation of on-cells) that becomes overt when the analgesic action is terminated.

In some ways this result parallels the anecdotal experience of many physicians who use analgesics on a long-term basis for treating headache. Although analgesics may give short-term relief, in some individuals their frequent use can induce a situation that leads to an overall worsening of pain. This so-called analgesic rebound headache may actually represent a form of physical dependence that subsides over time when the analgesic drug is terminated.

There is another category of neuron in the RVM that projects to the dorsal horn. This type of neuron, the neutral cell, shows no consistent response to noxious stimuli or to opioid administration. The majority of serotonergic neurons in the RVM are neutral cells.[47] In view of the evidence that serotonergic neurons in the RVM contribute to pain modulation, it is likely that some neutral cells play an important, but as yet undetermined, role in controlling pain transmission neurons.

It is important to note that, besides the PAG–RVM–DLPT circuit described in the preceding section, there are other descending inputs to dorsal horn nociceptive neurons. For example, there are direct projections from the somatosensory cortex, the hypothalamus, and the subnucleus reticularis dorsalis of the medulla.[48,49] Any of these pathways could contribute to the clinical variability of pain and to the demonstrated modulatory effects of mood, expectation, and attention on pain intensity and tolerance. Furthermore, there is evidence that in addition to descending control, ascending brain stem pathways can modulate thalamic nociceptive neurons.

To summarize, although pain pathways may be modulated at multiple sites and there are several candidate efferent pathways for modulatory control, the most completely described pain-modulating circuit includes the PAG, DLPT, and RVM in the brain stem. Through descending projections, this circuit controls both spinal and trigeminal dorsal horn pain transmission neurons and contributes to the analgesic effect of exogenous opioid administration, PAG electrical stimulation, and possibly tricyclic antidepressants. Endogenous opioid and biogenic amine neurotransmitters are involved in the modulatory actions of this circuit, which exerts bidirectional control of pain through on-cells that facilitate and off-cells that inhibit dorsal horn nociceptive neurons.

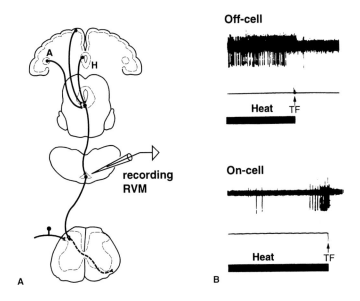

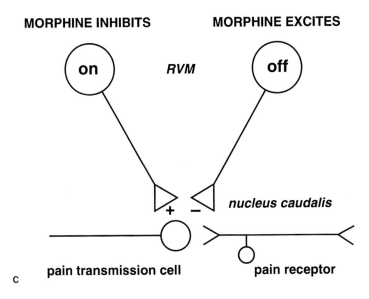

Figure 3.3   On- and off-cells in the rostral ventromedial medulla (RVM). A. Input from amygdala (A) and hypothalamus (H) via the periaqueductal gray to the RVM, which is the site of single-unit recording. B. Traces are a single 10-second oscilloscope sweep. Top three traces show an off-cell (top line), which pauses just before the tail flick (middle trace at arrow labeled TF) in response to noxious heat applied during a period indicated by third (thick) line. Lower three traces illustrate an on-cell, which has the opposite firing pattern. C. Both on- and off-cells control pain transmission through projections to nucleus caudalis.

Activation of Pain-Modulating Circuits: Pain, Stress, and Conditioned Fear

Perhaps the most important unanswered question about pain modulation is its physiologic function. To answer this question we need to know the circumstances under which it is activated. Early studies used exogenous opioids and electrical stimulation to demonstrate analgesia. When the neurotransmitters that mediate the actions of this pain modulation system were discovered, antagonists—e.g., naloxone (opioid), methysergide (serotonin), yohimbine (alpha$_2$-adrenergic)—were given to disrupt it. Although these antagonists reduce opioid- or stimulation-produced analgesia, they have little effect on baseline behaviors. The most striking example of this differential action is that despite the close and functionally significant association of endogenous opioids and pain-modulating circuits, giving massive doses of naloxone to animals or people does not by itself produce pain. On the other hand, if significant pain is already present, naloxone worsens it in animals[50] and humans.[51,52]

Animal studies indicate that, aside from pain, a variety of stressors can engage pain-modulating systems. One of the most robust stressors leading to the activation of the PAG–RVM opioid-mediated pain-modulating circuit is fear. Thus, rats become analgesic when they are exposed to the sight of a cat (instinctive fear) or when placed in an environment where they previously have been exposed to painful stimuli (learned fear). These analgesic effects are blocked by naloxone and by lesions of the PAG and RVM.[53,54]

Because emotional stress, anxiety, and sad mood in humans generally lead to increased pain, it seems paradoxical that in animals, fear is correlated with analgesia. In rats, the analgesia is part of a set of complex stereotyped defensive behaviors elicited by threat.[55] During these behaviors, responding to noxious stimuli would have a negative impact on survival; the rat's attention is probably more focused on the threat than on the stimulus used to assess its response to pain.

As might be expected, the variables associated with activation of pain-modulating circuits in humans are complex. Consistent with animal studies, an opioid-mediated analgesic effect is observed during postoperative pain[52] or in a somatically painless but emotionally stressful situation.[56] However, in addition to pain- and fear-related stress, attention and expectation powerfully alter human pain reports. Thus, the suggestion that an analgesic medication has been given causes analgesia in some patients with postoperative pain (i.e., the placebo effect). Under some circumstances, placebo analgesia is naloxone reversible.[57,58] This observation links the placebo analgesic effect to the brain stem circuit activated by pain and fear in rodents. Although placebo analgesia seems to occur only if the pain being treated has reached some minimum level of intensity,[59] the administration of a placebo treatment would, if anything, be expected to reduce fear and anxiety.

The complexity of the relationship of anxiety to pain was illustrated by a study of 100 normal volunteers exposed to the painful stimulus of immersing a hand in ice water.[60] Prior to immersion, different subjects were instructed that the ice water would either be very painful or not very painful. Subjects in another two groups had an electrode placed on one arm and were told that they would receive either a very painful electric shock or one that was not very painful. Subjects who were highly anxious about the ice water reported significantly more pain on hand immersion than either those who were not very anxious or those who were highly anxious about the electrical shock. Interestingly, those who were highly anxious about the shock tended to report lower overall pain levels than either of the two low-anxiety groups. Thus, expectation and attention apparently play a determining role in whether anxiety has a pronociceptive or analgesic effect on pain. The report that headache sufferers have high levels of fear of pain suggests that these experimental findings are clinically significant.[21]

CNS structures that underlie emotion are activated by noxious stimuli and project to brain stem pain-modulating circuits. The relationship between psychological factors and pain is complex, especially in humans, and is perhaps even more so in patients with chronic recurring headache. It is clear, however, that there is a powerful and bidirectional interaction: Attention, expectation, emotional stress, and affect are altered by and also modulate pain. Once this crucial point is accepted, it becomes critical to define the neural substrate through which psychological factors modulate pain. As it turns out, a tantalizing amalgam of clinical and animal neurobiology suggests some of the linkages between the brain regions that underlie emotion and both pain transmission and pain modulation circuits.

Anatomic Substrate of Emotion

A complete review of the relevant literature on the neurobiology of emotion is beyond the scope of this chapter. However, it is essential to point out the overlap and interconnection of the brain systems underlying emotion, pain, and pain modulation. Lesion and electrical stimulation studies have indicated that certain cortical and subcortical forebrain structures are critical for the expression and experience of emotional states. These include areas in or closely interconnected with the limbic system, such as the anterior cingulate, medial frontal, and anterior temporal cortices and the amygdala, hippocampus, and related thalamic and hypothalamic nuclei.[61] The amygdala is a major subcortical structure that is interconnected with most limbic cortical areas.

Recent positron emission tomographic (PET) studies of CNS activation by intense emotions have provided a strong boost to our knowledge about the neural substrates of emotion in human beings. PET studies in which strong emotional responses are provoked in "normal" volunteers and in phobic subjects show consistent activation in several limbic-associated forebrain structures during emotional responses. For example, the anterior cingulate is consistently activated by exposure of human subjects to feared objects (such as a nearby spider or snake)[62] and by induction of a sad mood.[63] Other areas that are consistently activated by dysphoria-inducing stimuli include the medial frontal lobe and the anterior temporal lobe. These areas of cortex are interconnected with each other and with subcortical limbic forebrain structures such as the amygdala, hypothalamus, and limbic-associated thalamic nuclei.

Noxious Stimuli and the Activation of Limbic Forebrain

Intense or persistent noxious stimuli produce anxiety and depression. Unpleasant feelings (dysphoria) are an essential part of the pain experience, and they have

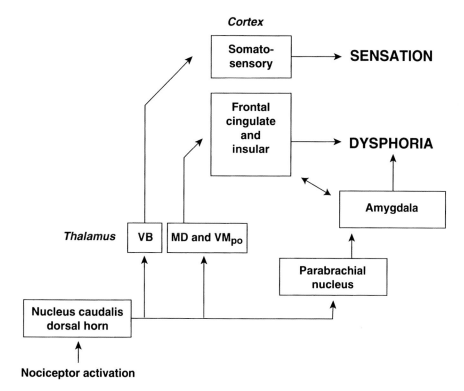

Figure 3.4 Central pathways for pain and dysphoria. Nociceptor stimulation (lower left) activates pain transmission neurons in nucleus caudalis or cervical dorsal horn. These neurons project to the thalamus or via the parabrachial nucleus to the amygdala. Thalamic nuclei that receive input from nociceptive spinothalamic tract neurons project to several cortical targets. The ventrobasal nucleus (VB) projects to somatosensory cortex and gives rise to the purely sensory aspects of pain (quality, intensity, location, time course). The dorsomedial (MD) and posterior ventrocaudal (VM$_{po}$) nuclei project to cingulate and insular regions of the frontal lobe. These latter regions, which are reciprocally connected to the amygdala, give rise to the unpleasantness or dysphoric aspects of pain.

an important role in the activation of pain-modulating circuits. Current evidence suggests that noxious stimuli activate pain-modulating circuits partly through connections to limbic forebrain areas.

Noxious stimuli activate several ascending pathways. One is the classic neospinothalamic pathway, which mediates the sensory discriminative aspects of pain via its projection to the ventrobasal thalamus and the somatosensory cortex. Lesions of this pathway block all normal pain sensation. Once the spinothalamic tract reaches the thalamus it splits to innervate several different nuclei (Figure 3.4). In addition to the ventrobasal thalamus, which projects to somatosensory cortex, spinothalamic neurons also project to the dorsal medial and ventrocaudal posterior thalamus.[64] From the dorsal medial thalamus, a projection has been demonstrated to the anterior cingulate in primates, and, in rodents, to the orbitofrontal cortex. In primates, the ventrocaudal thalamus projects to the anterior insula (medial frontal lobe).[64]

The clinical relevance of the primate anatomic studies is supported by PET studies of humans during application of noxious cutaneous stimuli. These studies show that, in addition to somatosensory thalamus and cortex, noxious stimuli activate the anterior cingulate and anterior insula.[65,66] Thus, some of the same limbic forebrain regions activated by elicitation of a strong emotional response such as fear or sadness are also activated by painful stimuli.[62,63] Given the proclivity of noxious stimuli to induce fear or anxiety, this overlap of neural substrates is not surprising.

In addition to the spinothalamic pathway, noxious stimuli can activate limbic structures through a midbrain relay that bypasses the thalamus. A massive projection of spinal and trigeminal nociceptive neurons terminates in the midbrain parabrachial nucleus and is relayed to the amygdala (see Figure 3.4). Noxious stimuli thus activate multiple pathways to the limbic forebrain structures whose activity is associated with emotional expression. Furthermore, those limbic structures may be activated by the anticipation of continued pain. In summary, both somatically induced pain and exteroceptively induced fear activate anatomically overlapping limbic forebrain structures including the anterior cingulate, medial frontal lobe, and amygdala.

Inputs to Brain Stem Pain-Modulating Circuits

Given that strong emotions have powerful effects on the perception of subsequent noxious stimuli, it is reasonable to propose that these limbic forebrain structures provide a major input to pain-modulating circuits. Our most extensive knowledge is of the PAG. The ventrolateral PAG receives direct projections from the central nucleus of the amygdala and from the orbital frontal/insular cortex (Figure 3.5)[55] The projections from the amygdala to the PAG are crucial for the opioid-mediated analgesic effects elicited by conditioned fear in rodents. In the rodent, nociceptive regions of the orbital frontal cortex project to PAG and contribute to its pain-modulating actions.[67] The key point is that through their projections to the PAG, limbic forebrain structures activated by stimuli that are noxious or produce emotional stress in other ways are positioned to modulate pain transmission neurons through a well-established brain stem circuit that exerts bidirectional control.

DO PAIN-MODULATING CIRCUITS CAUSE HEADACHE?

Although any ideas on the causal relationship of pain-modulating circuits to headache must be considered preliminary, the conjecture that headache can be triggered or exacerbated through the action of pain-modulating neurons is both reasonable and potentially testable. The idea that headaches in general and migraine in particular might be caused by dysfunction or deficiency of central pain-modulating circuits originated with Sicuteri.[68] Because of the evidence that serotonergic neurons contribute to pain-modulating circuits, a drop in plasma

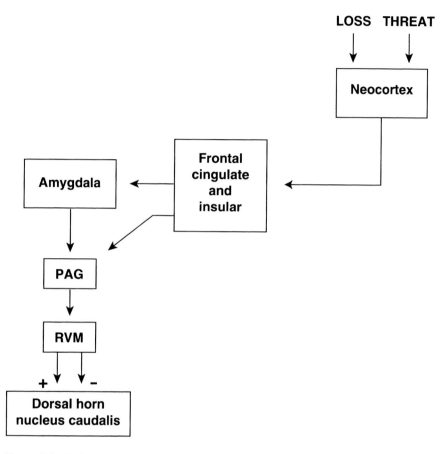

Figure 3.5   Pathways that mediate psychological influences on pain transmission. Limbic areas of cortex (cingulate and insular) project both directly and via the amygdala to the periaqueductal gray (PAG), which controls pain transmission neurons in nucleus caudalis via the rostral ventromedial medulla (RVM).

serotonin often precedes a migraine attack, depletion of serotonin can induce headaches and worsen pain in general, and serotonin agonists have a migraine-relieving action, Sicuteri and others have proposed that migraine represents a dysfunction of serotonergic neurons or receptors.[2,68,69]

The brain stem pain-modulating circuit described in this chapter has well-defined serotonergic links, both from the midbrain to the medulla and from the medulla to spinal and trigeminal pain transmission neurons. Although each class of medullary pain-modulating neuron receives serotonergic input,[70] the contribution to pain modulation of these serotonergic inputs to the RVM are unknown. On the other hand, the serotonergic terminals of RVM neutral cells in the dorsal horn (and trigeminal nucleus caudalis) are inhibitory. Because RVM neurons exert bidirectional control over pain transmission, a deficiency of serotonergic function could have two distinct pronociceptive actions: reducing serotonergic inhibition of pain transmission neurons and releasing the pain-facilitating on-cells from serotonergic inhibition.

The idea that some idiopathic headaches are correlated with a generalized shift toward facilitation of pain-modulating circuits receives some support from the observation that, in patients with chronic tension-type headaches, somatic pain thresholds and tolerance are reduced throughout the body.[71,72] There is also some evidence that specifically supports the involvement of the PAG-to-RVM pain-modulating circuitry in the etiology of idiopathic headache including migraine. One supportive observation is that implanting an electrode in the PAG may produce ipsilateral headache and other migrainous phenomena.[2] A second important observation is that during an attack of migraine without aura, strong PET activation is observed in the region of the contralateral ventrolateral PAG.[73] This region remains active immediately following abortion of the headache by sumatriptan, indicating that its activation is not secondary to the head pain.

SUMMARY

Mood alterations, anxiety, expectation, and attention exert powerful effects on subjectively experienced pain. In fact, attention and expectation may be sufficient to produce pain sensation in the absence of peripheral noxious stimuli. Pain transmission neurons at all levels of the neuraxis are under modulatory control from the somatosensory cortex and from limbic forebrain structures via the PAG and the RVM. These pain-modulating circuits are engaged by psychological factors, and they exert bidirectional control over pain transmission neurons. They contribute to pain reduction by opioid analgesics, serotonin agonists, tricyclic antidepressants, stress reduction, and placebo administration. Conversely, the same circuits (but different component neurons) could mediate the enhancement of pain by anxiety, expectation, depression, and analgesic rebound. The facilitatory control is particularly interesting because it offers the possibility of generating a pain signal by central activation of spinal neurons without input from peripheral nociceptors.

REFERENCES

1. Moskowitz MA, Macfarlane R. Neurovascular and molecular mechanisms in migraine headaches. Cerebrovasc Brain Metab Rev 1993;5:159.
2. Raskin NH. Headache (2nd ed). New York: Churchill Livingstone, 1988.
3. Beecher HK. The powerful placebo. JAMA 1955;159:1062.
4. Beecher HK. Measurement of Subjective Responses: Quantitative Effects of Drugs. New York: Oxford University Press, 1959.
5. White L, Tursky B, Schwartz GE. Placebo: Theory, research, and mechanisms. New York: Guilford, 1985.
6. Wall PD, Melzack R. Textbook of Pain (3rd ed). Edinburgh: Churchill Livingstone, 1994.
7. Livingston WK. Pain Mechanisms. New York: Macmillan, 1943.
8. Miron D, Duncan GH, Bushnell MC. Effects of attention on the intensity and unpleasantness of thermal pain. Pain 1989;39:345.

9. Bushnell MC, Duncan GH, Dubner R, Jones RL, et al. Attentional influences on noxious and innocuous cutaneous heat detection in humans and monkeys. J Neurosci 1985;5:1103.
10. Bayer TL, Baer PE, Early C. Situational and psychophysiological factors in psychologically induced pain. Pain 1991;44:45.
11. Fishbain DA, Goldberg M, Meagher BR, Steele R, et al. Male and female chronic pain patients categorized by DSM-III psychiatric diagnostic criteria. Pain 1986;26:181.
12. Merikangas KR, Angst J, Isler H. Migraine and psychopathology: Results of the Zurich cohort study of young adults. Arch Gen Psychiatry 1990;47:849.
13. Ziegler DK, Paolo AM. Headache symptoms and psychological profile of headache-prone individuals: A comparison of clinic patients and controls. Arch Neurol 1995;52:602.
14. Breslau N, Davis GC, Andreski P. Migraine, psychiatric disorders, and suicide attempts: An epidemiologic study of young adults. Psychiatry Res 1991;37:11.
15. Wells KB, Stewart A, Hays RD, Burnam MA, et al. The functioning and well-being of depressed patients: Results from the Medical Outcomes Study. JAMA 1989;262:914.
16. Zelman DC, Howland EW, Nichols SN, Cleeland CS. The effects of induced mood on laboratory pain. Pain 1991;46:105.
17. Taenzer P, Melzack R, Jeans ME. Influence of psychological factors on postoperative pain, mood, and analgesic requirements. Pain 1986;24:331.
18. Stewart WF, Linet MS, Celentano DD. Migraine headaches and panic attacks. Psychosom Med 1989;51:559.
19. DeBenedittis G, Lorenzetti A, Pieri A. The role of stressful life events in the onset of chronic primary headache. Pain 1990;40:65.
20. Gannon LR, Haynes SN, Cuevas J, Chavez R. Psychophysiological correlates of induced headaches. J Behav Med 1987;10:411.
21. Hursey KG, Jacks SD. Fear of pain in recurrent headache sufferers. Headache 1992;32:283.
22. Basbaum AI, Fields HL. Endogenous pain control systems: Brainstem spinal pathways and endorphin circuitry. Annu Rev Neurosci 1984;7:309.
23. Fields HL, Heinricher MM, Mason P. Neurotransmitters in nociceptive modulatory circuits. Annu Rev Neurosci 1991;14:219.
24. Fields HL, Basbaum AI. Central Nervous System Mechanisms of Pain Modulation. In PD Wall, R Melzack (eds), Textbook of Pain. New York: Churchill Livingstone, 1994;243.
25. Duncan GH, Bushnell MC, Bates R, Dubner R. Task-related responses of monkey medullary dorsal horn neurons. J Neurophysiol 1987;57:289.
26. Baskin DS, Mehler WR, Hosobuchi Y, Richardson DE, et al. Autopsy analysis of the safety, efficacy, and cartography of electrical stimulation of the central gray in humans. Brain Res 1986;371:231.
27. Pasternak GW, Standifer KM. Mapping of opioid receptors using antisense oligodeoxynucleotides: Correlating their molecular biology and pharmacology. Trends Pharmacol Sci 1995;16:344.
28. Taddese A, Nah S-Y, McCleskey EW. Selective opioid inhibition of small nociceptive neurons. Science 1995;270:1366.
29. Duggan AW, North RA. Electrophysiology of opioids. Pharmacol Rev 1983;35:219.
30. Grudt TJ, Williams JT. Mu-opioid agonists inhibit spinal trigeminal substantia gelatinosa neurons in guinea pig and rat. J Neurosci 1994;14:1646.
31. Kiefel JM, Rossi GC, Bodnar RJ. Medullary mu and delta opioid receptors modulate mesencephalic morphine analgesia in rats. Brain Res 1993;624:151.
32. Pan ZZ, Fields HL. Endogenous opioid-mediated inhibition of putative pain-modulating neurons in rate rostral ventromedial medulla. Neuroscience 1996; in press.
33. Roychowdhury SM, Fields HL. Endogenous opioids acting at a medullary mu opioid receptor contribute to the behavioral antinociception produced by GABA antagonism in the midbrain periaqueductal grey. 1996; in press.
34. LeBars D. Serotonin and Pain. In NN Osborne, M Hamon (eds), Neuronal Serotonin. New York: Wiley, 1988;171.
35. Beitz AJ. The sites of origin brainstem neurotensin and serotonin projections to the rodent nucleus raphe magnus. J Neurosci 1982;2:829.
36. Kwiat GC, Basbaum AI. The origin of brainstem noradrenergic and serotonergic projections to the spinal cord dorsal horn in the rat. Somatosens Mot Res 1992;9:157.
37. Clark FM, Proudfit HK. Projections of neurons in the ventromedial medulla to pontine catecholamine cell groups involved in the modulation of nociception. Brain Res 1991;540:105.
38. Barbaro NM, Hammond DL, Fields HL. Effects of intrathecally administered methysergide and yohimbine on microstimulation-produced antinociception in the rat. Brain Res 1985;343:223.

39. Bernard J-M, Kick O, Bonnet F. Comparison of intravenous and epidural clonidine for postoperative patient-controlled analgesia. Anaesth Analg 1995;81:706.
40. Taiwo YO, Fabian A, Pazoles CJ, Fields HL. Potentiation of morphine antinociception by monoamine reuptake inhibitors in the rat spinal cord. Pain 1985;21:329.
41. Fields HL, Malick A, Burstein R. Dorsal horn projection targets of on and off cells in the rostral ventromedial medulla. J Neurophysiol 1995;74:1742.
42. Mason P, Back SA, Fields HL. A confocal laser microscopic study of enkephalin-immunoreactive appositions onto physiologically identified neurons in the rostral ventromedial medulla. J Neurosci 1992;12:4023.
43. Heinricher MM, Morgan MM, Tortorici V, Fields HL. Disinhibition of off-cells and antinociception produced by an opioid action within the rostral ventromedial medulla. Neuroscience 1994;63:279.
44. Kim DH, Fields HL, Barbaro NM. Morphine analgesia and acute physical dependence: Rapid onset of two opposing, dose-related processes. Brain Res 1990;516:37.
45. Bederson JB, Fields HL, Barbaro NM. Hyperalgesia during naloxone-precipitated withdrawal from morphine is associated with increased on-cell activity in the rostral ventromedial medulla. Somatosens Mot Res 1990;7:185.
46. Kaplan H, Fields HL. Hyperalgesia during acute opioid abstinence: Evidence for a nociceptive facilitating function of the rostral ventromedial medulla. J Neurosci 1991;11:1433.
47. Potrebic SB, Fields HL, Mason P. Serotonin immunoreactivity is contained in one physiological cell class in the rat rostral ventromedial medulla. J Neurosci 1994;14:1655.
48. Holstege G. Direct and Indirect Pathways to Lamina I in the Medulla Oblongata and Spinal Cord of the Cat. In HL Fields, J-MB Besson (eds), Pain Modulation. Amsterdam: Elsevier, 1988;47.
49. Villanueva L, Bernard JF, Le Bars D. Distribution of spinal cord projections from the medullary subnucleus reticularis dorsalis and the adjacent cuneate nucleus: A Phaseolus vulgaris-leucoagglutinin study in the rat. J Comp Neurol 1995;352:11.
50. Jacob JJ, Tremblay EC, Colombel MC. Enhancement of nociceptive reactions by naloxone in mice and rats [in French]. Psychopharmacologia 1974;37:217.
51. Levine JD, Gordon NC, Jones RT, Fields HL. The narcotic antagonist naloxone enhances clinical pain. Nature 1978;272:826.
52. Gracely RH, Dubner R, Wolskee PJ, Deeter WR. Placebo and naloxone can alter post-surgical pain by separate mechanisms. Nature 1983;306:264.
53. Helmstetter FJ, Tershner SA. Lesions of the periaqueductal gray and rostral ventromedial medulla disrupt antinociceptive but not cardiovascular aversive conditional responses. J Neurosci 1994;14:7099.
54. Watkins LR, Cobelli DA, Mayer DJ. Classical conditioning of front paw and hind paw footshock induced analgesia (FSIA): Naloxone reversibility and descending pathways. Brain Res 1982;243:119.
55. Bandler R, Shipley MT. Columnar organization in the midbrain periaqueductal gray: Modules for emotional expression? Trends Neurosci 1994;17:379.
56. Pitman RK, van der Kolk BA, Orr SP, Greenberg MS. Naloxone-reversible analgesic response to combat-related stimuli in posttraumatic stress disorder: A pilot study. Arch Gen Psychiatry 1990;47:541.
57. Levine JD, Gordon NC, Fields HL. The mechanism of placebo analgesia. Lancet 1978;2:654.
58. Grevert P, Goldstein A. Placebo Analgesia, Naloxone, and the Role of Endogenous Opioids. In L White, B Tursky, GE Schwartz (eds), Placebo: Theory, Research and Mechanisms. New York: Guilford, 1985;332.
59. Levine JD, Gordon NC, Bornstein JC, Fields HL. Role of pain in placebo analgesia. Proc Natl Acad Sci U S A 1979;76:3528.
60. Al Absi M, Rokke PD. Can anxiety help us tolerate pain? Pain 1991;46:43.
61. LeDoux JE. Emotion. In SR Geiger (ed), Handbook of Physiology: A Critical, Comprehensive Presentation of Physiological Knowledge and Concepts. Bethesda, MD: American Physiological Society, 1987;419.
62. Rauch SL, Savage CR, Alpert NM, Miguel EC, et al. A positron emission tomographic study of simple phobic symptom provocation. Arch Gen Psychiatry 1995;52:20.
63. George MS, Ketter TA, Parekh PI, Horwitz B, et al. Brain activity during transient sadness and happiness in healthy women. Am J Psychiatry 1995;152:341.
64. Craig AD. Pain, Temperature, and the Sense of the Body ("Gemeingefuhl"). In O Franzen, R Johansson, L Terenius (eds), Somatosensory Function. Basel: Birkhauser, in press.
65. Talbot JD, Marrett S, Evans AC, Meyer E, et al. Multiple representations of pain in human cerebral cortex [see comments]. Science 1991;251:1355.

66. Berman J. Imaging pain in humans. Br J Anaesth 1995;75:209.
67. Hutchison WD, Harfa L, Dostrovsky JO. Ventrolateral orbital cortex and periaqueductal gray stimulation–induced effects on on- and off-cells in the rostral ventromedial medulla in the rat. Neuroscience 1996;70:391.
68. Sicuteri F. Headache: Disruption of Pain Modulation. In JJ Bonica, D Albe-Fessard (eds), Advances in Pain Research and Therapy. New York: Raven, 1976;871.
69. Marcus DA. Serotonin and its role in headache pathogenesis and treatment. Clin J Pain 1993;9:159.
70. Potrebic SB, Mason P, Fields HL. The density and distribution of serotonergic appositions onto identified neurons in the rat rostral ventromedial medulla. J Neurosci 1995;15:3273.
71. Schoenen J, Bottin D, Hardy F, Gerard P. Cephalic and extracephalic pressure pain thresholds in chronic tension-type headache. Pain 1991;47:145.
72. Langemark M, Bach FW, Jensen TS, Olesen J. Decreased nociceptive flexion reflex threshold in chronic tension-type headache. Arch Neurol 1993;50:1061.
73. Weiller C, May A, Limmroth V, Juptner M, et al. Brainstem activation in spontaneous human migraine attacks. Nature Med 1995;1:658.

4

New Targets for Antimigraine Drug Development

F. Michael Cutrer, Volker Limmroth, Christian Waeber,
Xian Yu, and Michael A. Moskowitz

Migraine is a syndrome of recurrent headache, nausea, vomiting, photophobia, phonophobia, and malaise. A significant portion of migraine sufferers also experience transient neurologic symptoms including visual or language disturbance, paresthesias, weakness, and vertigo. It has been estimated that migraine afflicts as many as 15.7% of women and 5.7% of men (see Chapters 5 and 6).[1] Yet despite its high prevalence, a firm understanding of migraine's underlying pathophysiology continues to elude investigators. One of the primary obstacles has been the paucity of experimental models that have been validated in humans. Models of neurogenic inflammation and cephalic pain have nonetheless provided important clues that have advanced our understanding of headache and targeted relevant receptor populations for new drug treatments. These animal models have also facilitated understanding of the actions of classical antimigraine medications. A clearer understanding of the number and types of receptor populations can promote the development of more potent and specific agents with fewer side effects.

ANATOMY OF THE TRIGEMINOVASCULAR SYSTEM

The trigeminal nerve and upper cervical spinal cord segments subserve the bulk of somatosensory function in the head (see Chapters 1 and 3). Epilepsy surgery performed more than 50 years ago provided important information about the origins of intracranial pain. In craniotomies performed on awake patients using only local anesthesia, it was found that electrical or mechanical stimulation of the meninges and meningeal blood vessels produced severe, penetrating headache, but that similar stimulation of brain parenchyma was essentially painless.[2] Meningeal and meningovascular sensory innervation is provided by trigeminal pseudounipolar neurons. Small-caliber C fibers originating within the trigeminal ganglia carry nociceptive information from meningeal vessels and project centrally, terminating within the trigeminal nucleus caudalis (TNC).[3] Activation of trigeminovascular fibers releases neuropeptides from the activated nerve terminals into dural vessel walls and evokes responses in areas of the brain associated with nociception.[4]

TRADITIONAL THEORIES OF MIGRAINE

The century-old debate surrounding migraine pathogenesis has focused on two theories. The vasogenic theory, articulated and developed by Wolff and colleagues during the late 1930s and early 1940s, considers migraine to be the result of abrupt changes in cerebrovascular caliber. According to this theory, the aura develops as a consequence of transient ischemia due to focal cerebrovascular vasoconstriction. The headache is thought to develop from rebound intracranial and extracranial vasodilation, which activates nociceptive fibers within the walls of engorged vessels.[5] The neurogenic theory, on the other hand, views migraine as a brain disorder, asserting that neuronal dysfunction accounts for both the neurologic symptoms and the vascular changes. There is general agreement that vascular changes occur within a migraine attack; however, controversy still surrounds the precise correspondence of the vascular changes and clinical symptoms and the question of whether vascular changes are necessary or even sufficient to provoke and sustain an attack. Proponents of the neurogenic theory argue that the neurologic symptoms develop from remote areas of brain and cannot be explained by spasm of a single vessel. Furthermore, they point out that the thirst, food craving, or affective changes that anticipate many headache attacks are unlikely to develop from vasoconstriction.

It is increasingly recognized that inflammatory processes within the meninges may be involved in the prolongation and intensification of head pain during a migraine attack. Neurogenic inflammation (NI), which results from the release of vasoactive, proinflammatory neuropeptides (substance P, neurokinin A, and calcitonin gene-related peptide) from the terminals of sensory neurons, has been observed in tissues such as the skin,[6,7] eye,[8] genitourinary tract,[9] joints,[10,11] and airways.[12,13] In general, NI is an adaptive response to real or threatened tissue injury. Plasma extravasation and edema formation facilitate dilution and removal of foreign substances such as bacteria, toxins, or other chemicals. In addition, NI increases blood flow and mast cell activation and promotes rapid delivery of nutrient substrates and local cellular immune response.

TWO ANIMAL MODELS OF HEADACHE

Animal models have been developed that investigate two aspects of headache pathophysiology. The first model, the trigeminal stimulation model, is a quantitative measure of neurogenic inflammation within the dura mater caused by chemical or electrical stimulation of trigeminovascular fibers. The second model measures the expression of the immediate early gene c-*fos* within the trigeminal nucleus caudalis after noxious chemical stimulation of the meninges.

Model 1: Trigeminovascular Extravasation—A Model of Neurogenic Inflammation

Electrical stimulation of the trigeminal ganglion or intravenous injection of the irritant capsaicin activates small-caliber C fibers and releases neuropeptides from nerve terminals in the meninges of rodents. With stimulation, neuropeptide (i.e., calcitonin gene-related peptide) levels increase in draining venous effluent.[14] Once released, the neuropeptides initiate a cascade of events known collectively as NI, which includes (1) an increase in leakage of plasma from meningeal vessels; (2) vasodilation; (3) the formation of endothelial microvilli, endothelial vesicles, and vacuoles, specifically within postcapillary venules[15]; (4) activation and degranulation of mast cells[16]; and (5) platelet aggregation.

The leakage of radiolabeled albumin from meningeal blood vessels is used to estimate NI. Electrical stimulation (5 Hz, 5 ms, 0.6–1.0 mA, 5 minutes) of the trigeminal ganglia on one side is preceded or followed by a femoral vein injection of ^{125}I-albumin. Ten minutes later, the animals are perfused to remove residual labeled albumin from the intravascular compartment, and the dural tissues from both the stimulated and unstimulated sides are harvested. The residual radioactivity from extravasated plasma on the stimulated side is then compared with that on the unstimulated side, and the comparison is expressed as a ratio. The effect of a test drug on this ratio is assessed.

Prejunctional Blockade of Extravasation: Serotonin Receptors

The application of molecular biological techniques to the study of 5-hydroxytryptamine (5-HT) receptors has uncovered 14 different subtypes over the past few years.[17] Functional effects assigned to a specific receptor 5 years ago might now be explained by other receptor subtypes. Sumatriptan-mediated responses provide a good example. In 1989, the effect of sumatriptan was thought to be mediated solely by the 5-HT_{1D} receptor. However, the cloning and characterization of the 5-HT_{1F} receptor subtype, which displays an even higher affinity for sumatriptan,[18] and the existence of two different 5-HT_{1D} receptor isoforms, suggests the need to reconsider that conclusion.

The analysis of messenger RNAs contained in different tissues using the polymerase chain reaction or Northern blots can provide circumstantial evidence for the involvement of a given subtype. Thus far, such techniques have shown that 5-HT_{1B} receptors seem to predominate in human and bovine cerebral blood vessels,[19] whereas the human and guinea-pig trigeminal ganglia contain predominantly 5-HT_{1D} messenger RNA.[20] The use of a specific 5-HT_{1D} receptor antagonist, GR-127,935, provides a more direct indication that 5-HT_{1D} receptors inhibit NI. Pretreatment with this compound abolishes the effect of sumatriptan in guinea pigs.[21] Unfortunately, the affinity of GR-127,935 for 5-HT_{1F} receptors is not known; hence the involvement of this receptor cannot be determined. GR-127,935 does not discriminate between 5-HT_{1D} and 5-HT_{1B} receptors. In the absence of a more selective antagonist, we have tested the effect of sumatriptan on dural plasma extravasation in knockout mice lacking 5-HT_{1B} receptors.[*] In these mutant mice, sumatriptan does not block neurogenic

---

[*]Humans, as well as guinea pigs, rats, and mice, possess two subtypes of 5-HT_{1D} receptors, termed 5-HT_{1D} and 5-HT_{1B}. Although the pharmacologic properties of 5-HT_{1D} receptors in all species are similar, a single mutation in the 5-HT_{1B} gene in rats and mice results in a considerable alteration of the pharmacologic profile of the corresponding receptor. This receptor has thus been termed 5-HT_{1B} (see Chapter 2).

inflammation, which indicates that sumatriptan acts exclusively on 5-HT_{1B} and not 5-HT_{1D} or 5-HT_{1F} receptors in this species.[21] Obviously, species differences are of great importance to 5-HT_{1D} receptors.

5-Carboxamidotryptamine (5-CT) and the sumatriptan derivative CP-122,288 inhibit plasma protein extravasation with more than 1,000 times the potency of sumatriptan in rats, mice, and guinea pigs (Figure 4.1A).[22] However, the affinity of these drugs for 5-HT_{1D} and 5-HT_{1B} receptors is comparable with that of sumatriptan, suggesting that they act at another receptor subtype or through a different mechanism.[23] This hypothesis has recently been confirmed. Pretreatment with the antagonist GR-127,935 does not affect the response to 5-CT and CP-122,288 in guinea pigs.[21] Moreover, both drugs retain their potency in 5-HT_{1B} knockout mice (Figure 4.1B).[21] It is thus likely that receptor binding sites other than 5-HT_{1D} (or 5-HT_{1B}) are important. None of the 14 cloned 5-HT receptors is an ideal candidate, however, and further studies are needed to clarify this point.[24] Because CP-122,288 inhibits plasma extravasation at doses far lower than those required to constrict cerebral blood vessels, it might represent a remarkably potent medication without vasoconstrictor side effects.

Although presynaptic 5-HT receptors represent the most promising therapeutic targets, the same model has identified other potentially important receptor sites. These sites include alpha$_2$-adrenergic, histamine H_3, somatostatin, and mu-opioid receptors.[25] It is noteworthy that all these receptors (including 5-HT_{1D} receptors) are located outside the blood–brain barrier.

Postjunctional Blockade of Extravasation: Substance-P Antagonism

Because of the importance of substance P to peripheral and central pain mechanisms, treatment with an NK1-receptor antagonist might be useful in migraine. The novel nonpeptide NK1-receptor antagonist RPR 100,893, but not its enantiomer, significantly and dose-dependently inhibited plasma protein extravasation in dura mater when given intravenously 30 minutes prior to electrical stimulation.[26] Furthermore, it reduced plasma leakage when given orally, at doses of 100 mg per kg, 60 minutes prior and 10, 40, and 80 minutes after stimulation. With oral administration, RPR 100,893 dose-dependently inhibited capsaicin-induced plasma protein extravasation with a median effective dose of 7.4 mg per kg for dura and 82 mg per kg for conjunctiva.

Gamma-Aminobutyric Acid Receptor

There is strong clinical evidence that the anticonvulsant valproic acid (2-propyl-pentanoic acid) is effective in the prophylactic treatment of migraine.[27–29] Valproic acid inhibits gamma-aminobutyric acid (GABA) aminotransferase,[30] which metabolizes GABA and activates the GABA-synthetic enzyme glutamic acid decarboxylase,[31] suggesting a potential role for GABA in migraine therapy.

When tested in the trigeminal stimulation model, valproic acid attenuated plasma extravasation in clinically relevant dosages (≥ 3 mg per kg). This effect was reversed by bicuculline, a GABA$_A$ antagonist, but not by a GABA$_B$ antagonist, phaclofen.[32] Furthermore, the effect of valproic acid was mimicked by the

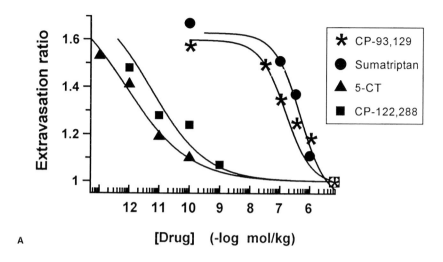

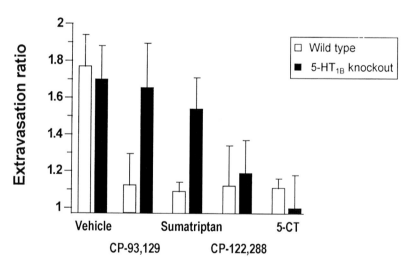

Figure 4.1 A. Inhibition of plasma protein extravasation within the meninges by a series of 5-HT–receptor agonists. Sumatriptan and the 5-HT$_{1B}$–selective agonist CP-93,129 have comparable potencies in this model. The very high potency and the shallow dose-response curves of both 5-CT and CP-122,288 suggest that their effect might be mediated by a receptor other than 5-HT$_{1B}$. Data are expressed as the ratio of extravasated tracer on the stimulated side versus the nonstimulated side. B. Effects of various 5-HT$_{1B/1D}$ agonists on the dural extravasation in control mice and in knockout mice lacking 5-HT$_{1B}$ receptors. CP-93,129 and sumatriptan (both 1 mmol per kg IV), as well as CP-122,288 and 5-CT (both 1 nmol per kg IV), inhibit extravasation to the same extent in control mice. Only CP-122,288 and 5-CT retain their effectiveness in mice lacking 5-HT$_{1B}$ receptors. The lack of effect of CP-93,129 and sumatriptan in knockout mice indicates that their action is mediated mainly by 5-HT$_{1B}$ receptors. Therefore, the molecular target or targets of CP-122,288 and 5-CT remain to be characterized.

GABA$_A$ agonist muscimol, but not by the GABA$_B$ agonist baclofen, suggesting a GABA$_A$-receptor–mediated mechanism.[32] Unlike sumatriptan, valproic acid attenuates substance P–induced plasma extravasation in animals neonatally treated with capsaicin, suggesting that the relevant GABA$_A$ receptor is not located on afferent C fibers.[32] Preliminary studies suggest the importance of nerve fibers projecting from the sphenopalatine ganglion.[33]

The GABA$_A$ receptor is a complex of macromolecular proteins that form a transmembrane chloride ion channel with binding sites for barbiturates, benzodiazepines, picrotoxin, and anesthetic steroids as well as GABA. Further studies suggest that agents that bind to these modulatory sites on the GABA$_A$ receptor complex also decrease plasma extravasation.[33] For example, the benzodiazepines zolpidem, CL218.872, and diazepam all decrease plasma extravasation in a dose-dependent manner.

The steroid modulatory site may be of particular significance in headache pathogenesis because of the association of migraine with hormonal changes accompanying menarche, the menstrual cycle, and menopause. However, the manner in which hormones might influence the induction, severity, or treatment of headache remains unclear. Progesterone decreased plasma extravasation dose-dependently in female ovariectomized and male rats (Figure 4.2).[33] In contrast, the progesterone-receptor agonist promegestone, which is not metabolized, did not block protein extravasation even at high dosages, suggesting that plasma extravasation is not modulated by the hormonal (progesterone) receptor. Progesterone's effects were reversed by the GABA$_A$ antagonist bicuculline (10 mg per kg) but not by the GABA$_B$ antagonist phaclofen (100 mg per kg), indicating a GABA$_A$-dependent mechanism. Progesterone and its A-ring–reduced metabolites (neurosteroids) allosterically modulate GABA action on GABA$_A$ receptors. The naturally occurring neurosteroids allopregnanolone (3α-hydroxy-5α-pregnan-20-one [THP]) and tetrahydroxydeoxycorticosterone (3α,21-dihydroxy-5α-pregnan-20-one [THDOC]), as well as the synthetic steroid alphaxalone, proved to be very potent in this model. Allopregnanolone completely blocked plasma extravasation. This response was reversed by the GABA$_A$ antagonist bicuculline, but not by the GABA$_B$ antagonist phaclofen. The enantiomer of allopregnanolone, 3β-hydroxy-5α-pregnan-20-one, was inactive (Figure 4.3). The epimer of THP (3α-hydroxy-5α-pregnan-20-one), 3β-hydroxy-5α-pregnan-20-one, was inactive in this model, suggesting a stereoselective mechanism.[33]

We tested the efficacy of bicuculline-methiodide, a quaternary nitrogen derivative that is unable to pass the blood–brain barrier. The effects of progesterone and its metabolites were reversed by bicuculline-methiodide, suggesting that the receptor does not require penetration of the blood–brain barrier.[33]

Plasma and brain allopregnanolone levels correlate with progesterone in rats as well as in humans. Because high concentrations of both are observed during the menstrual cycle, pregnancy, or stress,[34] it has been suggested that neuroactive steroids, via central GABA$_A$ receptors, may mediate the analgesic, anxiolytic, or both effects associated with pregnancy or stress.[35,36] Because pregnancy, menopause, and stress affect the clinical presentation of migraine, progesterone and its metabolites in particular may be important in headache modulation. The possibility that endogenous neurosteroids modulate meningeal inflammation and affect the clinical course of migraine through GABA$_A$ receptors outside the blood–brain barrier deserves further investigation.

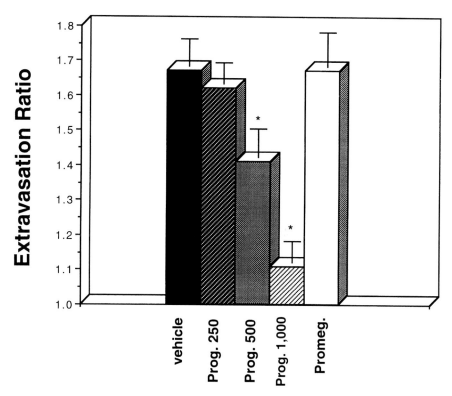

Figure 4.2 Progesterone (Prog.) decreased dural plasma extravasation in a dose-dependent manner. Progesterone (250, 500, and 1,000 μg) was given subcutaneously to male Sprague Dawley rats 55 minutes before electrical stimulation of the trigeminal ganglion. Dosages ≥ 500 μg decreased plasma extravasation significantly ($^*P < 0.05$), whereas promegestone (Promeg.), a nonmetabolizing agonist of the progesterone receptor, was inactive, indicating that the observed effects were not mediated through the progesterone receptor. Similar results were observed in female ovariectomized rats (data not shown).

Hormones have been used in the abortive and prophylactic treatment of headache for more than 60 years. Progesterone and closely related steroids have been evaluated in more than 500 patients in at least 12 clinical trials, all of them suggesting some efficacy.[37–41] Only a single study of six patients reported contradictory data.[42] Endocrine (hypertension, glucose intolerance, weight gain) and central nervous system (sedation, tremor, psychiatric) side effects, however, limit the direct use of hormones in headache treatment. Brain-impermeant drugs may avoid these side effects.

Model 2: C-*fos* Expression in Trigeminal Nucleus Caudalis

The second model of headache measures the expression of c-*fos*, an immediate early gene, as a semiquantitative marker of cephalic head pain. Expression of

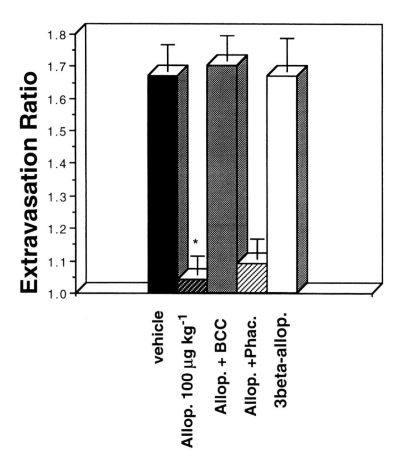

Figure 4.3   The progesterone metabolite and neurosteroid allopregnanolone (Allop.), but not its enantiomer, decreased plasma extravasation by activation of GABA$_A$ receptors. Allopregnanolone (100 μg per kg; $^*P < 0.01$) completely blocked plasma extravasation. This response was reversed by the GABA$_A$ antagonist bicuculline (BCC) (10 μg per kg) but not by the GABA$_B$ antagonist phaclofen (Phac.) (100 μg per kg). The enantiomer of allopregnanolone, 3β-hydroxy-5α-pregnan-20-one (1,000 μg per kg), was inactive. Similar results were observed in female ovariectomized rats (data not shown).

c-*fos* is widely used as a nonspecific indicator of neuronal activation[43] and can be induced in the brain by a variety of stimuli.[44,45] C-*fos*–like immunoreactivity (c-*fos*-LI) within the dorsal horn of the spinal cord (lamina I, II$_o$) is a well-characterized marker of painful peripheral stimulation. Noxious somatic, visceral, and articular stimulation results in an increase in c-*fos*-LI in lamina I, II$_o$ of rat dorsal horn.[46] Morphine pretreatment reduced formalin injection–evoked c-*fos* expression within the dorsal horn in a dose-dependent and naloxone-reversible manner.[47] C-*fos*-LI within lumbar spinal cord after hind-paw formalin injection correlates with the results of behavioral testing.[48]

C-*fos*-LI can be evoked within lamina I, II_o of the TNC (an area analogous to the dorsal horn in the spinal cord) by stimulating meningeal nociceptive neurons using intracisternal irritants. A small catheter is placed through the atlanto-occipital membrane into the cisterna magna of anesthetized rats or guinea pigs. Five and one-half hours later, either drug or vehicle is administered (intravenously or intraperitoneally). Six hours after catheter placement, a chemical stimulus (either autologous blood or a dilute capsaicin solution) is injected into the cisterna magna. Two hours later (at the peak of c-*fos* expression), animals are overdosed and perfused via the ascending aorta. The brain stems and attached spinal cords are then dissected, sectioned (50 μm), and processed immunohistochemically. The cells exhibiting c-*fos*-LI are then counted in every third 50-μm section at three sampling levels within the TNC (−0.225, −2.475, and −6.975 from obex).[49]

Previously, Nozaki et al. demonstrated that intracisternal injection of autologous blood would induce c-*fos* expression within lamina I, II_o of the TNC.[50] The number of cells expressing c-*fos* corresponded to the amount of injectate and was reduced after destruction of unmyelinated fibers by neonatal capsaicin treatment or by surgical trigeminal transection.

Several compounds known to block neurogenic inflammation and migraine headaches also attenuate c-*fos*-LI selectively within the TNC. Sumatriptan, dihydroergotamine, or morphine pretreatment[51] significantly decreased c-*fos* expression in TNC after intracisternal blood or carrageenan injection. CP-122,288 (a sumatriptan analogue that potently blocks neurogenic inflammation) attenuates c-*fos* expression in the TNC at very low doses ($\geq$ 100 pmol per kg)[52] after intracisternal capsaicin. The nonpeptide NK1-receptor antagonist RPR 100,893 also attenuates c-*fos*-LI in the TNC at doses of greater than or equal to 1 μg per kg while its enantiomer, RPR 103,253 (100 μg per kg), is inactive.[49]

Gamma-Aminobutyric Acid in C-*fos*

Just as in NI, GABA-receptor agonists block c-*fos* expression within the TNC. We examined the effects of valproic acid (which increases endogenous GABA) on c-*fos*-LI 2 hours after intracisternal injection of the irritant capsaicin. Valproic acid at clinically relevant doses reduced labeled cells by 52% selectively within lamina I, II_o of the TNC (Figure 4.4).[53] Pretreatment with bicuculline (30 μg per kg intraperitoneally), a $GABA_A$ antagonist, but not phaclofen, a $GABA_B$ antagonist, reversed the effect of valproic acid and increased c-*fos*–positive cells within lamina I, II_o, suggesting the importance of $GABA_A$ receptors (Figure 4.5).[53] Somewhat paradoxically, bicuculline by itself (30 μg per kg intraperitoneally) decreased the number of labeled cells, indicating that more than a single GABA-ergic mechanism can suppress c-*fos* expression. As noted previously, valproic acid is useful in the prophylactic treatment of migraine. Butalbital, one of the most widely used treatments, may well bind to barbiturate modulatory sites within the $GABA_A$-receptor complex.

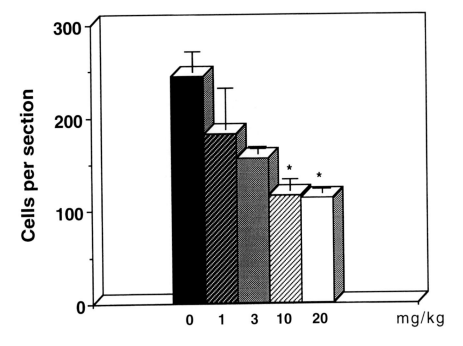

Figure 4.4   Pretreatment with valproate dose-dependently decreased the number of c-*fos*–like immunoreactive cells within lamina I, II_o of the trigeminal nucleus caudalis evoked by intracisternal capsaicin injection. Vehicle or valproate 1, 3, 10, or 20 mg per kg was injected 30 minutes prior to capsaicin and the animals were killed 120 minutes later. (*$P < 0.01$ as compared with vehicle-treated group.)

CONCLUSIONS

During the past decade, we have developed two animal models to aid in our understanding of the actions of antimigraine drugs. One is a model of meningeal neurogenic inflammation following activation of innervating primary afferent fibers. The second measures expression of the c-*fos* gene product within the TNC as a semiquantitative indicator of activation within the cephalic nociceptive system. Evidence from these two experimental animal models suggests three possible therapeutic targets: (1) prejunctional receptors on sensory terminals that prevent release of proinflammatory neuropeptides; (2) postjunctional receptors that can be blocked by selective antagonists; and (3) $GABA_A$ receptors, which may reside on parasympathetic fibers or within nucleus caudalis, that suppress NI and cephalic pain (Figure 4.6). By characterizing one or more of these potential sites, it may be possible to obtain new antimigraine drugs with fewer cardiovascular or central nervous system side effects.

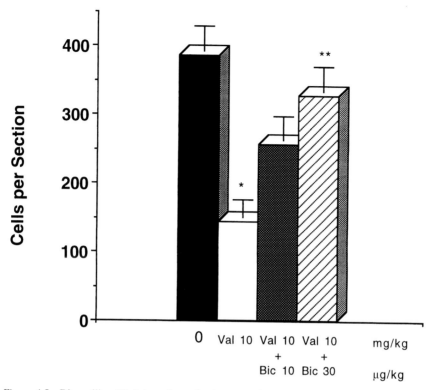

Figure 4.5   Bicuculline (Bic) dose-dependently reversed valproate (Val)-induced suppression of c-*fos*–immunoreactive cells per 50-μm section within trigeminal nucleus caudalis (lamina I, II$_o$) after intracisternal capsaicin injection. C-*fos*-LI was significantly higher in animals receiving bicuculline (30 μg per kg) plus valproate (10 mg per kg) than in those receiving valproate alone (**P < 0.01). Vehicle (solid bar), valproate, 10 mg per kg intraperitoneal (clear bar), bicuculline, 10 μg per kg intraperitoneal, plus valproate, 10 mg per kg (stippled bar), or bicuculline, 30 μg per kg intraperitoneal, plus valproate, 10 mg per kg (hatched bar) were injected intraperitonealy 40 (bicuculline) or 30 (vehicle or valproate) minutes prior to intracisternal capsaicin, and the animals were killed 120 minutes later (*P < 0.05). Only valproate, 10 mg per kg injection, gave results significantly different from those obtained with vehicle-treated controls.

Acknowledgments

The work described here was supported in part by NS 21558 (MAM) and K08 NS 01803 (FMC) of the NINDS, the Deutsche Forschungsgemeinschaft Li 617 (VL), and the British Migraine Trust (CW). M.A.M. is the recipient of a Bristol-Myers Unrestricted Research Award in Neuroscience.

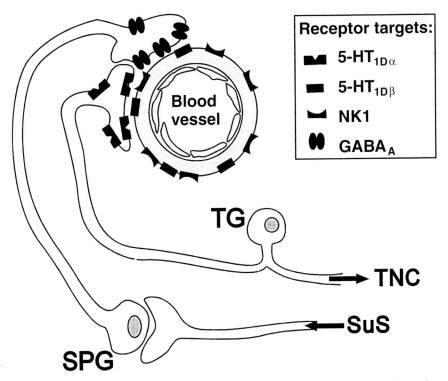

Figure 4.6 Schematic representation of the potential sites of action of different drugs that inhibit neurogenic inflammation in the guinea pig dura mater. While 5-HT$_{1D\beta}$ receptors have been identified in the vascular smooth muscle cells, where they mediate constriction, prejunctional 5-HT$_{1D\alpha}$ receptors inhibit neuropeptide release from trigeminovascular fibers. The relevance of one or the other subtype of 5-HT$_{1D}$ receptors to migraine treatment is debated (see text for details). Released neuropeptides, including substance P, act on binding sites located on the blood vessel; blockade of NK1 receptors has also been shown to inhibit neurogenic inflammation. GABA$_A$ receptors are an additional site that has recently been shown to inhibit neurogenic inflammation in rats. These receptors are likely to be located on parasympathetic sphenopalatine ganglion (SPG) neurons, because the inhibitory effect of GABA$_A$ agonists or modulators disappears in rats 2 weeks after the ablation of the SPG. (TG = trigeminal ganglion; TNC = trigeminal nucleus caudalis; SuS = superior salivatory nucleus.)

REFERENCES

1. Stewart WF, Lipton R, Celentano DD, Reed ML. Prevalence of migraine headache in the United States. JAMA 1992;267:64.
2. Ray, BS, Wolff HG. Experimental studies on headache: Pain-sensitive structures of the head and their significance in headache. Arch Surg 1940;41:813.
3. Mayberg MR, Zervas NT, Moskowitz MA. Trigeminal projections to supratentorial pial and dural blood vessels in cats demonstrated by horseradish peroxidase histochemistry. J Comp Neurol 1984;223:46.
4. Strassman A, Mason P, Moskowitz M, Maciewicz R. Response of brainstem trigeminal neurons to electrical stimulation of the dura. Brain Res 1986;379:242.

5. Wolff HG. Headache and Other Head Pain (2nd ed). New York: Oxford University Press, 1963.
6. Anderssen RGG, Anderson C, Grundstroem N, Lindren BR. Neurogenic inflammation. Acta Derm Venereol 1988;68(Suppl):35S.
7. Gliski W, Glinska-Ferenz M, Pierozyska-Dubowska M. Neurogenic inflammation induced by capsaicin in patients with psoriasis. Acta Derm Venereol 1991;71:51.
8. Krootila K, Uusitalo H, Palkama A. Effect of topical and intracranial methysergide on calcitonin gene-related peptide–induced irritative changes in the rabbit's eye. J Ocul Pharm Ther 1992;8:121.
9. Maggi CA, Giuliani S. The neurotransmitter role of calcitonin gene-related peptide in the rat and guinea pig ureter: Effect of a calcitonin gene-related peptide antagonist and species-related differences in the action of omega conotoxin on calcitonin gene-related peptide from primary afferents. Neuroscience 1991;43:261.
10. Levine JD, Dardick SJ, Roisen MF, Helms C, et al. Contribution of sensory afferents and sympathetic efferents to joint injury in experimental arthritis. J Neurosci 1986;6:3423.
11. Smith GD, Harmar AJ, McQueen DS, Seckl JR. Increase in substance P and CGRP, but not somatostatin content of innervating dorsal root ganglia in adjuvant monoarthritis in the rat. Neurosci Lett 1992;137:257.
12. Barnes PJ. Neuropeptides in human airways: Function and clinical implications. Am Rev Respir Dis 1987;136:77S.
13. Solway J, Leff AR. Sensory neuropeptides and airway function. J Appl Physiol 1991;71:2077.
14. Buzzi MG, Carter WB, Shimizu T, Heath H III, et al. Dihydroergotamine and sumatriptan attenuate levels of CGRP in plasma in rat superior sagittal sinus during electrical stimulation of the trigeminal ganglion. Neuropharmacology 1991;30:1193.
15. Dimitriadou V, Buzzi MG, Theoharides TC, Moskowitz MA. Ultrastructural evidence for neurogenically mediated changes in blood vessels of the rat dura mater and tongue following antidromic trigeminal stimulation. Neuroscience 1992;48:187.
16. Dimitriadou V, Buzzi MG, Moskowitz MA, Theoharides TC. Trigeminal sensory fiber stimulation induces morphological changes reflecting secretion in rat dura mater mast cells. Neuroscience 1991;44:97.
17. Branchek TA. More serotonin receptors? Curr Biol 1993;3:315.
18. Adham N, Kao H-T, Schechter LE, Bard J, et al. Cloning of another human serotonin receptor (5-HT_{1F}): A fifth 5-HT_1 receptor subtype coupled to inhibition of adenylate cyclase. Proc Natl Acad Sci U S A 1993;90:408.
19. Hamel E, Fan E, Linville D, Ting V, et al. Expression for the serotonin 5-hydroxytryptamine-1D beta receptor subtype in human and bovine cerebral arteries. Mol Pharmacol 1993;44:242.
20. Rebeck GW, Maynard KI, Hyman B, Moskowitz MA. Selective 5-$HT_{1D\alpha}$–receptor expression in trigeminal ganglia: Implications for antimigraine drug development. Proc Natl Acad Sci U S A 1994;91:3666.
21. Yu X, Cutrer FM, Moskowitz MA, Waeber C. The 5-HT_{1D} receptor antagonist GR-127,935 prevents inhibitory effects of sumatriptan but not CP-122,288 and 5-CT on neurogenic plasma extravasation within guinea pig dura mater. Neurophamacology, submitted.
22. Lee WS, Moskowitz MA. Conformationally restricted sumatriptan analogues CP-122,288 and CP-122,638 exhibit enhanced potency against neurogenic inflammation in dura mater. Brain Res 1993;626:303.
23. Waeber C, Moskowitz MA. [^{3}H]sumatriptan labels both 5-HT_{1D} and 5-HT_{1F} receptor binding sites in the guinea pig brain: An autoradiographic study. Naunyn Schmiedebergs Arch Pharmacol 1995;352:263.
24. Hoyer D, Clarke DE, Fozard JR, Hartig PR, et al. VII International Union of Pharmacology classification of receptors for 5-hydroxytryptamine (serotonin). Pharmacol Rev 1994;46:157.
25. Matsubara T, Moskowitz MA, Huang Z. UK-14,394, R(-)-a-methylhistamine and SMS 201-995 block plasma protein leakage within dura mater by prejunctional mechanism. Eur J Pharmacol 1992;224:145.
26. Lee WS, Moussaoui SM, Moskowitz MA. Blockade by oral or parenteral RPR 100893 (a nonpeptide NK1-receptor antagonist) of neurogenic plasma protein extravasation within guinea-pig dura mater and conjunctiva. Br J Pharmacol 1994;112:920.
27. Hering R, Kuritzky A. Sodium valproate in the prophylactic treatment of migraine: A double-blind study versus placebo. Cephalalgia 1992;12:81.
28. Jensen R, Brinck T, Oleson J. Sodium valproate has a prophylactic effect in migraine without aura: A triple-blind, placebo-crossover study. Neurology 1994;44:647.
29. Coria F, Sempere AP, Duarte J, Claveria LE, et al. Low-dose sodium valproate in the prophylaxis of migraine. Clin Neuropharmacol 1994;17:569.

30. Godin Y, Heiner L, Mark J, Mandel P. Effects of di-n-propylacetate, an anticonvulsive compound, on GABA metabolism. J Neurochem 1969;16:869.

31. Löscher W. Valproate induced changes in GABA metabolism at the subcellular level. Biochem Pharmacol 1981;30:364.

32. Lee WS, Limmroth V, Ayata C, Cutrer FM, et al. Peripheral GABA$_A$ receptor mediated effects of sodium valproate on dural plasma extravasation to substance P and trigeminal stimulation. Br J Pharmacol 1995;116:1661.

33. Limmroth V, Lee WS, Moskowitz MA. GABA$_A$-receptor mediated effects of progesterone, its ring-A metabolites, and synthetic neuroactive steroids on neurogenic edema in the rat meninges. Br J Pharmacol, in press.

34. Paul SM, Purdy RH. Neuroactive steroids. FASEB J 1992;6:2311.

35. Majewska MD. Neurosteroids: Endogenous bimodal modulators of the GABA$_A$ receptor. Mechanism of action and physiological significance. Prog Neurobiol 1992;38:379.

36. Purdy RH, Morrow AL, Moore PH Jr., Paul SM. Stress-induced levels of gamma-aminobutyric acid type A receptor–active steroids in the rat brain. Proc Natl Acad Sci U S A 1991;88:4553.

37. Blakie NH, Hossack JC. The treatment of migraine with emmenin: A preliminary report. Can Med Assoc J 1932;27:45.

38. Gray LA. The use of progesterone in nervous tension states. South Med J 1941;34:1004.

39. Singh I, Singh I, Singh D. Progesterone in the treatment of migraine. Lancet 1947;1:745.

40. Lundberg PO. Prophylactic treatment of migraine with flumedroxone. Acta Neurol Scand 1968;45:309.

41. Bradley WG, Hudgson JB, Foster JB, Newell DJ. Double-blind controlled trial of a micronized preparation of flumedroxone (Demigran) in prophylaxis of migraine. BMJ 1968;3:531.

42. Sommerville BW. The role of progesterone in menstrual migraine. Neurology 1971;21:853.

43. Morgan JI, Curran T. Stimulus-transcription coupling in the nervous system: Involvement of the inducible proto-oncogenes *fos* and *jun*. Annu Rev Neurosci 1991;14:421.

44. Morgan JI, Curran T. Role of ion flux in the control of c-*fos* expression. Nature 1986;322:552.

45. Morgan JI, Cohen DR, Hempstead JL, Curran T. Mapping patterns of c-*fos* expression in the central nervous system after seizure. Science 1987;237:192.

46. Menetrey D, Gannon A, Levine JD, Basbaum AI. The expression of c-*fos* protein in presumed-nociceptive interneurons and projection neurons of the rat spinal cord: Anatomical mapping of the central effects of noxious somatic, articular, and visceral stimulation. J Comp Neurol 1989;258:177.

47. Presley RW, Menetrey D, Levine JD, Basbaum AI. Systemic morphine suppresses noxious stimulus–evoked *fos* protein–like immunoreactivity in the rat spinal cord. J Neurosci 1990;10:323.

48. Gogas KR, Presley RW, Levine JD, Basbaum AI. The antinociceptive action of supraspinal opioids results from an increase in descending inhibitory control: Correlation of nociceptive behavior and c-*fos* expression. Neuroscience 1991;42:617.

49. Cutrer FM, Moussaoui S, Garret C, Moskowitz MA. The nonpeptide NK1 antagonist RPR 100893 decreases c-*fos* expression in trigeminal nucleus caudalis following noxious chemical meningeal stimulation. Neuroscience 1995;64:741.

50. Nozaki K, Boccalini P, Moskowitz MA. Expression of c-*fos*–like immunoreactivity in brain stem after meningeal irritation by blood in the subarachnoid space. Neuroscience 1992;49:669.

51. Nozaki K, Moskowitz MA, Boccalini P. CP-93,129, sumatriptan, dihydroergotamine block c-*fos* expression within rat trigeminal nucleus caudalis caused by chemical stimulation of the meninges. Br J Pharmacol 1992;106:409.

52. Cutrer FM, Schoenfeld D, Limmroth V, Panahian N, et al. The sumatriptan analog, CP-122,288 decreases c-*fos* expression in trigeminal nucleus following chemical stimulation of the meninges. Br J Pharmacol 1995;114:987.

53. Cutrer FM, Limmroth V, Ayata G, Moskowitz MA. Attenuation by valproate of c-*fos* immunoreactivity in trigeminal nucleus caudalis induced by intracisternal capsaicin. Br J Pharmacol 1996;116:3199.

II
Clinical Issues for the Migraine Population

5
Epidemiology and Comorbidity of Migraine

Richard B. Lipton and Walter F. Stewart

Although migraine has been recognized since 3,000 BC, our views of migraine epidemiology have changed dramatically over the last decade.[1–3] Recent epidemiologic studies have clarified our understanding of the scope and distribution of the public health problem posed by migraine.[2–4] These findings have implications for both clinical practice and public health policy.[5]

Epidemiologic studies can contribute to our understanding of migraine from several perspectives. The methods used by epidemiologists can clarify the demarcation between migraine and other primary headache disorders.[2,3] They can also be used to assess the reliability, validity, and generalizability of various case definitions.[6–10] Studies of migraine prevalence provide one measure of the scope of the migraine problem. The impact of illness on individuals and society can be addressed by measuring quality of life, work loss, and health care use in population-based samples. Examination of sociodemographic, familial, and environmental risk factors helps to identify groups at highest risk for migraine and may ultimately provide clues to disease mechanisms or preventive strategies. The natural history of migraine as it unfolds across the life span has not been well examined. Epidemiologic studies have identified a number of conditions that are comorbid with migraine; comorbidity must be considered in formulating treatment plans and may provide insights into the mechanisms of disease.[11] Finally, epidemiologic studies are an important prelude to public health interventions designed to improve diagnosis and treatment.[5]

Population-based studies identify people with migraine whether or not they are seeking care; using epidemiology methods, individuals are actively screened to identify migraine sufferers. Only 15–30% of active migraine sufferers see a doctor each year.[12,13] Most migraine studies are clinic-based, yet less than 15% of migraine sufferers ever consult neurologists, and fewer than 2% consult headache specialists.[12–14] As a consequence, clinic-based studies suffer from substantial selection bias. Factors that predispose individuals to consult specialists may be mistaken for attributes of the disease.

Recent epidemiologic studies have employed the criteria of the International Headache Society (IHS).[15–19] These criteria are more complete, explicit, and rigorous than criteria used in past studies.[2,3,20] This chapter reviews the epidemiology of migraine, emphasizing the population-based studies that use the criteria proposed by the IHS.

MIGRAINE CASE DEFINITION

For clinical practice and epidemiologic research, it is important to have a reliable and valid case definition of migraine.[3,6,7,8] One definition of reliability requires that independent diagnostic evaluations yield consistent diagnostic results. Validity refers to the relationship between the assigned diagnosis and the underlying biology of the disorder. In the absence of a true diagnostic gold standard, it is difficult to study validity. Validity is supported by the creation of diagnostic groups that include members with common risk factors, natural histories, treatment responses, profiles, and biological markers.

Many case definitions for migraine have been proposed. Although different definitions have emphasized different features, some so-called criteria are poorly specified. For example, the criteria of the Ad Hoc Committee on Classification of Headache (1962) do not specify the features or combinations of features required to establish or exclude a diagnosis, but only which features are usually present.[20] Such a lack of clarity in case definition will invariably lead to unreliability in diagnosis.

Some authors have included family history as a defining feature of migraine.[21,22] Information provided by a patient about headache in relatives is often inaccurate.[23] In addition, some studies have included family history as part of the migraine definition and then investigated the prevalence of headache in first-degree relatives of migraine sufferers, inescapably overestimating familial aggregation. Family history, in our view, should be a confirmatory, not a diagnostic, criterion.

Efforts to assess definitions of migraine empirically have attempted to distinguish migraine from tension-type headache based on specific symptom constellations. Such work is often intended to test the "spectrum" or "continuum" concept, the idea that migraine and tension-type headache exist as polar ends on a continuum of severity, varying more in degree than in kind.[24–26] The alternative model views migraine and tension-type headache as distinct entities that happen to differ in severity.

Waters examined the associations between his three "key features" of migraine (warning, unilateral pain, and nausea or vomiting) in a sample of women between the ages of 20 and 64 and found that as headache intensity increased, migrainous symptoms occurred together more frequently.[26,27] He concluded: "The distribution of the headache severity extends as a continuous spectrum from mild attacks, which usually have neither unilateral distribution nor warning nor nausea, to severe headaches which are frequently accompanied by the three migraine features." Other authors have provided empirical support for the continuum concept.[24,28]

There is ongoing debate regarding the relationship between migraine and tension-type headache.[19,24,26] In our view, the available data do not distinguish the opposing models. Progress requires the development of testable predictions that are compatible with only one model. Much of the epidemiologic work assumes that migraine is a distinct disorder. If the continuum concept is correct, the current literature describes the epidemiology of the upper tail of a distribution of severity rather than the epidemiology of a distinct disorder.

To improve the classification of headache disorders, in 1988 the IHS published its criteria for a broad range of headache disorders.[19] The criteria, based on international expert consensus, are much more explicit than the prior consensus criteria. They clearly indicate the features required to confirm or exclude particular headache diagnoses. Empirical assessment of the criteria is an area of active research. In one study, four clinicians reviewed videotapes of structured interviews and then assigned diagnoses based on IHS criteria. The overall level of agreement was moderate, as reflected by the kappa statistic of 0.74.[29] Other studies have also examined the performance of the IHS criteria.[3,9,10] Conflicting results have been obtained with respect to the comprehensiveness of the criteria. Analysis of a population-based study revealed the criteria to be comprehensive in that virtually all headache types can be classified[30]; however, in clinic-based studies, substantial numbers of patients could not be classified. Particularly problematic for the IHS criteria is the classification of chronic daily headaches evolving from migraine.[31–34] As data emerge, the IHS criteria will be reviewed and perhaps revised. Despite their limitations, the IHS criteria represent an important advance in headache classification.

Migraine headaches were formerly divided into two major varieties: classic and common, based on the presence or absence of an aura (the complex of focal neurologic symptoms preceding or accompanying an attack). The IHS criteria identify seven subtypes of migraine.[19] Common migraine was renamed "migraine without aura" (designated 1.1), and classic migraine was termed "migraine with aura" (designated 1.2).

SOME EPIDEMIOLOGIC TERMS

Many epidemiologic studies have examined migraine prevalence. *Prevalence* refers to the proportion of a given population that has migraine over a defined period of time. *Lifetime prevalence* refers to the proportion of individuals who have ever had the condition. *Period prevalence* refers to the proportion of individuals who have had at least one attack within some defined interval, usually within 1 year of the time of ascertainment. Prevalence increases as the period selected for study increases. Prevalence is an important measure of the burden of disease.

Incidence refers to the onset of new cases of a disease in a defined population over a given period of time. To conduct a migraine incidence study, one must first eliminate from study anyone in the population who has migraine. Migraine-free individuals are then followed to determine the rate of development of new cases.

There is a mathematical relationship between incidence and prevalence. Prevalence is determined by the product of average incidence and average duration of disease. In a given population, the prevalence of migraine may increase because either incidence or duration of disease is increasing. (Duration here refers not to the duration of an individual attack but to the period of a person's life over which attacks occur.)

MIGRAINE INCIDENCE

Migraine incidence should be estimated by defining a target population, excluding all current and former migraine sufferers, and then following subjects without migraine to determine the rate of onset of new cases. In the follow-up period, a person followed for 1 year contributes 1 person-year at risk for migraine. Person-years at risk become the denominator of the incidence fraction. Once a person develops migraine, he or she no longer contributes person-years at risk to the denominator. Incidence is typically expressed as new cases per 1,000 person-years at risk. Incidence studies are typically time-consuming, costly, and difficult to conduct, especially for episodic diseases.[35]

Cross-sectional data can be used to derive incidence estimates. Stewart et al. used data on reported age of migraine onset to estimate the age-specific incidence profile of migraine.[36] The phenomenon of "telescoping" complicates these estimates: People tend to report events in the past at a time closer to the present than when they actually occurred.[37] It is a ubiquitous source of error in research based on recall. The researchers developed statistical methods to correct for the effects of telescoping. An additional problem is that people may not reliably report the characteristics of headache from the remote past. Stewart et al. used case definitions intended to circumvent the problems of unreliable reporting.

The estimates of age- and sex-specific incidence rates for the onset of migraine with and without aura were based on 392 male and 1,018 female subjects with migraine (Figure 5.1). Among male subjects, age-specific incidence of migraine with aura peaks around 5 years of age at 6.6 per 1,000 person-years; the peak for migraine without aura was 10 per 1,000 person-years between 10 and 11 years of age. New cases of migraine were uncommon in men in their 20s. In women, the incidence of migraine with aura peaked between ages 12 and 13 (14.1 per 1,000 person-years); migraine without aura peaked between ages 14 and 17 (18.9 per 1,000 person-years). Thus, migraine begins earlier in male than in female subjects and earlier for migraine with aura than for migraine without aura.

Stang et al. conducted a migraine incidence study using very different methods.[38] They used the linked medical records system in Olmstead County, MN, to identify migraine sufferers who sought medical care for headaches. Migraine diagnoses were assigned based on medical records review. They found a lower incidence than Stewart et al.,[36] perhaps because many people with migraine do not consult doctors or receive a medical diagnosis.[12–14,39] The peaks they identified occurred later than those identified by Stewart et al., perhaps because medical diagnosis occurs substantially after the age of onset in some people. The linked medical records system is an ideal method for studying conditions that are completely ascertained by the health care system. Stang et al. point out that it is less than ideal for migraine because it is a disorder for which many people do not consult a health professional.[38] Their study provides an excellent method for examining both the spectrum of migraine seen in the doctor's office and health care use for migraine.

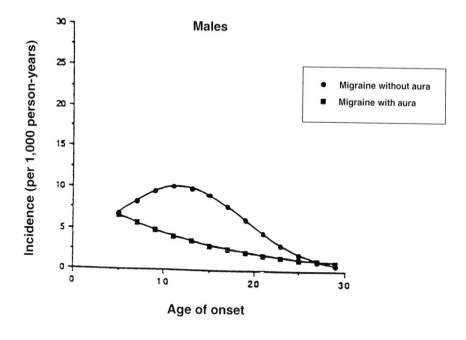

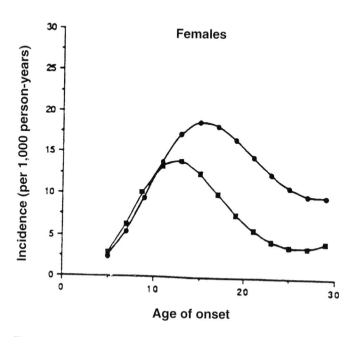

Figure 5.1 Age- and sex-specific incidence of migraine. (Reprinted with permission from WF Stewart, MS Linet, DD Celentano, M Van Natta, et al. Age- and sex-specific incidence rates of migraine with and without visual aura. Am J Epidemiol 1993;34:1111.)

PREVALENCE

The published estimates of migraine prevalence have varied widely.[2,3,40] We conducted a meta-analysis to identify the factors accounting for the variation in prevalence.[40] We reviewed 58 published population-based headache prevalence studies and identified 24 studies that met inclusion criteria for a meta-analysis.[40] We included only population-based studies that reported prevalence in clearly defined age and gender groups. In addition, the studies had to define migraine directly by ascertaining migraine symptoms and then assigning a diagnosis using operational diagnostic criteria. Reasons for excluding each of the 34 studies not included in the meta-analysis are summarized elsewhere.[40]

Despite the enormous range of results among the studies, the meta-analysis showed that 70% of the variation in estimated prevalence is accounted for by differences in the definitions of migraine and in the age and gender distribution of the study samples.[40] In particular, the studies that used the definition introduced by Waters and coworkers[26] tended to give the highest prevalence estimates. The results of the meta-analysis have been fully presented elsewhere.[40]

Based on these results, one might expect more stable prevalence estimates from the studies that used the IHS criteria. Because many migraineurs do not consult doctors and are not medically diagnosed, studies based on medical diagnosis and self-diagnosis will underestimate migraine prevalence. Studies that use medical records or survey questions about medical diagnosis or self-report will therefore yield lower prevalence estimates than those that systematically assess headache features and use them to assign diagnoses. Migraine prevalence varies strikingly with age, gender, race, and income. If study samples differ in terms of these covariates, considerable variation in prevalence can be expected.

Summary of Selected Studies

Rasmussen et al. conducted the first epidemiologic study using the operational diagnostic criteria of the IHS.[15] The study sampled 1,000 men and women, 25–64 years old, residing in Copenhagen. The sample was invited to have a general health examination, and 76% participated. Headache diagnoses were assigned using an in-person assessment by a physician. In men, the lifetime prevalences were 93% for any kind of headache, 8% for migraine, and 69% for tension-type headache. For women, the lifetime prevalences were 99% for all headache, 25% for migraine, and 88% for tension-type headache. The 1-year period prevalence of migraine was 6% in men and 15% in women; the 1-year period prevalence of tension-type headache was 63% and 86%, respectively.

In the American Migraine Study, questionnaires were mailed to 15,000 households selected to be representative of the U.S. population.[16] A questionnaire was completed by each household member with severe headache. The basis for migraine diagnosis differed from the IHS criteria in that the lifetime number of previous migraine attacks and headache duration were not considered. Subjects with daily headaches were not eligible to receive a migraine diagnosis. Migraine prevalence was 17.6% for women and 6% for men. These results closely paralleled the estimates of Rasmussen et al.

In a nationwide study of migraine epidemiology in France, Henry and coworkers reported that the prevalence of migraine according to IHS criteria was 11.9% in women and 4.0% in men.[17] The study included 4,204 subjects, aged 15 or older, who were selected using the quota method. The quota method constructs a sample representative of a particular population by selecting participants based on certain characteristics. This method facilitates projections to that target population, for example, the population of a particular country. In general, samples are constructed to be representative of the target population in terms of covariates that influence prevalence, such as age, gender, socioeconomic status, etc. In the study conducted by Henry et al., diagnoses were assigned based on lay interviews using a validated algorithm. For the group that included "borderline migraine," prevalence estimates were 17.6% for female and 6.1% for male subjects, remarkably close to the findings of Stewart et al. A number of other recent studies in Western Europe and the United States have examined the prevalence of migraine.[3,18,41–43]

Sociodemographic Variables

Most studies report that the prevalence of migraine varies by age and gender. A number of reports have demonstrated that before puberty, migraine prevalence is higher in boys than in girls; prevalence increases more rapidly in girls than in boys as adolescence approaches.[22,44–50] This prevalence profile is consistent with data on gender- and age-specific incidence.[36] The American Migraine Study revealed increasing prevalence in both men and women over the age of 12. Prevalence increases until approximately age 40, after which it declines (Figure 5.2).[16,40,44] These dramatic age effects account for some of the variation in prevalence estimates from study to study.

The gender ratio (the ratio of migraine prevalence in female to that in male subjects) also varies with age (Figure 5.3). The American Migraine Study demonstrated that the gender ratio increases from menarche to about age 42, and then begins to decline.[16,44] Cyclic hormonal changes associated with menses may account for some aspects of the migraine prevalence ratio.[51] The onset of the rising phase corresponds to the onset of menses. The declining phase may correspond with decreasing estrogen levels before and after menopause. However, hormonal factors cannot account for all of the gender differences; prevalence remains substantially higher in women than men even at the age of 70, well beyond the time that cyclic hormonal changes can be considered a factor.

Physician- and clinic-based studies have suggested that migraine is associated with high intelligence and social class. Bille did not demonstrate an association between migraine prevalence and his measure of intelligence in schoolchildren.[22,45] Epidemiologic studies in adults using intelligence testing and occupation as measures of socioeconomic status do not confirm the direct relationship between migraine and social class or intelligence.[52] In the American Migraine Study, migraine prevalence was inversely related to social class and intelligence.[16] Migraine prevalence fell as household income increased. An analysis of data from the National Health Interview Study (NHIS) confirmed that migraine prevalence is highest in low-income groups.[53] In that study, prevalence was lowest for middle-income groups and began to rise in the high-income

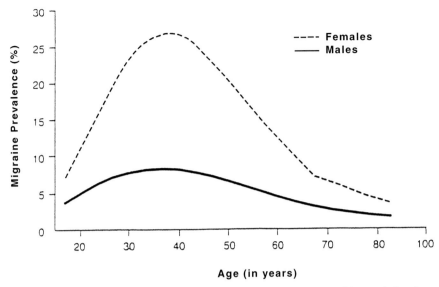

Figure 5.2   Age- and sex-specific prevalence of migraine. (Reprinted with permission from RB Lipton, WF Stewart. Migraine in the United States: Epidemiology and health care use. Neurology 1993;43[Suppl 3]:6.)

group. Because the study relied on self-reported migraine and because migraine awareness rises with income, differential ascertainment by income level may account for this relationship in higher-income groups. A population-based study in Kentucky[42] and a managed care–based study[53] have confirmed this inverse relationship in the United States.

In the American Migraine Study, individuals from high-income groups were much more likely to report a medical diagnosis of migraine than were those with lower income.[39] Migraine appears to be a disease of high-income groups in the doctor's office, but not in the community. As Waters suggested, people from higher-income households are more likely to consult physicians and are therefore disproportionately included in clinic-based studies.[26]

There are several possible explanations for the higher migraine prevalence in the lower socioeconomic groups. It may be a consequence of a circumstance associated with both low income and migraine, such as poor diet, poor medical care, or stress.[16] It may also reflect social selection; i.e., migraineurs may have lower incomes because migraine interferes with educational and occupational function, causing loss of income or interference with the ability to rise out of low-income groups.

The relation of migraine and socioeconomic status requires further study. Outside the United States, some studies have not found a relationship between migraine prevalence and social class.[3,15,18,26,27,54] The relationship may be influenced by patterns of medical consulting behavior and access to medical care in different countries.

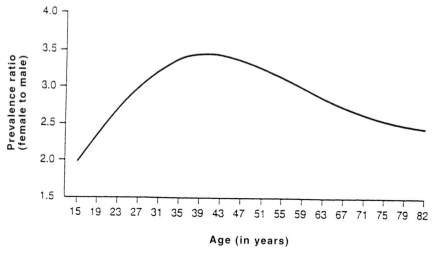

Figure 5.3 Female-to-male prevalence ratio of migraine by age. (Reprinted with permission from RB Lipton, WF Stewart. Migraine in the United States: Epidemiology and health care use. Neurology 1993;43[Suppl 3]:6.)

Is Migraine Prevalence Increasing?

Several lines of evidence suggest that the prevalence of migraine may be increasing.[55] According to a report from the Centers for Disease Control, migraine prevalence in the United States increased 60%, from 25.8–41.0 per 1,000 persons, between 1981 and 1989. These results were derived from the NHIS. Because that survey asks respondents whether they have migraine headache, it misses migraine sufferers who are not aware of their diagnosis. And because the study defines migraine by self-reported diagnosis, improved recognition of migraine over time could produce this result. For example, if increased medical consultation produced increased rates of physician diagnosis or if rising public awareness improved self-diagnosis, an apparent increase in prevalence might occur without a true increase in prevalence.

Lending credibility to the Centers for Disease Control findings, an increase in migraine prevalence was also observed in Rochester, MN, during an earlier observation period.[38] In addition, Sillanpaa reported that the prevalence of migraine in schoolchildren appears to be rising.[50] We are not aware of any major changes in migraine awareness or in patterns of diagnosis during the 1980s that could account for these findings.

If the prevalence of migraine is rising, the increase could be a result of an increasing incidence of disease, an increasing duration of disease, or both. Because the NHIS includes a representative sample of the United States population and Sillanpaa provided evidence for increasing prevalence in Finland, the data imply a problem that is international in distribution. If that is the case, it will be important to identify internationally distributed risk factors that contribute to the increase in migraine prevalence.

COMORBIDITY OF MIGRAINE

Originally coined by Feinstein,[56] the term *comorbidity* is now used to refer to the greater than coincidental association of two conditions in the same individual.[11] Migraine is comorbid with a number of neurologic and psychiatric disorders including stroke, epilepsy, depression, and anxiety disorders. Understanding the comorbidity of migraine is potentially important from a number of different perspectives.[11]

First, the occurrence of comorbidity has implications for the diagnosis of headache disorders. Migraine has substantial symptomatic overlap with several of the conditions comorbid with it. For example, both migraine and epilepsy can cause transient alterations of consciousness as well as headache. Both migraine and depression can cause changes in mood or behavior in addition to head pain. This problem of differential diagnosis is well recognized. Less well recognized is the problem of concomitant diagnosis. When two conditions are comorbid, the presence of migraine should increase, not reduce, the index of suspicion for epilepsy, depression, and anxiety disorders. Clinicians should be aware that migraine patients may well have more than one disease.

Second, once recognized, comorbidity has important implications for treatment. Although the presence of comorbid conditions may impose therapeutic limitations, they also create therapeutic opportunities. For example, when migraine and depression occur together, a beta-blocker may be a suboptimal treatment choice because of its potential to exacerbate depression. On the other hand, antidepressant therapy may successfully treat both conditions with a single drug. When migraine and epilepsy occur together, an antidepressant may be suboptimal because of its capacity to lower seizure threshold. The antimigraine, antiepileptic agent divalproex sodium may prevent attacks of both migraine and epilepsy.

Finally, the study of comorbidity may provide epidemiologic clues about the fundamental mechanisms of migraine. When comorbidity occurs, several different causal explanations should be considered. One possibility is a spurious association. Two disorders may occur together due to chance or methodologic artifact. Because migraine is common, coincidental associations are likely. As a consequence, controlled studies are essential. A more subtle problem may arise because of patterns of referral and methods of identifying cases. For example, if migraine patients with asthma are more likely to be referred to specialists (because of the contraindication to beta-blockers), a study conducted in a specialist's office may overestimate the association between migraine and asthma.[11] This bias, often referred to as Berkson's bias, is an issue in hospital- and clinic-based studies.[57] To avoid the problem, comorbidity is best studied in population-based samples.

There are also a number of models that could account for genuine comorbidity.[11] The simplest model is based on unidirectional causation. This model states that conditions A and B are comorbid because A causes B or B causes A. For example, one (false) hypothesis is that migraine and depression occur together because depression develops as a response to recurrent headache pain. An alternative causal model states that conditions occur together because of shared environmental or genetic risk factors. For example, head injury is a risk factor for both epilepsy and migraine and may account for some of the relationships between them. An inherited abnormality in a neurotransmitter system could potentially account for the relationship between migraine and depression.

Unfortunately, migraine and the conditions comorbid with it are biologically heterogeneous. Migraine occurs in several different clinical forms and in patients with different risk factor profiles and genetic diatheses. Depression, anxiety, epilepsy, and stroke also occur in multiple forms that may reflect different mechanisms. The complexities of migraine and its comorbid conditions make simple causal links unlikely. Perhaps independent genetic and environmental risk factors converge to produce changes in the brain that give rise to migraine and its comorbid conditions with increased probability.

Regardless of mechanisms, comorbidity is of great importance from the perspective of diagnosis and treatment. This section reviews the evidence on the comorbidity of migraine with stroke, epilepsy, depression, and anxiety disorders.

Migraine and Stroke

Both migraine and stroke are chronic neurologic disorders associated with alterations in cerebral blood flow, focal neurologic deficits, and headache. The relationships between migraine and stroke are complex. Headaches have been associated with stroke as ictal, preictal, and postictal phenomena.[58] Migraine aura, if prolonged, may give rise to stroke in a condition termed true migrainous infarction.[19,58]

The task of clarifying the relationships between stroke and migraine can be approached both at the epidemiologic level and at the clinical level. A better understanding ultimately requires a systematic classification for the various migraine-stroke syndromes and an assessment of risk for these syndromes in population-based samples. The causal relationship between migraine and stroke may be difficult to disentangle in individual patients.

Although a number of studies have examined migraine as a risk factor for stroke, most such studies have been limited. Methodologic problems include selection of stroke cases, selection of controls, ascertainment and definition of migraine (most studies did not use IHS criteria), and identification and adjustment for confounders and effect modifiers. The underdiagnosis of migraine makes studies of the relationship between migraine and stroke difficult. There is good evidence that many people with migraine never receive a medical diagnosis.[13,39] As headaches often remit in midlife,[16] many people who develop stroke later in life no longer accurately recall their headaches. Thus, it may be difficult to accurately identify a history of migraine in late-onset stroke patients and in control subjects.

A number of hospital series have attempted to estimate the proportion of all stroke attributable to migraine using case-by-case clinical review. In patients under the age of 50, 1–17% of strokes were attributed to migraine.[58–60] The association between migraine and stroke appears more often for migraine with aura and for stroke within the posterior circulation.[60–62] Bougousslavsky et al. reported that among patients with stroke, if the stroke occurred during the migraine attack, only 9% had arterial lesions; if the stroke was remote from the migraine attack, 91% had an arterial lesion.[63] This finding supports the idea that mechanisms other than traditional arterial disease may underlie migrainous infarction.

A number of case-control studies have examined migraine as a risk factor for stroke. The Collaborative Group for the Study of Stroke in Young Women compared hospitalized stroke patients with both hospital-based and community controls.[64] The study found a twofold increase in the risk of stroke for women with migraine when compared with community controls but not when compared with hospital controls.[64] Henrich and Horowitz found an association between migraine and stroke in a hospital-based case-control study, but differences disappeared after adjusting for stroke risk factors.[65]

Tzourio et al. reported that in women under age 45, migraine was associated with a fourfold increase in the risk of stroke; the risk became even greater in women who smoked.[66,67] These studies did not examine the relationship between migraine and stroke at the time of the attack, making inferences about causal mechanisms difficult.

In a longitudinal study, Henrich et al. estimated that the incidence of cerebral migrainous infarction was 3.36 per 100,000; if subjects with other stroke risk factors are excluded, estimates fall to 1.44 per 100,000.[68] Overall rates of ischemic stroke in the population under age 50 range from 6.5 per 100,000 to 22.8 per 100,000.[69] Interpretation of these data requires estimation of the relative risk in migrainous and nonmigrainous populations, stratified by migraine type (with and without aura), with adjustment for potential confounders.

To better understand the relationship between migraine and stroke, Welch has proposed a classification system that recognizes four types of relationships between migraine and stroke: coexistent stroke and migraine, stroke with clinical features of migraine, migraine-induced stroke, and uncertain classification.[58] For coexistent stroke and migraine, "a clearly defined stroke syndrome must occur remotely in time from a typical migraine attack."[58] It may be not be possible to establish the presence or absence of a causal relationship in an individual case. At least some cases may be coincidentally related; some cases may be linked by underlying risk factors such as mitral valve prolapse or an antiphospholipid antibody syndrome.

In stroke with clinical features of migraine, Welch indicates that "a structural lesion that is unrelated to migraine pathogenesis presents with clinical features of a migraine attack."[58] He identifies two subtypes: symptomatic and migraine mimics. In the symptomatic group, established structural disease causes episodes typical of migraine with aura. Arteriovenous malformations that masquerade as migraine provide an example. In migraine mimics, stroke is accompanied by headache and other neurologic symptoms and signs that resemble migraine.

In migraine-induced stroke, the neurologic deficit of the stroke must be identical to the neurologic symptoms of prior migraine attacks. In addition, the stroke must occur in the course of a typical migraine attack, and other causes of stroke must be excluded.

In the group with uncertain classification, migraine and stroke appear to be related but causal attribution is difficult. For example, a patient may have a typical migraine with aura, take a vasoactive drug such as ergotamine, and then have a cerebral infarction. When this rare sequence occurs, it is not clear whether the stroke is a consequence of the migraine itself, the treatment, or an interaction of the two. To clarify the causal mechanisms, we would have to compare the rates of stroke in close proximity to migraine with aura, in groups with and without vasoactive treatment. Both migraine-like headaches and stroke may be associated with systemic vasculitides, antiphospholipid antibody syndrome, mitochondrial encephalopathies, and oral contraceptive use. The classification of stroke and migraine under such conditions may be difficult.

Migraine and Epilepsy

A large body of evidence suggests that migraine and epilepsy are comorbid. In their summary of 13 studies that examined the prevalence of epilepsy in persons with migraine, Andermann and Andermann[70] reported a median prevalence of 5.9% (range, 1–17%). This greatly exceeds the 1-year period prevalence of epilepsy in the population—approximately 0.5%.[71] The prevalence of migraine in persons with epilepsy has been reported to range from 8–23%.[70] Andermann and Andermann pointed out that the lack of appropriate control groups, variation in case definitions, and small sample size make many of these studies difficult to interpret.[70]

Ottman and Lipton[72–74] used the Epilepsy Family Study of Columbia University to explore the comorbidity of migraine and epilepsy. The study sample comprised 1,923 probands with epilepsy, 88 relatives with epilepsy, and 1,316 relatives without epilepsy. Among the probands, the prevalence of a history of migraine was 24%. Among relatives with epilepsy, 26% had a history of migraine. In the control relatives without epilepsy, the prevalence of a history of migraine was 15%. Using the relatives without epilepsy as the control group, the relative risk of migraine in probands with epilepsy was 2.4 (95% confidence interval [CI] 2.0–2.9). The risk of migraine was similarly elevated in the epileptic relatives of probands with epilepsy.

The risk of migraine in probands with epilepsy did not differ by age of epilepsy onset. The risk was elevated in patients with partial and generalized seizures. Although migraine risk was highest in probands with a history of head trauma (relative risk [RR] 4.1, 95% CI 2.9–5.7), it was also elevated in idiopathic epilepsy (RR 2.3, 95% CI 1.9–2.7) and in other symptomatic epilepsy (RR 2.6, 95% CI 1.9–2.8). The risk of migraine was also elevated in probands with and without a family history of epilepsy.

The reasons for the comorbidity of migraine and epilepsy are uncertain. Migraine risk is elevated both before and after seizure onset, a fact that defeats simple notions of unidirectional causation. Migraine risk cannot be counted solely as a cause or solely as a consequence of epilepsy. Because migraine risk is elevated in individuals with posttraumatic epilepsy, and because head injury is also a risk factor for both disorders, it appears that shared environmental risk factors may contribute to comorbidity.[75,76] However, known environmental risk factors cannot fully account for the comorbidity because migraine risk is also elevated in individuals with idiopathic epilepsy. Nor can shared genetic risk factors completely account for comorbidity, because migraine risk is elevated in probands both with and without a positive family history of epilepsy.

Ottman and Lipton, based on the ideas of Welch,[77,78] postulated that an altered brain state may increase the risk of both migraine and epilepsy and so account for the comorbidity of these disorders.[72] Genetic or environmental risk factors may increase neuronal excitability or decrease the threshold for attacks of both types. Reduction in brain magnesium[78] or alterations in neurotransmitters provide plausible potential substrates for this alteration in neuronal excitability.[79]

Regardless of mechanisms, the association between migraine and epilepsy has implications for clinical practice. When treating patients for migraine or epilepsy, it is important to maintain a heightened index of suspicion for the other disorder. Differentiating migraine and epilepsy can be difficult,[70,80] because both conditions are characterized by episodes of neurologic dysfunction. Headache without other neurologic features is rare as a manifestation of epilepsy. The most difficult diagnostic issue is differentiating between migraine with aura and partial complex seizure. If the aura is brief (< 5 minutes) and associated with alteration of consciousness, automatisms, and other positive motor features (tonic-clonic movements), epilepsy is more likely. If the aura is of long duration (> 5 minutes) and has a mix of positive (scintillations, tingling) and negative features (visual loss, numbness), migraine is more likely.

Treatment strategies for patients with comorbid migraine and epilepsy should take into account the presence of comorbid disease. For example, in the treatment of migraine, drugs that lower seizure threshold should be used cautiously. These drugs include the tricyclic antidepressants, selective serotonin reuptake inhibitors, and neuroleptics. On the other hand, it is sometimes advantageous to treat both migraine and epilepsy with a single drug. Divalproex sodium has well-established efficacy in both migraine and epilepsy.[81]

Migraine, Major Affective Disorders, and Anxiety

A series of studies have examined the comorbidity of migraine and various psychiatric disorders.[82] Clinic-based studies report that migraine prevalence is increased in patients with major depression and that the prevalence of major depression is increased in patients with migraine.[83,84] Clinic-based studies are subject to Berkson's bias, as previously discussed.[57] Several population-based studies have examined the comorbidity of migraine, major depression, panic disorder, and other psychiatric disorders.[41,85–88]

In a population-based telephone interview survey (the Washington County Study), Stewart et al. reported on the relationship of migraine to panic disorder and panic attacks.[86] They examined the frequency of migraine attacks in the 1-week period prior to a telephone interview in men and women with a history of panic disorder. The relative risk of migraine headache in that week in persons with a history of panic disorder was 7.0 for men and 3.7 in women.

In a subsequent analysis, Stewart et al.[87] examined the influence of panic disorder on consulting behavior for headache. They found that 14.2% of women and 5.8% of men reporting a headache in the previous 12 months had consulted a doctor for headache. An unexpectedly high proportion of those who had consulted a physician for headache had a history of panic disorder. Of those who had recently seen a physician, 15.0% of women and 12.8% of men between the ages of 24 and 29 years had panic disorder. Comorbid psychiatric disease is apparently associated with seeking care for headache disorders.

Merikangas et al.[85] studied the comorbidity of migraine with specific psychiatric disorders in a sample of almost 500 adults, aged 27–28, residing in Zurich, Switzerland. One-year rates of anxiety and affective disorders were elevated in persons with migraine. Comparing persons with and without migraine, the odds ratios were elevated for depression (odds ratio [OR] 2.2, 95% CI 1.1–4.8), bipolar spectrum disorders (OR 2.9, 95% CI 1.1–8.6), generalized anxiety disorder (OR 2.7, 95% CI 1.5–5.1), panic disorder (OR 3.3, 95% CI 0.8–13.8), simple phobia (OR 2.4, 95% CI 1.1–5.1), and social phobia (OR 3.4, 95% CI 1.1–10.9). In this sample, major depression and anxiety disorders commonly occurred together. In persons with all three disorders, Merikangas and coworkers suggest that the onset of anxiety generally precedes the onset of migraine, whereas the onset of major depression most often follows the onset of migraine.

Breslau and coworkers[41,89–92] studied the psychiatric comorbidity of IHS-defined migraine in a sample of more than 1,000 young adults, aged 21–30 years, in southeastern Michigan. They conducted a cross-sectional and then a longitudinal study. Lifetime rates of affective and anxiety disorders were elevated in persons with migraine. After adjusting for sex, the odds ratios were 4.5 for major depression (95% CI 3.0–6.9), 6.0 for manic episode (95% CI 2.0–18.0), 3.2 for any anxiety disorder (95% CI 2.2–4.6), and 6.6 for panic disorder (95% CI 3.2–13.9).[91] In general, the associations were stronger between migraine with aura and various psychiatric disorders than for migraine without aura.

Breslau et al.[92] subsequently reported on a prospective study of migraine and major depression in the same cohort. Comparing subjects with and without migraine, the relative risk for the first onset of major depression during the follow-up period was 4.1 (95% CI 2.2–7.4). Comparing subjects with and without major depression, the relative risk for the first onset of migraine during the follow-up period was 3.3 (95% CI 1.6–6.6). This bidirectional influence of each condition on the risk for the other is incompatible with simple unidirectional causal models.[92] Migraine is neither simply a cause nor simply a consequence of depression.

In summary, recent population-based studies demonstrate an association between migraine and major depression. The longitudinal studies show a bidirectional influence, from migraine to subsequent onset of major depression and from major depression to first migraine attack. Furthermore, these epidemiologic studies indicate that persons with migraine have increased prevalence of bipolar disorder, panic disorder, and anxiety disorders.[82]

Migraine and Personality Characteristics

The relationships between migraine and personality characteristics have been discussed far more often than they have been systematically studied.[82] The idea of a migraine personality first grew out of clinical observations of the highly selected patients seen in subspecialty clinics. Many early authors have described migraineurs as perfectionistic, rigid, competitive, frustrated, and overly sensitive.[93,94]

Many investigators used personality scales such as the Minnesota Multiphasic Personality Inventory (MMPI) or the Eysenck Personality Questionnaire (EPQ).[95–98] The EPQ is a well-standardized measure that includes four scales: psychoticism (P), extroversion (E), neuroticism (N), and lie (L). Many of the studies using these measures have been limited by several factors.[86,87] Because the MMPI studies are usually clinic-based, their findings are of limited generalizability and subject to selection bias. Most studies have used historical norms instead of concurrent controls. Many have not used explicit diagnostic criteria for migraine. Despite these limitations, most studies show elevation of the neurotic triad, although the elevation is often not statistically significant.[82]

In the first population-based case-control study of personality in migraine, Brandt et al.[99] used the Washington County Migraine Prevalence Study sample. Subjects received the EPQ and the 28-item version of the General Health Questionnaire, following detailed telephone interviews. Migraineurs had higher scores than controls on the EPQ N scale, indicating that they were more tense, anxious, and depressed than the control group. Women with migraine scored significantly higher than controls on the P scale, indicating that they were more hostile, less interpersonally sensitive, and out of step with their peers.

Merikangas et al.[88] investigated the cross-sectional association between personality, symptoms, and headache subtypes as part of a prospective longitudinal study of 19- and 20-year-old subjects in Zurich, Switzerland. Migraineurs scored higher on indicators of neuroticism than did nonmigraine subjects.

Most of the population-based studies of migraine and personality have generally not controlled for drug use, headache frequency, and headache-related disability. Nor have they controlled for major psychiatric disorders (such as major depression or panic disorder), which, as we have discussed, occur more commonly in migraineurs. Because major psychiatric disorders are associated with both migraine and with personality disorders, confounding may alter the measured associations between those disorders and migraine.[82]

Breslau and Andreski[93] assessed the association between migraine and personality, adjusting for the co-occurrence of psychiatric disorders, using their epidemiologic study of young adults in Detroit. They reported an association between migraine and neuroticism, which remained significant after controlling for sex and history of major depression and anxiety disorders. Differences between migraine sufferers and controls cannot, then, be accounted for by *prior* depression and anxiety.

PUBLIC HEALTH SIGNIFICANCE

Migraine is a public health problem of enormous scope that has an impact both on the individual sufferer and on society.[100] The American Migraine Study estimates that there are 23 million U.S. residents with severe migraine headache.[16] Among them, 25% of women experience four or more severe attacks per month; 35% experience one to three severe attacks per month; 40% experience one, or less than one, severe attack per month. Similar frequency patterns were observed for men.

In the American Migraine Study, more than 85% of the women and more than 82% of the men with severe migraine had some headache-related disability. About one-third were severely disabled or needed bed rest. In addition to the disability related to attacks, many migraineurs live in fear, knowing that at any time an attack could disrupt their ability to work, care for their families, or meet social obligations.

In addition to its impact on the individual sufferer, migraine has an enormous impact on society. An American survey of 40,000 households (representing 112,000 persons) found that 5.5 days of restricted activity per 100 person-years were due to headache.[101] In Washington County, 8% of male and 14% of female subjects missed all or part of a day of work or school in the 4-week period prior to the interview.[13] Annual lost productivity due to migraine in the United States costs more than 1 billion dollars per year[53] and may cost as much as 17 billion dollars per year.[102]

Migraine has a marked impact on health care use. The National Ambulatory Medical Care Survey conducted from 1976–1977 found that 4% of all visits to physicians' offices (more than 10 million visits per year) were for headache.[103] Migraine also results in major use of emergency rooms and urgent care centers.[104] Vast amounts of prescription and over-the-counter medications are taken for headache disorders.

PROGNOSIS

Although cross-sectional data provide detailed information about prevalence, longitudinal epidemiologic data are relatively sparse. Bille followed a cohort of children with severe migraine for up to 37 years.[22,44] As young adults, 62% were migraine-free for more than 2 years, but after 30 years only 40% continued to be migraine-free, suggesting that migraine is often a lifelong disorder. Hockaday reported similar long-term remissions.[105] For 15 years, Fry collected information on migraine patients in his general practice in Kent.[106] His data showed a tendency for the severity and frequency of attacks to decrease as the patients got older. After 15 years, 32% of the men and 42% of the women no longer had migraine attacks. Waters noted a similar decrease in migraine prevalence.[26,52]

Clinic-based studies suggest that there is a subgroup of migraine sufferers afflicted with a syndrome variously called chronic daily headache evolving from migraine, transformed migraine, or malignant migraine, in which attacks increase in frequency over a number of years until a pattern of daily headache evolves.[51,107–109] In subspecialty clinics, about 80% of patients with this disorder are overusing acute headache medication. Medication overuse is believed to contribute to the accelerating pattern of pain through a mechanism that has been termed rebound headache. When the cycle of medication overuse is broken, headaches often improve.[110] However, this process of acceleration occurs in the absence of medication overuse in about 20% of subspecialty clinic patients, suggesting that there is a subgroup of migraine sufferers with a progressive condition.

CONCLUSION

Large, population-based epidemiologic studies in Denmark, the United States, France, Canada, and elsewhere have used the IHS criteria to shed light on the descriptive epidemiology of migraine. Although migraine is a remarkably common cause of temporary disability, many migraineurs, even those with disabling headache, have never consulted a physician for the problem. Prevalence is highest in women, in persons between the ages of 25 and 55, and, at least in the United States, in individuals from low-income households. Nonetheless, migraine occurs with high prevalence outside these groups at highest risk. The prevalence of migraine may be increasing in the United States, but this is not certain. Longitudinal studies are required to better determine the incidence and natural history of migraine as well as the life course of comorbid conditions.

REFERENCES

1. Patterson SM, Silberstein SD. Headache in the arts and literature. Headache 1993;33:76.
2. Lipton RB, Silberstein SD, Stewart WF. An update on the epidemiology of migraine. Headache 1994;34:319.
3. Rasmussen BK. Epidemiology of headache. Cephalalgia 1995;15:45.
4. Linet MS, Stewart WF. Migraine headache: Epidemiologic perspectives. Epidemiol Rev 1984;6:107.
5. Lipton RB, Amatniek JC, Ferrari MD, et al. Migraine: Identifying and removing barriers to care. Neurology 1994;44(Suppl 6):56.
6. Lipton RB, Stewart WF, Merikangas K. Reliability in headache diagnosis. Cephalalgia 1993;13(Suppl 12):29.
7. Merikangas KR, Whitaker AE, Angst J. Validation of diagnostic criteria for migraine in the Zurich longitudinal cohort study. Cephalalgia 1993;13(Suppl 12):47.
8. Merikangas KR, Frances A. Development of diagnostic criteria for headache syndromes: Lessons from psychiatry. Cephalalgia 1993;13(Suppl 12):34.
9. Mortimer J, Kay J, Jaron A. Epidemiology of headache and childhood migraine in an urban general practice using ad hoc, Vahlquist, and IHS criteria. Dev Med Childhood Neurol 1992;34:1095.
10. Metsahonkala L, Sillanpaa M. Migraine in children: An evaluation of the IHS criteria. Cephalalgia 1994;14:285.
11. Lipton RB, Silberstein SD. Why study the comorbidity of migraine. Neurology 1994;44:4.
12. Lipton RB, Stewart WF. Medical consultation for migraine. Neurology 1994;44(Suppl 2):199.
13. Stang PE, Osterhaus JT, Celentano DD. Migraine: Patterns of health care use. Neurology 1994;44(Suppl 4):47.
14. Linet MS, Stewart WF, Celentano DD, Siegler D, et al. An epidemiologic study of headache among adolescents and young adults. JAMA 1989;261:2211.
15. Rasmussen BK, Jensen R, Schroll M, Olesen J. Epidemiology of headache in a general population: A prevalence study. J Clin Epidemiol 1991;44:1147.
16. Stewart WF, Lipton RB, Celentano DD, Reed ML. Prevalence of migraine headache in the United States. JAMA 1992;267:64.
17. Henry P, Michel P, Brochet B, Dartigues JF, et al. A nationwide survey of migraine in France: Prevalence and clinical features in adults. Cephalalgia 1992;12:229.
18. Gobels H, Petersen-Braun M, Soyka D. The epidemiology of headache in Germany: A nationwide survey of a representative sample on the basis of the headache classification of the International Headache Society. Cephalalgia 1994;14:97.
19. Headache Classification Committee of the International Headache Society. Classification and diagnostic criteria for headache disorders, cranial neuralgias, and facial pain. Cephalalgia 1988;8(Suppl 7):1.
20. Friedman AP, Finley KH, Graham JR. Classification of headache. Arch Neurol 1962;6:173.
21. Vahlquist B. Migraine in children. Int Arch Allergy 1955;7:348.
22. Bille B. Migraine in school children. Acta Paediatr Scand 1962;51(Suppl 136):1.
23. Ottman R, Hong S, Lipton RB. Validity of family history data on severe headache and migraine. Neurology 1993;43:154.
24. Featherstone HJ. Migraine and muscle contraction headaches: A continuum. Headache 1985;24:194.
25. Raskin NH. Headache (2nd ed). New York: Churchill Livingstone, 1988.
26. Waters WE. Headache. Littleton, MA: PSG, 1986.
27. Waters WE. Headache and Migraine in General Practitioners, the Migraine Headache and Dixarit. Proceedings of a symposium held at Churchill College, Cambridge, Boehringer Ingelheim Brachnell, 1972.
28. Celentano DD, Stewart WF, Linet MS. The relationship of headache symptoms with severity and duration of attacks. J Clin Epidemiol 1990;43:983.
29. Granella E, D'Alessandro R, Manzoni GC, et al. International Headache Society Classification: Interobserver reliability in the diagnosis of primary headaches. Cephalalgia 1994;14:16.

30. Rasmussen BK, Jensen R, Olesen J. A population-based analysis of the diagnostic criteria of the International Headache Society. Cephalalgia 1991;11:129.
31. Solomon S, Lipton RB, Newman LC. Evaluation of chronic daily headache: Comparison to criteria for chronic tension-type headache. Cephalalgia 1992;12:365.
32. Sandrini G, Manzoni GC, Zanferrari C, Nappi G. An epidemiologic approach to nosography of chronic daily headache. Cephalalgia 1993;13(Suppl 12):72.
33. Mathew NT. Transformed migraine. Cephalalgia 1993;13(Suppl 2):78.
34. Silberstein SD, Lipton RB, Solomon S, Mathew NT. Transformed migraine: Proposed criteria. Headache 1994;34:1.
35. Cummings RG, Kelsey JL, Nevitt MC. Methodologic issues in the study of frequent and recurrent health problems. Ann Epidemiol 1990;1:49.
36. Stewart WF, Linet MS, Celentano DD, Van Natta M, et al. Age- and sex-specific incidence rates of migraine with and without visual aura. Am J Epidemiol 1993;34:1111.
37. Brown NR, Rips LJ, Shevelle SK. The subjective dates of natural events in very long term memory. Cognitive Psychol 1985;17:139.
38. Stang PE, Yanagihara T, Swanson JW, et al. Incidence of migraine headaches: A population-based study in Olmstead County, Minnesota. Neurology 1992;42:1657.
39. Lipton RB, Stewart WF, Celentano DD, Reed ML. Undiagnosed migraine: A comparison of symptom-based and self-reported physician diagnosis. Arch Intern Med 1992;152:1273.
40. Stewart WF, Simon D, Schechter A, Lipton RB. Population variation in migraine prevalence: A meta-analysis. J Clin Epidemiol 1995;48:269.
41. Breslau N, Davis GC, Andreski P. Migraine, psychiatric disorders, and suicide attempts: An epidemiological study of young adults. Psychiatry Res 1991;37:11.
42. Kryst S, Scherl E. A population-based survey of the social and personal impact of headache. Headache 1994;34:344.
43. Pryse-Phillips W, Findlay H, Tugwell P, Edmeads J, et al. A Canadian population survey on the clinical epidemiologic and societal impact of migraine and tension-type headache. Can J Neurol Sci 1992;19:333.
44. Lipton RB, Stewart WF. Migraine in the United States: Epidemiology and health care use. Neurology 1993;43(Suppl 3):6.
45. Bille B. Migraine in Children: Prevalence, Clinical Features, and a 30-Year Follow-up. In MD Ferrari, X Lataste (eds), Migraine and Other Headaches. New Jersey: Parthenon, 1989.
46. Sillanpaa M. Prevalence of migraine and other headache in Finnish children starting school. Headache 1976;15:288.
47. Sillanpaa M. Prevalence of headache in prepuberty. Headache 1983;23:10.
48. Sillanpaa M. Changes in the prevalence of migraine and other headaches during the first seven school years. Headache 1983;23:15.
49. Sillanpaa M, Piekkala P, Kero P. Prevalence of headache at preschool age in an unselected child population. Cephalalgia 1991;11:239.
50. Sillanpaa M. Headache in Children. In J Olesen (ed), Headache Classification and Epidemiology. New York: Raven, 1994;273.
51. Silberstein SD, Merriam G. Estrogens, progestins, and headache. Neurology 1991;41:786.
52. Waters WE. Migraine: Intelligence, social class, and familial prevalence. BMJ 1971;2:77.
53. Stang PE, Sternfeld B, Sidney S. Migraine headache in a pre-paid health plan: Ascertainment, demographics, physiological and behavioral factors. Headache 1996;36:69.
54. D'Alessandro R, Benassi G, Lenzi PL, et al. Epidemiology of headache in the Republic of San Marino. J Neurol Neurosurg Psychiatry 1988;51:21.
55. Prevalence of chronic migraine headaches: United States, 1980–1989. MMWR 1991;40:331.
56. Feinstein AR. The pretherapeutic classification of comorbidity in chronic disease. J Chronic Dis 1970;23:455.
57. Berkson J. Limitations of the application of four-fold table analysis to hospital data. Biometrics Bull 1946;2:47.
58. Welch KMA. Relationship of stroke and migraine. Neurology 1994;44(Suppl 7):33.
59. Alvarez J, Matias-Guiu J, Sumalla J, et al. Ischemic stroke in young adults. I: Analysis of etiological subgroups. Acta Neurol Scand 1989;80:29.
60. Tatemichi TK, Mohr JP. Migraine and Stroke. In HJM Barnett, BM Stein, JP Mohr, FM Yarsu (eds), Stroke: Pathophysiology, Diagnosis, and Management. New York: Churchill Livingstone, 1986;845.
61. Bougousslavsky J, Regli F. Ischemic stroke in adults younger than 30 years of age: Cause and prognosis. Arch Neurol 1987;44:479.

62. Rothrock J, North J, Madden K, et al. Migraine and migrainous stroke: Risk factors and prognosis. Neurology 1993;43:2473.
63. Bougousslavsky J, Regli F, Van Melle G, et al. Migraine stroke. Neurology 1988;38:223.
64. Collaborative Group for the Study of Stroke in Young Women. Oral contraceptives and stroke in young women. JAMA 1975;281:718.
65. Henrich JB, Horowitz RI. A controlled study of ischemic stroke risk in migraine patients. J Clin Epidemiol 1989;42:773.
66. Tzourio C, Tehindrazanarivelo A, Iglesias S, et al. Case-control study of migraine and risk of ischaemic stroke. BMJ 1993;307:289.
67. Tzourio C, Tehindrazanarivelo A, Iglesias S, et al. Case-control study of migraine and risk of ischaemic stroke in young women. BMJ 1995;310:830.
68. Henrich JB, Sandercock PAG, Warlow CP, Jones LN. Stroke and migraine in the Oxfordshire Community Stroke Project. J Neurol 1986;233:257.
69. Kittner SJ, McCarer RJ, Sherwin RW, et al. Black-white differences in stroke risk among young adults. Stroke 1993;24(Suppl 1):113.
70. Andermann E, Andermann FA. Migraine-Epilepsy Relationships: Epidemiological and Genetic Aspects. In FA Andermann, E Lugaresi (eds), Migraine and Epilepsy. Boston: Butterworth, 1987;281.
71. Hauser WA, Annegers JF, Kurland LT. Prevalence of epilepsy in Rochester, Minnesota: 1940–1980. Epilepsia 1991;32:429.
72. Ottman R, Lipton RB. Comorbidity of migraine and epilepsy. Neurology 1994;44:2105.
73. Lipton RB, Ottman R, Ehrenberg BL, Hauser WA. Comorbidity of migraine: The connection between migraine and epilepsy. Neurology 1994;44(Suppl 7):28.
74. Ottman R, Lipton RB. Is the comorbidity of epilepsy and migraine due to a shared genetic susceptibility? Neurology 1996, in press.
75. Schechter A, Stewart WF, Celentano DD, et al. An epidemiologic study of migraine and head injury (abstract). Neurology 1990;40(Suppl 1):345.
76. Annegers JF, Grabow JD, Groover RV, et al. Seizures after head trauma: A population study. Neurology 1980;30:683.
77. Welch KMA. Migraine: A behavioral disorder. Arch Neurol 1987;44:323.
78. Welch KMA, Barkley GL, Tepley N, D'Andrea G. Magnetoencephalographic Studies of Migraine: Evidence for Central Neuronal Hyperexcitability. In FC Rose (ed), New Advances in Headache Research, Vol. 2. London: Smith Gordon, 1991;127.
79. Olesen J. Synthesis of Migraine Mechanisms. In J Olesen, P Tfelt-Hansen, KMA Welch (eds), The Headaches. New York: Raven, 1993;247.
80. Marks DA, Ehrenberg BL. Migraine-related seizures in adults with epilepsy, with EEG correlation. Neurology 1993;43:2476.
81. Jensen R, Brinck T, Olesen J. Sodium valproate has a prophylactic effect in migraine without aura. Neurology 1994;44:647.
82. Silberstein SD, Lipton RB, Breslau N. Migraine: Association with personality characteristics and psychopathology. Cephalalgia 1995;15:1.
83. Marchesi C, De Ferri A, Petrolini N, et al. Prevalence of migraine and muscle tension headache in depressive disorders. J Affective Disord 1989;16:33.
84. Morrison DP, Price WH. The prevalence of psychiatric disorder among female new referrals to a migraine clinic. Psychol Med 1989;19:919.
85. Merikangas KR, Angst J, Isler H. Migraine and psychopathology: Results of the Zurich cohort study of young adults. Arch Gen Psychiatry 1990;47:849.
86. Stewart WF, Linet MS, Celentano DD. Migraine headaches and panic attacks. Psychosom Med 1989;51:559.
87. Stewart WF, Schechter A, Liberman J. Physician consultation for headache pain and history of panic: Results from a population-based study. Am J Med 1992;92:35S.
88. Merikangas KR, Stevens DE, Angst J. Headache and personality: Results of a community sample of young adults. J Psychiatric Res 1993;27:187.
89. Breslau N. Migraine, suicidal ideation, and suicide attempts. Neurology 1992;42:392.
90. Breslau N, Davis GC. Migraine, major depression, and panic disorder: A prospective epidemiologic study of young adults. Cephalalgia 1992;12:85.
91. Breslau N, Davis GC. Migraine, physical health, and psychiatric disorders: A prospective epidemiologic study of young adults. J Psychiatric Res 1993;27:211.
92. Breslau N, Davis GC, Schultz LR, et al. Migraine and major depression: A longitudinal study. Headache 1994;7:387.
93. Breslau N, Andreski P. Migraine, personality, and psychiatric comorbidity. Headache, in press.

94. Wolff HG. Personality features and reactions of subjects with migraine. Arch Neurol Psychiatry 1937;37:895.

95. Sternbach RA, Dalessio DJ, Junzel M, et al. MMPI patterns in common headache disorders. Headache 1980;20:311.

96. Kudrow L, Sutkus GJ. MMPI pattern specificity in primary headache disorders. Headache 1979;19:18.

97. Weeks R, Baskin S, Sheftell F, et al. A comparison of MMPI personality data and frontalis electromyographic readings in migraine and combination headache patients. Headache 1983;23:75.

98. Invernizzi G, Gala C, Buono M, et al. Neurotic traits and disease duration in headache patients. Cephalalgia 1989;9:173.

99. Brandt J, Celentano D, Stewart WF, et al. Personality and emotional disorder in a community sample of migraine headache sufferers. Am J Psychiatry 1990;147:303.

100. Ziegler DK. Headache: Public health importance. Neurol Clin 1990;8:781.

101. Black ER. Acute conditions: Incidence and associated disability. United States, July 1976–June 1977. Vital and Health Statistics, ser. 10, no. 125, DHEW publication no. 78-1553. Washington, D.C.: U.S. Government Printing Office, 1978.

102. Osterhaus JT, Gutterman DL, Plachetka JR. Health care resources and lost labor costs of migraine headaches in the United States. Pharmacoeconomics 1992;2:67.

103. National Center for Health Statistics. Advance data. Vital and Health Statistics of the United States. Department of Health, Education, and Welfare, PHS publication no. 53. Hyattsville, MD: National Center for Health Statistics, 1979.

104. Celentano DD, Stewart WF, Lipton RB, Reed ML. Medication use and disability among migraineurs: A national probability sample. Headache 1992;32:223.

105. Hockaday JM. Definitions, Clinical Features, and Diagnosis of Childhood Migraine. In JM Hockaday (ed), Migraine in Children. London: Butterworth, 1988;5.

106. Fry J. Profiles of Disease. Edinburgh: Livingstone, 1966.

107. Mathew NT, Stubits E, Nigam MP. Transformation of episodic migraine into daily headache: Analysis of factors. Headache 1982;22:66.

108. Mathew NT, Reuveni U, Perez F. Transformed or evolutive migraine. Headache 1987;27:102.

109. Silberstein SD, Lipton RB, Solomon S, Mathew NT. Classification of daily and near daily headaches. Proposed revisions to the IHS criteria. Headache 1994;34:1.

110. Silberstein SD, Silberstein JR. Chronic daily headache: Long-term prognosis following inpatient treatment with repetitive IV DHE. Headache 1992;32:439.

6

Classification of Migraine

Jes Olesen and Birthe Krogh Rasmussen

The headache classification published by an ad hoc committee of the National Institutes of Health in 1962[1] was quickly adopted in the United States as well as in parts of western Europe. At the time it represented an advance, but progress in the understanding of the various headache disorders has rendered that classification system obsolete. Furthermore, it did not define various headache disorders in operational terms, but only provided short descriptions that were open to individual interpretation. Scattered attempts were made to operationalize these diagnostic criteria for clinical trials,[2,3] but none gained international acceptance. In 1985 the International Headache Society (IHS) appointed a headache classification committee, and in 1988 the first international headache classification including operational diagnostic criteria for all headache disorders was published.[4] That classification was endorsed by all the national headache societies represented in the IHS and also very quickly by the World Federation of Neurology. The World Health Organization accepted the major principles of the new classification, which have been used in the recently published International Classification of Diseases (ICD-10)[5] and the ICD-10's neurologic adaptation.[6] The ICD-10 and especially its neurologic adaptation[5,6] closely follow the IHS classification, and a so-called diagnostic guide for headache presently in publication provides a crosswalk between these two coding systems and brings the operational diagnostic criteria of the IHS together with the ICD-10 code numbers.

The complete international headache classification has been translated into German, French, Italian, Spanish, Turkish, Portuguese, Russian, Thai, and Chinese. Essentials of the document have been translated into Slovenian, Danish, Swedish, Japanese, and a number of other languages. A Swiss abbreviated version including German, Italian, and French terms is also available.

TAXONOMY AND PREVIOUSLY USED TERMS

In the past, headache taxonomy was bewildering. Many old terms have remained in use despite lack of agreement about their exact meanings. The terms *classic*

Table 6.1   International Headache Society classification of migraine

1. Migraine
   1.1   Migraine without aura
   1.2   Migraine with aura
      1.2.1   Migraine with typical aura
      1.2.2   Migraine with prolonged aura
      1.2.3   Familial hemiplegic migraine
      1.2.4   Basilar migraine
      1.2.5   Migraine aura without headache
      1.2.6   Migraine with acute onset aura
   1.3   Ophthalmoplegic migraine
   1.4   Retinal migraine
   1.5   Childhood periodic syndromes that may be precursors to or associated with
      migraine
      1.5.1   Benign paroxysmal vertigo of childhood
      1.5.2   Alternating hemiplegia of childhood
   1.6   Complications of migraine
      1.6.1   Status migrainosus
      1.6.2   Migrainous infarction
   1.7   Migrainous disorder not fulfilling above criteria

migraine and *classical migraine* were used interchangeably and both with variable meaning. Some used the terms only when patients had sensory or motor auras. *Hemiplegic migraine* was sometimes used when patients had hemiparesis, but it was more often used when patients had hemisensory symptoms. Nonexperts often confused the words *classical* and *typical,* thus a patient could have a diagnosis of classical common migraine. These discrepancies became even more pronounced in areas where English was not spoken. The Headache Classification Committee of the IHS created a standardized nomenclature and new terms when necessary. *Common migraine* became migraine without aura, and *classic/classical migraine* became migraine with aura. The latter now includes the following previously used terms: migraine accompagné, hemiplegic, complicated, ophthalmic, hemisensory, aphasic, basilar, and confusional migraine.

The IHS classification is hierarchically constructed. It contains 13 diagnostic groups, which are subdivided to allow for coding up to a four-digit level. Thus, it is possible to use the classification at different levels of sophistication. Doctors in general practice can code just to one or two digits, whereas specialists and research centers can also code the third and fourth digits. Table 6.1 gives the subgroupings of migraine according to the IHS classification.

CURRENT CLASSIFICATION OF MIGRAINE

The subtypes of migraine are classified according to their clinical features and according to current concepts of pathophysiology. Migraine without aura is characterized by normal cerebral blood flow and the absence of neurologic symptoms, whereas migraine with aura is associated with typical changes in regional cerebral blood flow. Migraine with aura encompasses all forms of migraine that are preceded by neurologic symptoms originating from the brain or brain stem. Some of the subgroupings under migraine with aura are new; others have been recognized for a long time. A number of old terms were abandoned. Ophthalmoplegic migraine was recognized as a separate form of migraine because of a markedly different clinical picture and pathophysiology, possibly caused by retro-orbital granulomatous inflammation. Retinal migraine was also regarded as separate due to its presumed origin in the retina. Good studies to substantiate its existence are lacking. Finally, a mixed group of childhood periodic syndromes that may be precursors to or associated with migraine and complications of migraine were recognized. In order to make the classification exhaustive, the condition 1.7, "migrainous disorder not fulfilling above criteria," was included.

OPERATIONAL DIAGNOSTIC CRITERIA

The difficulty with an operational headache diagnosis is the lack of abnormalities found in routine laboratory investigations. The headache diagnoses must be made exclusively on the basis of information provided by the patient. During the twentieth century, various sophisticated techniques have been developed to measure such quantities as regional cerebral blood flow and transcranial Doppler. However, these tests mainly show changes during attacks, so they are not generally accessible for diagnostic use. The criteria of the IHS, therefore, depend largely on the headache history and on the exclusion of organicity by physical and neurologic examinations and laboratory tests. The IHS has used the principles developed by the American Psychiatric Society to create operational diagnostic criteria for psychiatric disorders.[7] The operational diagnostic criteria for migraine with and without aura are given in Table 6.2. Each set of criteria consists of a number of letter headings, A, B, C, etc. The requirements under each letter heading must be fulfilled for a diagnosis to be made of, say, migraine without aura. Each letter heading may consist of several characteristics, not all of which must be fulfilled. Features present only in 50% of patients, for example, can thus be included. This pertains to the characteristics of both headache and associated symptoms. Note that under C it is required only that pain characteristics fulfill two out of the four criteria. Most neurologists have seen typical migraine patients whose pain was bilateral and not pulsating. Such patients have migraine according to the IHS classification as long as the two other features of criterion C are fulfilled. It is similar for criterion D: although most patients have nausea, vomiting, or both during migraine attacks, an occasional patient will have absolutely typical migraine but without gastrointestinal symptoms. The diagnosis is accepted if the patient has photophobia as well as phonophobia. The purpose of criterion E is to rule out intracranial disease. It is rather lengthy, but as such it serves to protect patients from overinvestigation. It specifies that laboratory investigations are not necessary to rule out organic disorder in the great majority of headache patients.

The operational diagnostic criteria constitute the most important part of the headache classification. However, short descriptions of the disorders are also

Table 6.2 Diagnostic criteria for migraine with and without aura

---

Migraine without aura
- A. At least five attacks fulfilling B–D
- B. Headache attacks lasting 4–72 hours (untreated or unsuccessfully treated)
- C. Headache has at least two of the following characteristics:
    1. Unilateral location
    2. Pulsating quality
    3. Moderate or severe intensity (inhibits or prohibits daily activities)
    4. Aggravation by walking stairs or similar routine physical activity
- D. During headache at least one of the following:
    1. Nausea, vomiting, or both
    2. Photophobia and phonophobia
- E. At least one of the following:
    1. History and physical and neurologic examinations do not suggest one of the disorders listed in groups 5–11*
    2. History and/or physical and/or neurologic examinations do suggest such a disorder, but it is ruled out by appropriate investigations
    3. Such a disorder is present, but migraine attacks do not occur for the first time in close temporal relation to the disorder

Migraine with aura
- A. At least two attacks fulfilling B
- B. At least three of the following four characteristics:
    1. One or more fully reversible aura symptoms, indicating focal cerebral cortical and/or brain stem dysfunction
    2. At least one aura symptom develops gradually over more than 4 minutes or, two or more symptoms occur in succession
    3. No aura symptom lasts more than 60 minutes. If more than one aura symptom is present, accepted duration is proportionally increased
    4. Headache follows aura with a free interval of less than 60 minutes (it may also begin before or simultaneously with the aura)
- C. At least one of the following:
    1. History and physical and neurologic examinations do not suggest one of the disorders listed in groups 5–11*
    2. History and/or physical and/or neurologic examinations do suggest such a disorder, but it is ruled out by appropriate investigations
    3. Such a disorder is present, but migraine attacks do not occur for the first time in close temporal relation to the disorder

---

*Disorders listed in groups 5–11 refer to the headache associated with (1) head trauma, (2) vascular disorders, (3) nonvascular intracranial disorder, (4) substance use or withdrawal, (5) noncephalic infection, (6) metabolic disorder, or (7) cranium, neck, eyes, ears, nose, sinuses, teeth, mouth, or other facial or cranial structures.

given. They are more readable and are intended for use in textbooks and teaching. The short description of migraine without aura, for example, is as follows: "Idiopathic, recurring headache disorder manifesting in attacks lasting 4 to 72 hours. Typical characteristics of headache are unilateral location, pulsating quality, moderate or severe intention, aggravation by routine physical activity, and association with nausea, photo- and phonophobia."

HOW TO USE THE INTERNATIONAL
HEADACHE SOCIETY CLASSIFICATION

The fact that a single patient frequently has more than one type of headache has not been acknowledged in most previous classification systems, in which patients have been categorized as having, for example, either migraine or tension-type headache. In the IHS classification system, patients receive a diagnosis for each distinct form of headache. This results in a precise description of patients with coexistence of different types of headaches. It should be noted that diagnoses must follow changes in the headache pattern of individual patients over time, and they may require repeated adjustments. Some patients indicate that they have many different forms of headaches, even if they are all varieties of a single diagnosis according to the IHS classification. Other patients believe that their different forms of headaches are just variations of the same diagnosis. Careful history taking must clarify how many different forms of headaches the patient has and which criteria they fulfill. The diagnosis "combination headache" has been abandoned. Patients who would previously have been so diagnosed are now classified as having two diagnoses: migraine and tension-type headaches. The various subforms of tension-type headaches and of cluster headaches are mutually exclusive, but the subforms of migraine are not. A patient can thus have more than one migraine diagnosis, for example, migraine without aura and migraine with aura. If a patient receives two diagnoses, which is the more important one? And how do we assess the severity of the headache disorder? It is recommended that the estimated number of headache days per year be included in brackets after each diagnosis to add a quantitative aspect to the headache diagnosis. Not all headache episodes in a patient can or should be diagnosed. Atypical episodes are frequent because of early treatment, lack of ability to remember symptoms exactly, and other factors. The patient should be asked to describe typical untreated or unsuccessfully treated episodes. It should be decided which set of diagnostic criteria these episodes fulfill and whether the required number of episodes have been experienced. Then the number of days per year on which that particular type of headache occurs should be estimated, including treated attacks and less typical attacks believed to be of the same type. With respect to the severity of the headache, the classification distinguishes between mild, moderate, and severe pain intensity. A mild pain does not inhibit daily activities; a moderate pain inhibits but does not prevent daily activities; and a severe pain suspends daily activities.

In unclear cases it is recommended that the patient be asked to keep a diagnostic headache diary.[8] Prospective recording of symptoms will usually make the diagnosis more precise. If a particular form of headache fulfills two sets of criteria, the diagnosis mentioned first in the classification should be coded for.

SCIENTIFIC EVALUATION OF THE INTERNATIONAL
HEADACHE SOCIETY CLASSIFICATION

The primary headaches constitute disease entities characterized by a clustering of specific combinations of symptoms. It is intuitively evident that the explicit diagnostic criteria for all headache disorders of the IHS[4] represent a substantial improvement over previous diagnostic systems. Nevertheless, the criteria require systematic field testing. There are some fundamental requirements of a classification; one is that it should be generalizable, which means it should be applicable in diverse settings (headache clinics, general practices, general populations, etc.). The IHS criteria are derived from expert consensus. As such they are mostly based on experience with highly selected migraine patients and therefore might be expected to be most relevant in a specialist practice or in a hospital setting. However, in recent years the IHS criteria have been used in several studies from the general population and have been found to be highly applicable.[9–11] Another basic requirement of the ideal classification system is that of exhaustiveness. The classification is exhaustive if it is possible to classify all headaches according to diagnostic criteria. This was recently shown to be the case in a large population-based study.[10] In the Danish population study, only two of 740 normal Danes were referred to group 13, "headache not classifiable."

The criteria should also be reliable, which means that they have a low interobserver variability and that individuals receive the same diagnoses when repeatedly diagnosed according to the criteria. The repeatability of the criteria when applied to the same individual at different times may, however, be influenced by the episodic nature of headaches and by changes in the types of headaches that occur over time. Thus, poor repeatability may be due to unreliable criteria or to actual changes in the individual. Few studies of interobserver reliability are currently available. Granella et al.[12] found that when clinicians reviewed videotaped interviews, the agreement rate for classification of migraine at both the one- and two-digit levels was substantial (kappa 0.74 and 0.65, respectively). In another study of the reliability of the IHS criteria, the clinical records of 100 consecutive outpatients were evaluated by two neurologists.[13] Interobserver agreement in the application of the IHS criteria of migraine was almost perfect (kappa 0.88), and similar results emerged for the subgroupings of migraine without aura (kappa 0.78) and migraine with aura (kappa 0.90).[13] In concordance, two blinded observers always made the same IHS diagnoses when interpreting the records of prospective diagnostic headache diaries recorded by patients from a headache clinic.[8]

Finally, there is the requirement of validity, which means that the diagnosis reflects the underlying biological disorder. However, it is very difficult to evaluate the validity of the headache classification, because no gold standard exists. Nonetheless, a number of approaches have been used to study the validity of the classification. Some have compared the IHS diagnoses with the diagnoses of expert clinicians. The diagnostic process of expert clinicians is characterized by a kind of pattern recognition—all experts know that they can recognize a migraine patient, but the exact criteria used to diagnose may vary considerably from one expert to another and even for the same expert from case to case. Furthermore, the studies that have attempted to evaluate the validity of the criteria by comparing the diagnoses they yield with those made by expert clinicians[14,15] have employed the IHS criteria via nonvalidated questionnaires or lay interviews. Thus, any inability of the criteria to classify individual headache types in these studies could be due to the limitations (poor validity, reliability, etc.) of the questionnaires or lay interviews or to those of the diagnostic criteria themselves. In an earlier study, the utility of a self-administered headache questionnaire based on the IHS criteria was analyzed by comparison of its results to

data obtained by a clinical interview in which physicians applied
ria to make diagnoses in the same subjects.[16] The limitations of diag
tionnaires were illustrated. Because of a substantial number of mis
misclassified cases, and unclassifiable cases, the questionnaire was f
be valid for diagnosing headache according to the IHS criteria. One c ... main
problems in diagnosing headaches by a questionnaire is probably the frequent
coexistence of different headache forms. The respondents cannot distinguish
between the different types when answering the many questions. Another important problem concerns the episodic nature of headache: reporting tends to be
biased toward the more recent or more severe attacks.

Two previous studies[11,17] have validated the criteria by comparison with diagnoses obtained using the former Ad Hoc Committee classification of headache.[1]
In a Danish study of a clinical sample of about 80 headache sufferers, Iversen et
al.[17] found a good correlation between the two classification systems, whereas
Merikangas et al.,[11] in the Zurich cohort study, found lower prevalence rates of
migraine employing the Ad Hoc Committee criteria compared with the IHS criteria (the agreement rate between the two classifications was not presented).
The Zurich study suggests that the criteria may be too unrestrictive when applied
to a nonclinic sample. Contrarily, in France the IHS criteria have been found to
be too restrictive both in a general population and in a clinic sample.[14,15] In the
Danish study, the IHS criteria as well as the criteria of the Ad Hoc Committee
were applied by neurologists. In the Zurich study, it was nonphysicians who performed the headache interviews, and in the French studies, lay interviews or questionnaires were used. Therefore, it is tempting to suggest that the lower
applicability of the criteria in the studies from France and Zurich compared with
the Danish study are due to the limitations of the methods used for ascertaining
the diagnoses rather than to those of the diagnostic criteria.

In recent years, the IHS criteria have been used worldwide in several large,
multicenter, multinational, double-blind drug trials.[18-20] Those studies have
shown remarkably consistent response rates to the agent sumatriptan, reflecting
the homogeneity of the defined migraine group. The validity of the criteria is also
reflected in consistent epidemiologic profiles and homogeneous nosologic characteristics of the various headache types that have been found in several recent
epidemiologic studies employing the IHS diagnostic criteria.[9,14,21-23]

COEXISTING MIGRAINE AND TENSION-TYPE HEADACHES

The terms *tension-vascular headache, combined headache, combination
headache, mixed headache,* and *vascular and muscle-contraction headache* have
been used when migraine and tension-type headaches coexist in the same individual. This type of headache has never been precisely defined, and it has been
judged impossible to single out a suitable group of subjects who should receive
the diagnosis.[4,24] Headache sufferers include those who have pure migraine,
those with pure tension-type headache, and others who have migraine in combination with greater or lesser amounts of tension-type headache. The concept of
combination headache is arbitrary; therefore, patients with both migraine and
tension-type headache should instead have both diagnoses, as suggested in the

IHS classification. The term *interval headache* has also been widely used, usually referring to the headaches that occur in periods between real migraine attacks. Recent studies, both clinical and epidemiologic, have documented that this type of headache is probably just regular tension-type headache: Nosographic characteristics and physical findings of tension-type headache in migraineurs are very similar to those in nonmigraineurs.[24,25] Other authors consider this interval-type headache to be a kind of mild migraine, but their supportive evidence is based on the experience with clinic patients suffering from daily headaches.[26–31] Many such patients use medication excessively, a practice that may be at least partly responsible for some of the headaches.[32–34] After drug overuse has been eliminated or reduced, the clinical picture of these patients usually becomes much simpler and it becomes possible to describe them fully using only one or two diagnoses according to the IHS criteria. We believe that adherence to the IHS classification system, including a diagnostic breakdown of different headache types occurring in the same individual, is far more useful than labeling patients with mysterious and arbitrary diagnoses such as chronic daily headache. The diagnostic breakdown of different headache types is essential to the development of treatment strategies, and it is helpful in explaining to patients how to identify different headache types when self-medicating. It is clearly indispensable for research purposes.

With the aim of assessing and improving the reliability and validity of the IHS criteria, future work should focus on continued field testing in various settings. More precise operationalization including more explicit behavior-oriented criteria to define each individual headache feature can be expected to improve the reliability, sensitivity, and specificity of the IHS diagnostic criteria.

REFERENCES

1. Ad Hoc Committee on Classification of Headache. Classification of headache. JAMA 1962;179:717.
2. Olesen J, Krabbe AÆ, Tfelt-Hansen P. Methodological aspects of prophylactic drug trials in migraine. Cephalalgia 1981;1:127.
3. Tfelt-Hansen P, Olesen J. Methodological aspects of drug trials in migraine. Neuroepidemiology 1985;4:204.
4. Headache Classification Committee of the International Headache Society. Classification and diagnostic criteria for headache disorders, cranial neuralgias, and facial pain. Cephalalgia 1988;8(Suppl 7):1.
5. World Health Organization. International Classification of Diseases 10. Geneva: World Health Organization, 1992.
6. World Health Organization. International Classification of Diseases 10: Neurological adaptation. Geneva: World Health Organization, 1996, in press.
7. American Psychiatric Association. Diagnostic and Statistical Manual (DSM-III-R). Washington, D.C.: American Psychiatric Association, 1987.
8. Russell MB, Rasmussen BK, Brennum J, Iversen HK, et al. Presentation of a new instrument: The diagnostic headache diary. Cephalalgia 1992;12:369.
9. Rasmussen BK, Jensen R, Schroll M, Olesen J. Epidemiology of headache in a general population: A prevalence study. J Clin Epidemiol 1991;44:1147.
10. Rasmussen BK, Jensen R, Olesen J. A population-based analysis of the diagnostic criteria of the International Headache Society. Cephalalgia 1991;11:129.
11. Merikangas KR, Whitaker AE, Angst J. Validation of diagnostic criteria for migraine in the Zürich longitudinal cohort study. Cephalalgia 1993;13(Suppl 12):47.
12. Granella F, D'Alessandro R, Manzoni GC, et al. International Headache Society classification: Interobserver reliability in the diagnosis of primary headaches. Cephalalgia 1994;14:16.

13. Leone M, Filippini G, D'Amico D, Farinotti M, et al. Assessment of International Headache Society diagnostic criteria: A reliability study. Cephalalgia 1994;14:280.
14. Henry P, Michel P, Brochet B, et al. A nationwide survey of migraine in France: Prevalence and clinical features in adult. Cephalalgia 1992;12:229.
15. Michel P, Dartigues JF, Henry P, et al. Validity of the International Headache Society criteria for migraine. Neuroepidemiology 1993;12:51.
16. Rasmussen BK, Jensen R, Olesen J. Questionnaire versus clinical interview in the diagnosis of headache. Headache 1991;31:290.
17. Iversen HK, Langemark M, Andersson PG, Hansen PE, et al. Clinical characteristics of migraine and episodic tension-type headache in relation to old and new diagnostic criteria. Headache 1990;30:514.
18. Cady RK, Wendt JK, Kirchner JR, Sargent JD, et al. Treatment of acute migraine with subcutaneous sumatriptan. JAMA 1991;265:2831.
19. Subcutaneous Sumatriptan International Study Group. Treatment of migraine attacks with sumatriptan. N Engl J Med 1991;325:316.
20. The Oral Sumatriptan Dose-Defining Study Group. Sumatriptan: An oral dose–defining study. Eur Neurol 1991;31:300.
21. Stewart WF, Lipton R, Celentano DD, Reed ML. Prevalence of migraine headache in the United States. JAMA 1992;267:64.
22. Breslau N, Davis GC, Andreski P. Migraine, psychiatric disorders, and suicide attempts: An epidemiologic study of young adults. Psychiatry Res 1991;37:11.
23. Edmeads J, Findlay H, Tugwell P, Pryse-Philips W, et al. Impact of migraine and tension-type headache on life-style, consulting behaviour, and medication use: A Canadian population survey. Can J Neurol Sci 1993;20:131.
24. Rasmussen BK, Jensen R, Schroll M, Olesen J. Interrelations between migraine and tension-type headache in the general population. Arch Neurol 1992;49:914.
25. Langemark M, Olesen J, Poulsen DL, Bech P. Clinical characterization of patients with chronic tension headache. Headache 1988;28:590.
26. Silberstein SD, Lipton RB, Solomon S, Mathew NT. Classification of daily and near-daily headaches: Proposed revisions to the IHS criteria. Headache 1994;34:1.
27. Sanin LC, Mathew NT, Bellmeyer LR, Ali S. The International Headache Society (IHS) Headache Classification as applied to a headache clinic population. Cephalalgia 1994;14:443.
28. Manzoni GC, Granella F, Sandrini G, Cavallini A, et al. Classification of chronic daily headache by International Headache Society criteria: Limits and proposals. Cephalalgia 1995;15:37.
29. Mathew NT, Stubits E, Nigam MP. Transformation of episodic migraine into daily headache: Analysis of factors. Headache 1982;22:66.
30. Mathew NT, Reuveni U, Perez F. Transformed or evolutive migraine. Headache 1987;27:102.
31. Saper JR. The mixed headache syndrome: A new perspective. Headache 1982;22:284.
32. Lippman CW. Characteristic headache resulting from prolonged use of ergot derivatives. J Nerv Ment Dis 1955;121:270.
33. Saper JR. Migraine. II: Treatment. JAMA 1978;239:2480.
34. Martignoni E, Solomon S. The Complex Chronic Headache: Mixed Headache and Drug Overuse. In J Olesen, P Tfelt-Hansen, KMA Welch (eds), The Headaches. New York: Raven, 1993;849.

7
Genetic Evaluation of Migraine

Stephen J. Peroutka

In the early twentieth century it was said that "there are few maladies that cause in the aggregate as much suffering as migraine, and about which so little is known concerning either causes, mechanism, prevention or cure."[1] The same conclusion can still be drawn in the late twentieth century. A major problem confronting all physicians who treat migraine patients is that diagnostic and therapeutic approaches are not based on objective measures. However, a revolutionary advance in the understanding of migraine is imminent based on recent advances in the genetic analysis of this common disorder.

PAST STUDIES

Significant data have existed for many years to indicate that migraine is a genetically transmitted syndrome. The hypothesis that migraine is inherited was well established in the nineteenth century. Indeed, Liveing[2] noted the frequent occurrence of "megrim" within families and that the disorder was often transmitted from parent to child. The genetic basis of migraine has been supported by numerous studies.[1,3] Twin studies have demonstrated a definite, but relatively small, genetic component in migraine. Anecdotal evidence from experienced clinicians has consistently provided support for a genetic basis of migraine. Some authors have even considered a positive family history as a prerequisite for the diagnosis of migraine.[4]

To assess the parental frequency of migraine in probands with migraine, a recent study analyzed a total of 255 individuals with symptoms consistent with a diagnosis of migraine without aura as defined by the International Headache Society.[5] The parents of those individuals were also interviewed directly for the presence of migraine. In 91% of the parent sets, one or both parents met International Headache Society criteria for migraine without aura. These data are consistent with previous studies in the neurologic literature (Table 7.1). The 91% frequency of inheritance is consistent with a dominant mode of genetic transmission.

Table 7.1.   Summary of familial migraine data

Parental frequency (%)	Ascertainment method	Proposed inheritance pattern	Reference
91	Unknown	Dominant	Allan, 1928[1]
91	Direct interviews	Dominant	Peroutka and Howell, 1995[5]
80	Questionnaire from parents	None proposed	Bille, 1962[7]
78	Interview of probands	Recessive (70% penetrance)	Goodell et al., 1954[8]
73	Interview of probands	"Complicated" heredity	Dalsgaard-Nielsen, 1965[9]
68	Interview of probands	"Sex limited"	D'Amico et al., 1991[10]
56	Questionnaire from probands	Genetic heterogeneity	Devoto et al., 1986[6]

This type of direct interview study represents the first step in initiating a molecular genetic analysis of migraine. Nearly all previous family studies of migraine have relied on reports of the probands to diagnose migraine in their first-degree relatives. As shown in Table 7.1, the frequency of the parental history of migraine decreases as the ascertainment method becomes less direct. For example, the only study that directly interviewed parents identified a 91% parental history,[5] whereas only a 56% parental history was obtained when probands were asked to complete a questionnaire about their parents' headache history.[6] Intermediate inheritance rates (68–78%) have been observed in studies in which probands, but not their parents, were interviewed directly.[7–10]

The next step required in the genetic analysis of migraine is a molecular analysis of familial DNA samples. Prior to recent technical advances in molecular genetics, it was hardly possible even to consider migraine as a candidate disease for a formal molecular genetic analysis. The wide spectrum of clinical symptomatology, the likely role of environmental factors such as stress and diet, and, perhaps most important, the high prevalence of migraine within the general population are all factors that make the genetic analysis of migraine a daunting task. Nonetheless, a formal molecular genetic analysis of migraine is under way in a number of laboratories around the world. A linkage analysis of DNA markers can be expected to allow for a precise determination of the genetic bases of migraine.

CURRENT STUDIES

Human Genome Project

Molecular genetics was revolutionized in the 1980s by technical advances in gene mapping. In particular, the development of the polymerase chain reaction technique led to an exponential growth in the ability to generate data about the human genome, which is the entire complement of a human's genes. The availability of increasingly numerous DNA polymorphisms as markers, together with methods of linkage analysis, is proving to be a powerful method to identify the genes responsible for a variety of human disorders and traits. The technical capabilities of molecular geneticists provide for unique opportunities in medicine and pharmaceutic development.

The Human Genome Project is rapidly generating vast amounts of information concerning the location, but not necessarily the function, of specific genes. Robotic advances have occurred so quickly that mapping of the human genome can now be expected to be completed within a few years. Indeed, the technologic successes of these endeavors have far exceeded the expectations of only a few years ago. As of 1996, a detailed map of the human genome exists in the public domain. A complete map of the normal human genome is certain to enter the public domain within the next few years.

MELAS Syndrome

The era of the molecular genetic analysis of migraine began with the publication in 1990 of data that genetically linked a specific mutation in mitochondrial DNA with a rare clinical syndrome, designated the MELAS syndrome that can include migraine. The MELAS syndrome consists of a mitochondrial encephalomyopathy, lactic acidosis, and stroke-like episodes and is caused by an A-to-G point mutation in the mitochondrial gene encoding for tRNA[Leu(UUR)] at nucleotide position 3243.[11] Episodic migraine-like headaches are another common clinical feature of the syndrome, especially early in the course of the disease. The genetic pattern of mitochondrial disorders is unique because only mothers transmit mitochondrial DNA. Thus, all children of mothers with MELAS are affected with the disorder.

Other Mitochondrial Mutations and Migraine

At the International Headache Society meeting in 1995, another mitochondrial mutation potentially related to migraine was described. It was reported that 13 of 53 (26%) migraine patients in Japan displayed an A-to-G point mutation in the coding region for the ND4 subunit of the respiratory complex I, which is a mitochondrial protein.[12] This variant leads to a threonine-to-alanine amino acid replacement in the protein. This molecule is believed to be involved in mitochondrial oxidative phosphorylation. The possible significance of this observation cannot be determined until the allelic variant is evaluated in other laboratories.

Familial Hemiplegic Migraine

Data were published in 1993 that genetically linked a region of DNA on human chromosome 19 to the clinical diagnosis of familial hemiplegic migraine (FHM).[13]

That syndrome is characterized by recurring episodes of hemiparesis or hemiplegia during the aura phase of a migraine headache. Other associated symptoms may include hemianesthesia or paresthesia, hemianopic visual field disturbances, dysphasia, and variable degrees of drowsiness, confusion, or coma. In severe attacks, the symptoms can persist for days or weeks, but characteristically they last for only 30–60 minutes and are followed by a unilateral throbbing headache.

Joutel and colleagues[13] analyzed two large French pedigrees in which multiple members had FHM. A region of chromosome 19 was selected for genetic analysis because the same investigators had localized a gene for cerebral autosomal dominant arteriopathy with subcortical infarcts and leukoencephalopathy (designated CADASIL) to this chromosomal region. The investigators found that FHM was also statistically linked to the same region of chromosome 19. That is, a specific region of chromosome 19 was transmitted from individual to individual in a dominant pattern that coincided with a clinical diagnosis of hemiplegic migraine. The investigators were able to further localize the critical area to a 30 cM (i.e., a specific length of DNA) region of the genome. One of the two initial families also displayed concurrent nystagmus (in 16 of 20 FHM subjects) whereas no nystagmus or cerebellar findings were observed in the second linked family. The same investigators have also reported on seven additional families with FHM.[14] Strong evidence of linkage to chromosome 19 was found in only two of the seven families, one of which also had comorbid cerebellar dysfunction.

The linkage of FHM to chromosome 19 in families has been confirmed by other investigator groups. For example, in a study of five FHM families, three families reportedly were linked to chromosome 19.[15] However, in each of those three families, nonpenetrant individuals, individuals diagnosed with FHM who did not link, or both were reported. These unexpected clinical findings indicate either that the families' condition may not be linked to this specific region of chromosome 19 or that the clinical diagnoses were incorrect. A definitive evaluation of these data must await the identification of the FHM gene.

A family with FHM from the United States has also been reported to have a link to chromosome 19.[16] As shown in Figure 7.1, a chromosome 19 marker designated D19S394 cosegregates with the clinical diagnosis of FHM. Family members who carry allele 236 all suffer from FHM. Those family members who lack this specific marker do not have FHM. The affected family members also displayed significant cerebellar atrophy and marked nystagmus. The authors hypothesized that FHM may result from a neurodegeneration of brain stem structures involved in the autonomic regulation of cerebral blood flow. Interestingly, many structures in the cerebellum influence cerebral blood flow. The cerebellar vermis projects by way of the fastigial nucleus to cortical and brain stem regions, and prominent atrophy of this region is present in members of the pedigree. Research in animal models has demonstrated that the fastigial nucleus is involved in the regulation of regional cerebral blood flow. It is conceivable that cerebellar vermian atrophy alters the normal physiologic regulation of cerebral blood flow mediated by the fastigial nucleus, resulting in regional hypoperfusion and focal neurologic deficits as seen during the migraine aura. Further studies seem warranted to investigate the contribution of cerebellar structures to the pathogenesis of FHM.

In summary, the localization of a gene for FHM has now been reported by three independent groups. Interestingly, each group identified families with FHM and concurrent cerebellar findings. All four families with cerebellar dysfunction were

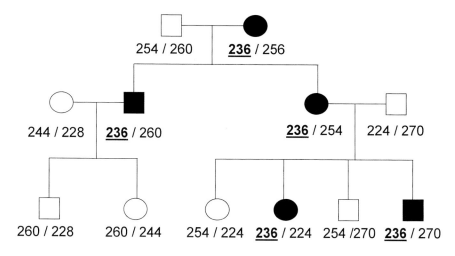

Figure 7.1   Linkage analysis of chromosomal marker D19S394 with the clinical diagnosis of familial hemiplegic migraine. (White square = male [unaffected]; white circle = female [unaffected]; black square = male [affected]; black circle = female [affected]).

found to link to chromosome 19. By contrast, 11 additional families without cerebellar dysfunction have been analyzed with a presumptive diagnosis of FHM. Only four of those 11 families (36%) show evidence of possible linkage to chromosome 19. It is possible that only FHM with concurrent cerebellar atrophy is linked to chromosome 19. The other linked FHM families may represent random statistical occurrences. Alternatively, all eight linked families may result from a genetic variant on chromosome 19, but the families with cerebellar findings may have a different genetic mutation than those families without cerebellar findings. Determination of the clinical variability resulting from molecular variations within the chromosome 19 locus must await the identification of the precise gene within this region of DNA that is responsible for the clinical expression of hemiplegic migraine.

Migraine with and Without Aura

A molecular genetic approach is being applied to the analysis of other types of vascular headache. For example, as shown in Table 7.2, it might be expected that cluster headache, migraine with aura, and migraine without aura will all prove to be genetically distinct from the gene defect underlying FHM. Alternatively, these other forms of vascular headache may be the result of different genetic defects in the same gene located on chromosome 19.

Association studies are another method of genetic analysis. Rather than analyzing family units in order to find stretches of DNA shared by all members with a given phenotype, association studies analyze the frequency with which certain

Table 7.2   Status of migraine genetics (as of late 1995)

Headache type	Prevalence (%)	Chromosome	Gene
MELAS syndrome	<0.0001	Mitochondria	tRNA[Leu(UUR)]
Familial hemiplegic migraine	<0.0001	19	?
Cluster headache	0.4	?	?
Migraine with aura	3.0	?	?
Migraine without aura	15.0	?	?

genetic markers occur in affected individuals versus control populations. For example, in a study of 112 unrelated migraine patients and a "healthy volunteer" control group, 11 genetic markers were analyzed.[17] Two of the markers were found to be present more frequently in the migraine group. An esterase D marker (designated 2-2), located near the $5-HT_{2A}$ receptor on chromosome 13, was present in 10% of the migraine subjects and 1.5% of the control group ($P < 0.0001$). A group-specific component marker (designated 1F-1F), located on chromosome 4, was present in 8.3% of the migraine subjects and 0.83% of the control group ($P < 0.0001$). The significance of these findings is somewhat difficult to assess because the source and characteristics of the control group were not well described in the publication.

However, a recent independent study did not confirm the positive association data in the $5-HT_{2A}$ receptor region. Specifically, the chromosomal DNA region overlapping the $5-HT_{2A}$ receptor (chromosome 13q13–q22) was analyzed for linkage to migraine.[18] A small subset of migrainous families did show slight statistical evidence for linkage, but there was no overall statistical evidence for linkage. In the same study, the $5-HT_{2C}$ receptor locus on chromosome Xq23–25 was also analyzed by linkage analysis,[18] but no statistical evidence for linkage was observed. In addition, the coding regions of the $5-HT_{2A}$ and $5-HT_{2C}$ receptor genes were also analyzed in migraine patients and unaffected controls using polymerase chain reaction and direct sequencing. No mutations were found in the deduced amino acid sequence of either receptor in the sample of migraineurs tested. These results indicate that mutations in the $5-HT_{2A}$ and $5-HT_{2C}$ receptors are not generally involved in the pathogenesis of migraine.[18]

FUTURE DIRECTIONS

As the genetic analysis of migraine proceeds in many laboratories around the world, it can be expected that Table 7.2 will be completed within the next few years. At that time, clinicians will have available a variety of DNA-based diagnostic tests that can accurately assess the status of the patient. Such tests could lead to a highly accurate prediction of drug dosage and responsivity for each individual genetic alteration. The ultimate hope, and one that is quite reasonable, is that knowledge of the molecular genetic basis of migraine will lead to more effective and safer medications than exist today.

DNA-Based Diagnostic Tests

Unlike many medical illnesses, migraine cannot currently be diagnosed by objective criteria. As a consequence, diagnoses are based solely on the clinical skills of the individual doctor. With headache, diagnosis is difficult and time-consuming; misdiagnosis occurs frequently among those who are not migraine experts. Such diagnostic errors can result in either the initiation of inappropriate therapy or the failure to appropriately treat the disorder.

Once the genes involved in migraine are identified, the information will be used to develop diagnostic, therapeutic, and gene therapy applications. Immediately upon identification of the pathologic gene, a DNA-based diagnostic test will become available to clinical researchers. Widely available commercial DNA-based diagnostic tests based on genetic information can be expected within 1 or 2 years following discovery of the gene.

DNA-Based Metabolic Monitoring Systems

The ability to diagnose *and* monitor migraine by providing an objective analysis of the genetic status of a patient will revolutionize clinical practice. The ability to objectively monitor the metabolic variation in migraine and related disorders will have a dramatic impact on the management of these conditions. This ability will render migraine management far more objective, much as blood pressure monitoring and serum glucose measurements have objectified the management of hypertension and diabetes. The value of the metabolic monitoring systems will be enhanced by their direct linkage to disease management recommendations.

Novel Pharmacologic and Gene Therapy Approaches

Knowledge of the genes involved in migraine is likely to lead to the development of novel therapeutic approaches to the disorder. The use of these new medications will be analogous to the current use of antibiotics. That is, patients will first be evaluated using a DNA-based test to determine their sensitivity to a range of medications. The specific medication and dosage will then be selected for use in an individual patient. Such an approach might be expected to result in 95–100% response rates rather than the approximately 70% efficacy rates achieved today.

In the twenty-first century, gene therapy may be an option for patients with severe and chronic migraine. However, gene therapies are still at least 5–10 years away as a practical solution to genetic problems. Nonetheless, identification of pathologic genes affecting migraine will provide incentive to develop this potentially curative treatment approach.

SUMMARY

As the genetic analysis of migraine proceeds, it can be expected that multiple genes for migraine will be identified within the next decade, allowing Table 7.2

to be completed. Then clinicians will have available a variety of accurate DNA-based diagnostic tests, which should lead to a highly accurate prediction of drug responsivity for each individual genetic alteration. Although it is clear that many drugs are highly successful in treating some patients with migraine, each fails to provide any relief for other patients with the same disorder. Because it appears that migraine can result from more than one genetic defect, it is reasonable to assume that the difference in response to drugs is, at least in part, dependent on the particular genotype of the patient. We can reasonably hope that knowledge of the molecular genetic basis of migraine will lead to more accurate diagnoses and to more effective and safer treatments.

Acknowledgments

I thank Tiffany A. Howell and Susan Price, MD, for their review of this manuscript.

REFERENCES

1. Allan W. Inheritance of migraine. Arch Intern Med 1928;42:590.
2. Liveing E. Megrim, Sick Headaches, and Allied Disorders. London: Churchill, 1873.
3. Russell MB, Hilden J, Sorensen SA, Olesen J. Familial occurrence of migraine without aura and migraine with aura. Neurology 1993;43:1369.
4. Sjaastad O, Stovner LJ. The IHS classification for common migraine: Is it ideal? Headache 1993;33:372.
5. Peroutka SJ, Howell TA. The Genetic Analysis of Migraine: Clinical Database Requirements. In F Rose (ed), Towards Migraine 2000. New York: Elsevier, 1996;35.
6. Devoto M, Lozito A, Staffa G, D'Alessandro R, et al. Segregation analysis of migraine in 128 families. Cephalalgia 1986;6:101.
7. Bille B. Migraine in school children. Acta Paediatr Scand 1962;51(Suppl 136):1.
8. Goodell H, Lewontin R, Wolff HG. Familial occurrence of migraine headache. Arch Neurol Psychiatry 1954;72:325.
9. Dalsgaard-Nielsen T. Migraine and heredity. Acta Neurol Scand 1965;41:287.
10. D'Amico D, Leone M, Macciardi F, et al. Genetic transmission of migraine without aura: A study of 68 families. Ital J Neurol Sci 1991;12:581.
11. Goto Y, Nonaka I, Horai S. A mutation in the tRNA[Leu(UUR)] gene associated with the MELAS subgroup of mitochondrial encephalomyopathies. Nature 1990;348:651.
12. Shimomura T, Kitano A, Marukawa H, Takahashi K. Mutation in platelet mitochondrial gene in patients with migraine. Cephalalgia 1995;15(Suppl 14):10.
13. Joutel A, Bousser M, Biousse V, et al. A gene for familial hemiplegic migraine maps to chromosome 19. Nat Genet 1993;5:40.
14. Joutel A, Ducros A, Vahedi K, et al. Genetic heterogeneity of familial hemiplegic migraine. Am J Hum Genet 1994;55:1166.
15. Ophoff RA, Van Eijk R, Sandkuul LA, et al. Genetic heterogeneity of familial hemiplegic migraine. Genomics 1994;22:21.
16. Elliott MA, Peroutka SJ, Welch S, May EF. Familial hemiplegic migraine, nystagmus, and cerebellar atrophy: Clinical description and chromosomal localization. Ann Neurol 1996;39:100.
17. Pardo J, Carredo A, Munoz I, et al. Genetic markers: Association study in migraine. Cephalalgia 1995;15:200.
18. Buchwalder A, Welch SK, Peroutka SJ. Exclusion of 5-HT$_{2A}$ and 5-HT$_{2C}$ receptor genes as candidate genes for migraine. Headache 1996;36:254.

III
CLINICAL ISSUES AFFECTING THE INDIVIDUAL

8
Drug Treatment of Migraine Attacks

Michel D. Ferrari and Joost Haan

GENERAL INTRODUCTION AND METHODOLOGIC ASPECTS

Migraine Attack

From the clinical practice point of view, migraine attacks may consist of four distinct phases: (1) the prodromal phase with premonitory symptoms, (2) the aura phase with transient neurologic signs and symptoms, (3) the headache phase with headache and associated symptoms including nausea, vomiting, and photophobia and phonophobia, and (4) the recovery phase, often associated with resting and sleeping.[1] It is important to recognize that only the headache phase symptoms can be treated. There is no treatment for the aura symptoms as they occur. For practical reasons it is even recommended to delay administration of antimigraine drugs until after the aura has stopped and the headache has begun, as discussed later in this chapter.

Evidence-Based Medicine

Medication for the treatment of acute migraine attacks can be divided into specific and nonspecific antimigraine drugs (Table 8.1). In both categories, there is a striking lack of international consensus with respect to drug preferences, doses, routes of administration, formulations, and combinations with other compounds such as caffeine and barbiturates. Although due in part to nationally and culturally dependent variables, this lack of consensus is largely the result of the limited number of well-designed, controlled clinical trials[2] that have been conducted with most drugs used in migraine. For the simple analgesics and nonsteroidal anti-inflammatory drugs (NSAIDs), only a few state-of-the-art clinical trials are available, and for the ergot alkaloids there has been no such trial at all. In fact, only for the latest antimigraine compound, sumatriptan, are there both scientific support for claims of its efficacy and recommendations on how to use it.

Table 8.1   Names, recommended doses per attack and per 24 hours, and formulations of acute antimigraine drugs with established or historically assumed efficacy against acute migraine

Drug	Recommended doses (mg)*	Doses per 24 hours/ formulations
Nonspecific compounds		
Simple analgesics		
Acetaminophen	500	2–6 tablets/suppositories
Nonsteroidal anti-inflammatory drugs		
Acetylsalicylic acid	500	2–6 tablets/suppositories
Naproxen	500	1–2 tablets/suppositories
Tolfenamic acid	200	1–2 tablets
Diclofenac	50–100	1–2 tablets/suppositories
Ibuprofen	600	1–2 tablets
Ketoprofen	100	1–2 suppositories
Prokinetic and antiemetic compounds		
Metoclopramide	20	1 suppository 30 minutes prior to analgesic
Domperidone	60	1 suppository 30 minutes prior to analgesic
Specific antimigraine drugs		
Sumatriptan	25–50–100	1–3 tablets; maximum 300 mg/ 24 hours
Sumatriptan	6	1–2 SC injections; maximum 12 mg/24 hours
Ergotamine	1–2	1–2 tablets/suppositories
Ergotamine	0.25–0.50	1–2 SC/IM injections
Dihydroergotamine	1	1–2 SC/IM/IV injections (preceded by 5 mg IV prochlorperazine)
Dihydroergotamine	0.5	2–4 intranasal puffs

*Except for sumatriptan, the recommended doses are approximations since no international consensus exists.

For this chapter, we have chosen to include only drugs for which there is some published evidence for efficacy. The ergot alkaloids, however, are included only for historical reasons and because of the vast clinical experience with them. Drug names, recommended dosages, and formulations are listed in Table 8.1. We have omitted quite a few drugs for which antimigraine efficacy has been claimed but not proven (for a review of those drugs, see Welch[3]).

Long-Term Consistency and Relative Values of Antimigraine Drugs

Although migraine is a chronic paroxysmal disorder, few data are available on the within-patient long-term consistency of the effects of drugs for treatment of acute migraine. Most clinical trials have tested compounds in only one attack per patient and some in up to three attacks. Only for sumatriptan have long-term efficacy and tolerability been studied.[4–8]

Similarly, little information is available on the relative value of the various drugs, mainly because of the paucity of comparator trials. Simply comparing absolute response rates of different drugs from different trials is misleading; trials differ widely with respect to study design, study population, and outcome measures. In the absence of sufficient comparative trials, the relative efficacy of different drugs can be tentatively estimated by comparing between trials the variation in response rates between the active compound and placebo.

Headache Recurrence

Though poorly recognized before the clinical trial program of sumatriptan, it is now well accepted that headache recurrence (i.e., return of the headache and associated symptoms within 24–48 hours after initial improvement following treatment) is a prominent feature of all antimigraine drugs used to treat attacks.[9] For the other compounds, formal clinical trial data on headache recurrence are lacking. Clinical experience, however, suggests differences between drugs with respect to time to recurrence, proportion of patients with recurrence, and response of the recurring headache to a repeated dose.

When assessing the efficacy of antimigraine drugs in treating attacks, it is important to distinguish between the *initial* amelioration of the headache symptoms within the first few hours after drug administration and the *duration* of the improvement. Physicians should warn patients of the risk of headache recurrence and advise them to take a repeated dose if the headache recurs.

Outcome Measures

Numerous parameters have been used for assessing the efficacy of antimigraine drugs. Since the introduction of sumatriptan, the most common, most robust, and clinically most relevant primary efficacy measure has come to be the proportion of patients with improvement of the headache from moderate or severe to mild or no pain within 2 or 4 hours (responders).[2,10] The proportion of responders with headache recurrence should be mentioned separately. New composite outcome measures, including initial response, recurrence rate, and use of additional (non-study) medication are also being developed. When reading results of clinical trials, it is important to be aware of which outcome measure has been used to avoid comparing apples and pears. Outcome measures such as average attack duration, average reduction in pain score, etc. are much less informative and often misleading.

Parenteral Drug Administration

During migraine attacks, oral drug resorption is usually impaired because of vomiting or gastrointestinal stasis and dilatation, even in patients who are not nauseated.[11,12] Parenteral drug administration is, therefore, usually preferred. The administration of a prokinetic and antiemetic drug 30 minutes prior to analgesic improves the oral resorption of simple analgesics and may combat the nausea (see Table 8.1). However, it is uncertain whether the procedure also results in improved clinical efficacy.

Choice of Drug and Dose

The choice of drug or drugs, dose, and route of administration depends on the characteristics, severity, variability, and frequency of the migraine attacks as well as on the specific preferences and contraindications of the patient. Not all attacks in a given patient are necessarily treated with the same drug or dose. Mild and moderate attacks may be treated with oral or parenteral analgesics or NSAIDs. Severe attacks usually respond better to parenteral sumatriptan or ergot alkaloids. Previous experience with a drug is important, but the opinion of a patient may be biased because of previous use of suboptimal doses. The appropriate drug and dose should be selected and titrated in a stepwise fashion, starting with the lowest likely effective dose and escalating the dose or changing the drug after treatment of two or three attacks, if necessary. The maximal tolerated and effective amount should then be taken in one dose, rather than using repeated smaller doses.[11]

SIMPLE ANALGESICS AND ACETYLSALICYLIC ACID

Many patients with mild or moderate attacks can manage their migraine headaches with paracetamol (acetaminophen) or aspirin (acetylsalicylic acid). Adverse events (AEs) are usually limited to mild dyspepsia or gastrointestinal hemorrhages (or both) for aspirin. Despite its slightly higher risk of causing (usually mild) side effects, the clinical impression is that aspirin, notably in an effervescent or parenteral form, is more effective in migraine than is paracetamol.

Both paracetamol and aspirin are often included in over-the-counter preparations, frequently in combination with caffeine, codeine, or both. Such combination preparations should generally be avoided. First, there is no evidence that the combination provides greater efficacy in treating migraine than the analgesic alone. Second, it is becoming more and more evident that too frequent use of such substances—especially caffeine, whether in over-the-counter preparations or in coffee—may increase the risk of so-called drug-dependent headache (discussed later in this chapter and in Chapter 12). Too frequent use of codeine may cause constipation, not to mention addiction.

Chronic use of analgesics (more frequent than 2 or 3 days per week), especially in combination preparations with caffeine, carries the risk of inducing analgesic-dependent headache (see Chapter 12). Such patients should be advised to abruptly stop using these compounds.[13] To prevent the syndrome, patients should be discouraged from regularly using analgesics more often than 2 or 3 days weekly.

ANTIEMETICS AND PROKINETIC DRUGS

Metoclopramide or domperidone, administered 30 minutes prior to the analgesic, improves the oral resorption of paracetamol and aspirin and may ameliorate the gastrointestinal manifestations of migraine (for review, see Tfelt-Hansen and Stewart Johnson[12]). However, despite improved resorption, there is no evidence that the administration of antiemetics results in improved antimigraine efficacy of the analgesics. Metoclopramide may cause acute dystonia in adolescents and especially in children. Domperidone may be used instead in this age group, because it does not easily cross the blood–brain barrier.

A recent study showed that MLAA, a combination of oral metoclopramide (10 mg) and lysine acetylsalicylic acid (1,620 mg, containing 900 mg of acetylsalicylic acid), was more effective than placebo and as effective as 100 mg of oral sumatriptan in treating the first study attack in a clinical trial.[14] In the second study attack, however, the efficacy of MLAA appeared to be much less, whereas the efficacy of sumatriptan was not reduced. Further trials should assess the long-term consistency of the antimigraine effect of MLAA.

NONSTEROIDAL ANTI-INFLAMMATORY DRUGS

The NSAIDs with established efficacy in migraine, along with the recommended doses, are listed in Table 8.1, in tentative order of choice (see Tfelt-Hansen and Stewart Johnson for review[15]). There are no convincing clinical studies to determine the relative efficacy of the listed NSAIDs and paracetamol and aspirin. The clinical impression is that NSAIDs, notably those that can be administered parenterally, are more efficacious than paracetamol and aspirin. The risk and severity of adverse events after NSAIDs, notably gastrointestinal symptoms and rectal burning (with suppositories), are also greater, however, making them drugs of second choice.

SUMATRIPTAN

Sumatriptan has been registered for migraine only since 1991, but it is already the most extensively investigated pharmacologic treatment for acute migraine. Worldwide, the drug is being used by millions of people. Accordingly, a wealth of both clinical trial and clinical practice data are available. At present a 6-mg subcutaneous formulation, using a subcutaneous autoinjector, and 25-, 50-, and 100-mg oral tablets are available. Beginning in 1997, intranasal and rectal formulations are expected to be on the market, for which preliminary data suggest response rates between those of the oral and subcutaneous formulations.

Pharmacology

Sumatriptan is a selective serotonin$_1$ (5-hydroxytryptamine$_1$; 5-HT$_1$) receptor agonist, with greatest affinity for 5-HT$_{1D}$ and 5-HT$_{1F}$ receptors. The drug crosses the blood–brain barrier poorly (for review of pharmacology, see Chapter 2 and references 9, 16–18). The antimigraine effect is believed to be mediated via one or more of the following mechanisms: (1) vasoconstriction of cerebral or meningeal and dural arteries; (2) peripheral neuronal inhibition, which blocks depolarization of sensory afferents of the trigeminal nerve, innervating the meninges and dura mater and blocking release of vasoactive neuropeptides within the dura mater; and (3) central neuronal inhibition within the trigeminal nuclei in the brain stem[9,16,18–24] (see also Chapters 1 and 2). Although sumatriptan constricts large cerebral arteries, including the middle cerebral and carotid arteries,[19,21] the drug does not affect regional cerebral blood flow (rCBF),[21,25,26] because the small vessels controlling the rCBF are not compromised.[22] However, in the acute phase of stroke, sumatriptan may affect rCBF and is therefore strictly contraindicated.

Pharmacokinetics

Following oral administration, the absorption of sumatriptan is limited and slow. The bioavailability is only 14%. Therapeutic plasma levels are reached after 30–60 minutes. Following subcutaneous administration, therapeutic plasma levels are reached after 10 minutes and the bioavailability is nearly 100%. For both formulations, plasma half-life is relatively short (approximately 2 hours).[16,18] Receptor binding is reversible. As a consequence, the biological effects of sumatriptan may last a relatively short time.

Clinical Use

Sumatriptan should be given only during the headache phase of migraine attacks. In attacks of migraine with aura, administration of sumatriptan must be delayed until the aura symptoms have disappeared and the headache phase has begun.[27] The reasons for this are threefold: (1) Sumatriptan has no ameliorating effect on the aura symptoms[27]; (2) when taken during the aura, although safe, sumatriptan appears to be less effective against the subsequent headache compared with when it is not given until during the headache phase[27]; and (3) aura may not always be followed by headache, so drug administration during the aura phase may be redundant and may contribute to the risk of drug-dependent headache.

To treat the attack, one dose of either oral (25-, 50-, or 100-mg tablets) or subcutaneous (6 mg per subcutaneous autoinjector) sumatriptan should be taken.[28] If the migraine symptoms do not improve following a first maximal dose of either 100 mg (orally) or 6 mg (subcutaneously), it is not useful to administer a second dose.[29] If, however, the headache and associated symptoms recur after initial improvement, a repeated dose can be taken and is usually effective.[30] Maximum recommended doses per 24 hours are 100 mg orally, 3 times, and 6 mg subcutaneously, twice.[28] Sumatriptan should not be administered too early.[6] It is probably wise for migraine patients to restrict their use of the drug to no more than 2 days per week, to reduce the risk of sumatriptan-dependent headache (discussed in the section on adverse events). However, for patients with cluster headache this precaution is probably not necessary.

Clinical Efficacy

Following oral administration, approximately 55% of patients experience significant clinical improvement within 2 hours, and up to 70% within 4 hours.

Following subcutaneous administration, the response rate is about 80% within 1 hour and 86% within 2 hours.[16,18,20] Thus, if patients do not respond to oral sumatriptan, there is still a considerable chance that subsequent attacks will respond to the subcutaneous formulation.

Headache Recurrence

In up to 40% of patients, the duration of sumatriptan's antimigraine action is too short, and the headache may return after a median time of 10 (subcutaneous) to 17 (oral) hours.[6,16,18,20,28] Repeated drug administration is usually effective to treat the recurring migraine headache, although the headache may recur yet again.[6] It should be noted that although it has been most thoroughly studied with sumatriptan, headache recurrence is a significant limitation of all drugs for acute migraine. The underlying mechanism of headache recurrence is unknown but may be related to the short plasma half-life and reversible receptor binding of the drugs. Patients whose attacks last longer than 1 day appear to be at greater risk of headache recurrence.[31]

Adverse Events

AEs following sumatriptan are rather frequent and quite marked.[6,16,18,20,28] In the vast majority of patients, however, the intensity of the AEs is mild, their nature insignificant, and their duration short (usually > 10–15 minutes). Onset is usually shortly after drug administration. The most frequent AEs include tingling, paresthesias, and warm and hot sensations in the head, neck, chest, and extremities. Less frequent AEs are dizziness, flushing, and neck pain or stiffness.

Of more relevance are the so-called chest symptoms, reported by up to 40% of patients who are specifically asked about them.[6] The chest symptoms consist mainly of a short-lived heaviness or pressure in the arms and chest, shortness of breath, anxiety, and palpitations. Rarely, patients report true chest pain. When patients are forewarned, these symptoms generally do not cause significant problems. However, they can sometimes closely mimic pectoral angina and thus may give rise to alarm, especially if patients have not been forewarned. In a small number of subjects, all with preexisting cardiovascular disease, use of sumatriptan was associated with myocardial ischemia or ventricular fibrillation.[18,20,32,33] Because sumatriptan may cause vasoconstriction of the peripheral and coronary arteries (usually short-lived and mild),[34,35] the drug is strictly contraindicated in subjects with cardiovascular disease.

The underlying mechanism of the chest symptoms produced by sumatriptan is unknown. Coronary vasoconstriction cannot be excluded in some patients, but seems an unlikely mechanism in the vast majority.[31] Other, less dangerous mechanisms, such as esophageal spasm,[36] pulmonary vasoconstriction, intercostal muscle spasm, or bronchospasm, seem more likely.[31–33]

The risk and severity of AEs is greater following subcutaneous compared with oral sumatriptan. Furthermore, whereas the subcutaneous dose is fixed at 6 mg, the oral dose can be adjusted to increase tolerability while maintaining efficacy. Patient acceptance of the adverse events is improved when they are preadvised about the risk and nature of the events.

Some patients have been reported to experience "sumatriptan-dependent headaches" while using sumatriptan on a daily basis, all of whom were previously abusing ergotamine or analgesics.[6] It is still too early to evaluate the true risk of misuse of sumatriptan. The clinical impression is that the risk is smaller than exists with ergotamine (discussed in the following section) but certainly not absent. Patients with a history of analgesic or ergotamine misuse seem at greater risk and should be strongly advised to restrict their use of sumatriptan to no more than 2 days per week.

Long-Term Consistency Within Patients

In the majority of patients, efficacy, headache recurrence, and chest symptoms are consistent over time and over multiple attacks. Within-patient consistency is greater with the subcutaneous formulation.[6] Thus, patients either always or hardly ever respond to sumatriptan, and they experience headache recurrence or chest symptoms either in every attack or very rarely.

Costs

Sumatriptan is a relatively expensive drug, especially when compared with the other antimigraine medications. So far there is little scientific pharmacoeconomic data to substantiate and support its price. On the other hand, even though formal comparator trials with other drugs are still insufficient, the clinical impression is that (especially subcutaneous) sumatriptan is the most effective antimigraine drug available. Many patients are extremely content with the drug because it is either the only effective medication or the most effective medication for their migraines.

Conclusions

Subcutaneous sumatriptan is, with little doubt, the most effective but also most expensive antimigraine drug available. Its principal advantage over other medications is the rapid, complete, and consistent relief of the headache and associated migraine symptoms experienced by the majority of patients. Major limitations, apart from the costs, include the invasive nature of administration; the high risk of headache recurrence, which makes repeated dosing often necessary as is the case with other drugs; and the occurrence of usually insignificant but sometimes frightening chest symptoms. For oral sumatriptan the pros and cons, in relation to other antimigraine medication, are lesser in extent.

ERGOT ALKALOIDS

For decades, ergotamine tartrate and (more recently) dihydroergotamine (DHE) were the only drugs available specifically for migraine. Despite this long history, few if any state-of-the-art controlled clinical trials have been conducted.[3,37-44] Placebo-controlled trials are lacking or of limited value. Most of our so-called knowledge is based on oral accounts of uncontrolled clinical practice experiences and a number of sometimes biased review papers summarizing the results of largely uncontrolled studies. As a consequence, there is a surprising lack of hard data on ergot alkaloids, a situation that contributes to striking differences between countries with respect to recommended doses, number of doses per attack, per day, and per week, routes of administration, formulations, and combinations with other compounds such as caffeine and barbiturates. The present recommendations, therefore, represent a compromise, taking into account all the mentioned limitations.

Pharmacology

The pharmacologic effects of the ergots are complex and various.[24,38,42-44] In part, this is due to their high affinity for a wide range of receptors, including 5-HT$_{1A}$, 5-HT$_{1D}$, 5-HT$_2$, and dopamine D$_2$ as well as alpha- and beta-adrenoceptors. In contrast to sumatriptan, the receptor binding of ergots is virtually irreversible. Their mechanisms of antimigraine action are probably similar to those of sumatriptan.

Pharmacokinetics

The bioavailability of ergots following oral or rectal administration is very poor (< 3%) and thus highly variable, both between and within subjects.[38,42-44] Consequently, there is no standard recommended dose. The dose should be individualized.[43] Plasma half-life is approximately 2 hours, but as a result of the irreversible receptor binding, the biological half-life (e.g., as measured with duration of vasoconstrictor action on peripheral vessels) may be considerably longer (>10 hours).[42,43] This difference may well explain why headache recurrence after ergots tends to be less frequent and to follow a longer latency compared with that following sumatriptan.[20,45]

Clinical Use

Major problems with the ergot alkaloids are the interindividual and intraindividual variability in pharmacokinetics and clinical responses and the lack of controlled clinical data. Dose recommendations, even in respectable standard textbooks, are thus not based on evidence. The most sensible approach is to start with the lowest recommended dose and have the patient try it for two or three attacks.[43] Depending on efficacy and side effects, the dose may be increased for each subsequent two or three attacks until an acceptable response is obtained. Ergots should be administered in one selected dose at the onset of the attack,[43] not divided into several portions, as unfortunately is often recommended. Ergots should preferably not be used more often than 1 day per week to prevent ergot-dependent headache (discussed below in a separate section).

Clinical Efficacy

The response rate of oral ergotamine seems to be in the same range as that of NSAIDs[3,15,37–39,41–43] and about 10% less compared with oral sumatriptan.[45] The response rate of rectal ergotamine may be slightly higher and less variable.[3,15,37–39,41–43] Intranasal administration, especially of DHE, has been purported to be quite effective,[39–41,44,46] but the published clinical trial data are so far unconvincing.[40,47,48] Based on the clinical impression from uncontrolled data and on "expert opinions" found in review papers, the response rate after intravenous, intramuscular, or subcutaneous administration of ergotamine, and notably DHE, may be substantial,[39–41,43,44] though it is probably still lower than with subcutaneous sumatriptan. Recently, however, a state-of-the-art study comparing subcutaneous DHE and subcutaneous sumatriptan, suggested similar efficacy for both compounds.[49] Sumatriptan, however, worked significantly faster but was associated with a higher proportion of headache recurrence. Pain relief rates were, at 1 hour, 57% (DHE) and 78% (sumatriptan, $P \leq 0.001$); at 2 hours, 73% (DHE) and 85% (sumatriptan, $P = 0.002$); and at 3 hours, 86% (DHE) and 90% (sumatriptan, P = not significant). Headache recurrence within 24 hours occurred in 18% of DHE-treated patients. Because far more patients in the DHE-treated group, compared with the sumatriptan-treated group, had a second injection because of initial inadequate response, it is not clear whether this difference is due to longer action of DHE or to the repeated dosage schema. Nausea and vomiting occurred more frequently after DHE, but chest symptoms were more frequent after sumatriptan.

Headache Recurrence

Except from one study,[45] no clinical trial data are available on the frequency and timing of headache recurrence after ergot alkaloids. The impression from clinical practice is that the frequency is marginally less and the latent time to recurrence some hours longer compared with sumatriptan.

Adverse Events

Side effects of ergots are frequent and various. They are often serious and may last several hours.[38–43,50] On incidental use, patients may complain of nausea and vomiting (the most common side effect, due to stimulation of dopamine D_2 receptors within the area postrema in the brain stem), diarrhea (possibly due to stimulation of dopamine D_2 receptors within the gut), muscle cramps, malaise, and potent vasoconstriction of peripheral blood vessels (due to stimulation of vascular adrenoceptor and 5-HT$_2$ receptors), causing cold and tingling fingers and toes.

Compared with sumatriptan, ergots have a much greater potency in contracting systemic, coronary, and cerebral arteries,[51] which precludes their use in patients with cardiovascular and cerebrovascular disease. A considerable number of case reports on myocardial and cerebral infarction in association with short-term or chronic (over)use of ergots, sometimes in patients without prior cardiovascular or cerebrovascular disease, have been published over the years.[39,41–43,50,52]

Ergotism is a rare, but life-threatening, complication of acute overdose or chronic overuse (usually more than 10 mg weekly) of ergotamine, associated with severe generalized vasospasm. Symptoms are acral cyanosis, necrosis of digits and extremities, intermittent claudication, and infarcts of various organs.[39,41–43,50,53–55] Vigorous treatment with direct-acting vasodilators (e.g., intravenous nitroglycerine) is then indicated.

Ergot-Dependent Headache

Ergot-dependent headache is a frequent complication of chronic recurrent use of ergots, characterized by (initially slowly) progressive increase over years of both migraine attack frequency and use of ergots.[39,42,43,50,53–55] Ultimately, patients suffer from daily migraine or migraine-like attacks, requiring daily use of ergots, which are often taken preventively before the headache begins (see also Chapter 12). This vicious circle can be stopped only by radical and abrupt withdrawal of the ergots, which initially causes severe withdrawal symptoms including profound headaches, nausea, vomiting, diarrhea, and malaise for 1–2 weeks, but which subsequently results in progressive amelioration and reduction of both the frequency and severity of attacks.[13,53–55] Patients who are using ergots 1 day per week or more, even in small quantities, are at significant risk of ergot-dependent headache. This risk is, in contrast to what has often been stated, independent of the total amount of ergots used.[53,54] Combination of ergots with caffeine seems to increase the risk of dependency.

Conclusions

Little is available in the way of evidence-based data on the clinical effects of ergot alkaloids. Their use in clinical practice is complicated, mainly because of the complex pharmacology and the high variability, both interindividually and intraindividually, of the pharmacokinetic profiles. A major advantage is that the direct costs of using ergot alkaloids are low. Ergots may be useful when the following considerations are taken into account: (1) they are contraindicated in patients with cardiovascular disease, (2) dosage and administration route should be individualized, (3) the rectal route is probably optimal next to the invasive routes, (4) use of ergots on more than 1 day per week should be discouraged, and (5) patients with more than one migraine-like attack per week should be checked for ergot-dependent headache; if it develops, the use of ergots should be stopped.

OPIOIDS

The use of narcotic analgesics in migraine is highly controversial. Again, few if any published controlled data can be consulted. Major disadvantages are the prominent side effects and the profound risk of inducing abuse and dependency.[56] In addition, there is no consensus as to the clinical efficacy of these compounds. Our personal opinion is that opioids are rarely if ever indicated in the treatment of acute migraine. It is our experience that patients who seem to require these compounds usually are having drug-dependent headaches. Once they have ceased to misuse analgesics or ergot alkaloids, such patients rarely require opioids.

FUTURE COMPOUNDS

At least nine different sumatriptan-like selective 5-HT_1–receptor agonists are currently in clinical development, but registration is not expected until 1998 or later. The newer compounds seem to have improved pharmacokinetic profiles after oral administration and claim to have better selectivity for cranial vessels over coronary arteries. Whether these promising properties will also result in clinical superiority and greater tolerability remains to be seen. Some of the new compounds, preclinical data show, at the likely clinical doses, have relative selectivity for neuronal rather than vascular receptors. If they prove to be effective, they could lead to a whole new line of antimigraine drugs devoid of vascular side effects[24] (see also Chapters 1 and 2).

SPECIAL SITUATIONS

The treatment of menstruation- and pregnancy-related attacks is discussed in Chapter 10. There is some suggestion that use of 50 mg of domperidone as soon as premonitory symptoms begin may block the full development of the migraine attack.[57] Practical problems with this approach are that few patients actually recognize premonitory symptoms (not to be confused with aura) and that few data exist on the sensitivity and specificity of these premonitory symptoms for the subsequent full development of the migraine attack. Only those patients in whom premonitory symptoms are virtually always followed by a full-blown migraine attack should be advised to take domperidone at this early stage.

Many physicians are uncertain about whether and how to treat the neurologic aura symptoms of attacks of migraine with aura, basilar migraine, or (familial) hemiplegic migraine. In general, aura symptoms cannot be treated. Only the headache and associated symptoms can be treated. Administration of antimigraine compounds during the aura symptoms is safe, but it seems to be associated with reduced efficacy against the headache phase symptoms and should therefore be avoided.

In childhood, migraine attacks tend to be shorter, and gastrointestinal symptoms may often prevail over the headache. Of the drugs listed in Table 8.1, many can be used in children as well, though of course with body weight–adjusted dosages. Sumatriptan has been formally investigated in only a few adolescents, and results have not been published. There is no relevant experience with sumatriptan in the even younger age group. Although they are sometimes used in the young, it is our opinion that ergots should not be prescribed for children.

REFERENCES

1. Headache Classification Committee of the International Headache Society (J Olesen, et al.). Classification and diagnostic criteria for headache disorders, cranial neuralgias and facial pain. Cephalalgia 1988;8(Suppl 7):1.
2. Tfelt-Hansen P, chairman, International Headache Society Committee on Clinical Trials in Migraine. Guidelines for controlled trials of drugs in migraine (1st ed). Cephalalgia 1991;11:1.
3. Welch KMA. Drug therapy of migraine. N Engl J Med 1993;329:1476.
4. Dahlöf C, Ekbom K, Persson L. Clinical experiences from Sweden on the use of subcutaneously administered sumatriptan in migraine and cluster headache. Arch Neurol 1994;51:1256.
5. Sheftell FD, Weeks RE, Rapoport AM, Siegel S, et al. Subcutaneous sumatriptan in a clinical setting: The first 100 consecutive patients with acute migraine in a tertiary care center. Headache 1994;34:67.
6. Visser WH, de Vriend RHM, Jaspers NMWH, Ferrari MD. Sumatriptan in clinical practice: A two-year review of 453 migraine patients. Neurology 1996;46:1.
7. Tansey MJB, Pilgrim AJ, Martin PM. Long-term experience with sumatriptan in the treatment of migraine. Eur Neurol 1993;33:310.
8. Rederich G, Rapoport A, Cutler N, Hazelrigg R, et al. Oral sumatriptan for the long-term treatment of migraine: Clinical findings. Neurology 1995;45(Suppl 7):S15.
9. Ferrari MD, Saxena PR. 5-HT$_1$ receptors in migraine pathophysiology and treatment. Eur J Neurol 1995;2:5.
10. Pilgrim AJ. Methodology of clinical trials of sumatriptan in migraine and cluster headache. Eur Neurol 1991;31:295.
11. Tfelt-Hansen P, Welch KMA. General Principles of Pharmacological Treatment. In J Olesen, P Tfelt-Hansen, KMA Welch (eds), The Headaches. New York: Raven, 1993;299.
12. Tfelt-Hansen P, Stewart Johnson E. Antiemetic and Prokinetic Drugs. In J Olesen, P Tfelt-Hansen, KMA Welch (eds), The Headaches. New York: Raven, 1993;343.
13. Hering R, Steiner TJ. Abrupt outpatient withdrawal of medication in analgesic-abusing migraineurs. Lancet 1991;337:1442.
14. Tfelt-Hansen P, Henry P, Mulder LJ, et al. The effectiveness of combined oral lysine acetylsalicylate and metoclopramide compared with oral sumatriptan for migraine. Lancet 1995;346:923.
15. Tfelt-Hansen P, Stewart Johnson E. Nonsteroidal Anti-Inflammatory Drugs in the Treatment of the Acute Migraine Attack. In J Olesen, P Tfelt-Hansen, KMA Welch (eds), The Headaches. New York: Raven, 1993;305.
16. Dechant KL, Clissold SP. Sumatriptan: A review of its pharmacokinetic properties, and therapeutic efficacy in the acute treatment of migraine and cluster headache. Drug 1992;43:776.
17. Hoyer D, Clarke DE, Fozard JR, et al. Seventh International Union of Pharmacology classification of receptors for 5-hydroxytryptamine. Pharmacol Rev 1994;46:157.
18. Plosker GL, McTavish D. Sumatriptan: A reappraisal of its pharmacology and therapeutic efficacy in the acute treatment of migraine and cluster headache. Drugs 1994;47:622.
19. Caekebeke JFV, Ferrari MD, Zwetsloot CP, et al. The antimigraine drug sumatriptan increases blood flow velocity in large cerebral arteries during migraine attacks. Neurology 1992;42:1522.
20. Ferrari MD, Saxena PR. Clinical and experimental effects of sumatriptan in humans. Trends Pharmacol Sci 1993;14:129.
21. Friberg L, Olesen J, Iversen HK, Sperling B. Migraine pain associated with middle cerebral artery dilation: Reversal by sumatriptan. Lancet 1991;338:13.
22. Humphrey PPA, Feniuk W. Mode of action of the antimigraine drug sumatriptan. Trends Pharmacol Sci 1991;12:444.
23. Humphrey PPA, Goadsby PJ. The mode of action of sumatriptan is vascular? A debate. Cephalalgia 1994;14:401.
24. Moskowitz MA. Neurogenic versus vascular mechanisms of sumatriptan and ergot alkaloids in migraine. Trends Pharmacol Sci 1992;13:307.
25. Ferrari MD, Haan J, Blokland JAK, et al. Cerebral blood flow during migraine attacks without aura and effect of sumatriptan. Arch Neurol 1995;52:135.
26. Scott AK, Grimes S, Ng K, et al. Sumatriptan and cerebral perfusion in healthy volunteers. Br J Clin Pharmacol 1992;33:410.
27. Bates D, Ashford E, Dawson R, et al. Subcutaneous sumatriptan during the migraine aura. Neurology 1994;44:1587.
28. Saxena PR, Tfelt-Hansen P. Sumatriptan. In J Olesen, P Tfelt-Hansen, KMA Welch (eds), The Headaches. New York: Raven, 1993;329.

29. The Subcutaneous Sumatriptan International Study Group (Ferrari MD, Melamed E, Gawel M, et al). Treatment of migraine attacks with sumatriptan. N Engl J Med 1991;325:316.
30. Ferrari MD, James MH, Bates D, et al. Oral sumatriptan: Effect of a second dose, and treatment of headache recurrence. Cephalalgia 1994;14:330.
31. Visser WH, Jaspers NMWH, de Vriend RHM, Ferrari MD. Chest symptoms after sumatriptan: A two-year clinical practice review in 735 consecutive migraine patients. Cephalalgia 1996, in press.
32. Chester AH, O'Neil GS, Yacoub MH. Sumatriptan and ischaemic heart disease. Lancet 1993;341:1419.
33. Hillis WS, MacIntyre PD. Sumatriptan and chest pain. Lancet 1993;341:1564.
34. MacIntyre PD, Bhargava B, Hogg KJ, Gemmill JD, et al. The effect of IV sumatriptan, a selective 5-HT$_1$–receptor agonist, on central haemodynamics and the coronary circulation. Br J Clin Pharmacol 1992; 34: 541.
35. MacIntyre PD, Bhargava B, Hogg KJ, Gemmill JD, et al. Effect of subcutaneous sumatriptan, a selective 5-HT$_1$ agonist, on the systemic, pulmonary, and coronary circulation. Circulation 1993;87:401.
36. Houghton LA, Foster JM, Whorwell PJ, Morris J, et al. Is chest pain after sumatriptan oesophageal in origin? Lancet 1994;344:985.
37. Dahlöf C. Placebo-controlled clinical trials with ergotamine in the acute treatment of migraine. Cephalalgia 1993;13:166.
38. Perrin VL. Clinical pharmacokinetics of ergotamine in migraine and cluster headache. Clin Pharmacokin 1985;10:334.
39. Quality Standards Subcommittee of the American Academy of Neurology. Practice parameter: Appropriate use of ergotamine tartrate and dihydroergotamine in the treatment of migraine and status migrainosus. Neurology 1995;45:585.
40. Scott AK. Dihydroergotamine: A review of its use in the treatment of migraine and other headaches. Clin Neuropharmacol 1992;15:289.
41. Silberstein SD, Young WB, for the Working Panel of the Headache and Facial Pain Section of the American Academy of Neurology. Safety and efficacy of ergotamine tartrate and dihydroergotamine in the treatment of migraine and status migrainosus. Neurology 1995;45:577.
42. Tfelt-Hansen P, Saxena PR, Ferrari MD. Ergot Alkaloids. In FA de Wolff (ed), Handbook of Clinical Neurology (Vol 65): Intoxications of the Nervous System, Part II. Amsterdam: Elsevier, 1995;61.
43. Tfelt-Hansen P, Johnson ES. Ergotamine. In J Olesen, P Tfelt-Hansen, KMA Welch (eds), The Headaches. New York: Raven, 1993;339.
44. Tfelt-Hansen P, Lipton RB. Dihydroergotamine. In J Olesen, P Tfelt-Hansen, KMA Welch (eds), The Headaches. New York: Raven, 1993;323.
45. The Multinational Oral Sumatriptan and Cafergot Comparative Study Group. A randomized, double-blind comparison of sumatriptan and cafergot in the acute treatment of migraine. Eur Neurol 1991;31:314.
46. Ziegler D, Ford R, Kriegler J, et al. Dihydroergotamine nasal spray for the acute treatment of migraine. Neurology 1994;44:447.
47. Gijsman HJ, Ferrari MD. Dihydroergotamine nasal spray. Neurology 1995;45:397.
48. Thrush D. Does Ergotamine Work for Migraine? In C Warlow, J Garfield (eds), Dilemmas in the Management of the Neurological Patient. Edinburgh: Churchill Livingstone, 1984;106.
49. Winner P, Ricalde O, Le Force B, Saper J, et al. A double-blind study of subcutaneous dihydroergotamine vs subcutaneous sumatriptan in the treatment of acute migraine. Arch Neurol 1996;53:180.
50. Meyler WJ. Side effects of ergotamine. Cephalalgia 1996;16:5.
51. Bax WA, Renzenbrink GJ, van Heuven-Nolsen D, et al. 5-HT receptors mediating contractions of isolated human coronary artery. Eur J Pharmacol 1993;239:203.
52. Galer BS, Lipton RB, Solomon S, Newman LC, et al. Myocardial ischemia related to ergot alkaloids: A case report and literature review. Headache 1991;31:446.
53. Saper JR. Ergotamine dependency: A review. Headache 1987;27:435.
54. Saper JR, Jones JM. Ergotamine tartrate dependency: Features and possible mechanisms. Clin Neuropharmacol 1986;9:244.
55. Tfelt-Hansen P, Aebelholt Krabbe A. Ergotamine abuse: Do patients benefit from withdrawal? Cephalalgia 1981;1:29.
56. Tfelt-Hansen P, Lipton RB. Miscellaneous Drugs. In J Olesen, P Tfelt-Hansen, KMA Welch (eds), The Headaches. New York: Raven, 1993;353.
57. Waelkens J. Warning symptoms in migraine: Characteristics and therapeutic implications. Cephalalgia 1985;5:223.

9
Preventive Treatment in Migraine

James W. Lance

There is no known cure for migraine. There may never be a complete cure, because migraine is a reaction of brain and blood vessels that depends on the same neurotransmitters that are responsible for components of perception, emotion, and personality. The object of preventive treatment is to adjust each person's lifestyle wherever possible to remove precipitating or aggravating factors, to promote mental and physical relaxation, and to reduce the frequency and severity of headache by prophylactic medication until natural remission takes place. If migraine headaches are infrequent and respond readily to treatment with sumatriptan, ergotamine, or other agents, prophylactic therapy is not indicated. When patients are subject to two or more headaches each month that are not aborted rapidly with treatment, the daily administration of preventive medication becomes worthwhile.

A drug is considered to be effective in prophylaxis if it has proven to be statistically significantly better than placebo in one or more double-blind controlled trials. Statistical efficacy does not necessarily equate with patient satisfaction. A significant reduction in headache frequency or in some headache index calculated from various components of the attacks may still leave a patient devastated by severe headaches. A more realistic criterion of efficacy is obtained by assessing patients as virtually headache-free, better than half improved, no change, or worse while on the medication being tried. Bear in mind that the results of clinical trials may be confounded by a lack of patient compliance.[1]

PHARMACOTHERAPY

This section considers drugs available for the prevention of migraine in groups according to their putative action.

β-Adrenergic Antagonists

β-Blocking agents have been used in the prophylaxis of migraine for 25 years and remain the first line of defense in nonasthmatic patients. Those without intrinsic sympathomimetic (agonist) activity have proven effective, but whether they act by β-blockade or by a 5-hydroxytryptamine$_1$ (5-HT$_1$) agonist effect remains an open question. They comprise the nonselective β-blockers propranolol, nadolol, and timolol as well as the selective β$_1$-blockers atenolol and metoprolol.[2] β-Blockers are best avoided in patients with a prolonged aura or severe focal neurologic symptoms because there have been reports of migrainous stroke with their use in such instances.[3]

Nonselective β-Blockers

Propranolol
Since propranolol was first reported to be efficacious in preventing migraine attacks,[4] there have been many confirmatory trials, cited by Pascual, Polo, and Berciano,[5] who studied the effect of dosage on response. Of 53 patients treated with low doses of 1 mg per kg body weight, commonly 20 mg three times daily, 39 experienced 50% or greater improvement in frequency and intensity of attacks. For nonresponders, the dose was increased progressively to 2–3 mg per kg in the eight patients who could tolerate it, producing a good response in six. Five patients could not continue with the low dosage, and four were unable to tolerate an increased dose; adverse effects were asthenia (seven patients), nausea (two patients), vomiting (one patient), and numbness of the lower limbs (one patient). Postural hypotension, muscle cramps, and vivid dreams have been encountered as side effects in reported series of treatment with propranolol and other β-blockers. A negative controlled trial of long-acting propranolol, 80 and 160 mg daily, in which neither formulation proved better than placebo, was reported by Al-Qassab and Findley.[6] The lack of side effects experienced by the patients in their trial raises questions about the bioavailability of this long-acting formulation. In a randomized crossover comparison between propranolol and amitriptyline, Ziegler et al.[7] found that propranolol reduced the severity but not the frequency of headaches and that the response did not correlate with blood levels of the drug.

Timolol
Timolol, 10 mg twice daily, proved to be as effective as propranolol, 80 mg twice daily, and better than placebo in a three-way double-blind crossover trial involving 96 patients.[8,9] Headache frequency per month was reduced from a baseline of approximately 6 to approximately 5 on placebo and approximately 3.5 on the active drugs, so significant disability still remained. The authors suggested starting patients on one-fourth of the previously mentioned dosage and increasing slowly.

Nadolol
Nadolol has a plasma half-life of 20–24 hours and is therefore administered only once daily. Sudilovsky et al.[10] studied 140 patients with classical and common migraine, comparing the effect of nadolol, 80–160 mg once daily, to that of propranolol, 80 mg twice daily. Of the 98 patients who completed the trial, all those on active medication had decreased blood pressure and heart rate. Headache days per month were reduced to half or less compared with baseline in approximately

30% of patients on propranolol and the lower dose of nadolol, and in about 60% of patients after 2 months on the higher dose of nadolol. Side effects were experienced by 4% of patients on nadolol and 9% of patients on propranolol.

Relatively Selective β_1-Blockers

Metoprolol

A double-blind parallel study of 71 patients taking metoprolol, 200 mg (slow-release formation), or placebo once daily was reported by Andersson et al.[11] The number of migraine days per month was reduced from about 8 to approximately 5.5 on the active drug but remained at the baseline level in those on placebo medication. Side effects, including insomnia and nightmares, were experienced equally by both groups. A clinical trial limited to patients with classical migraine (migraine with aura) was conducted by Kangasniemi et al.,[12] using the same dose and form of metoprolol in a crossover study against placebo. The monthly frequency of attacks was significantly reduced (1.8 versus 2.5) from a mean of 3.8 in the pretreatment phase, as was the average duration of attacks (6 versus 8 hours) compared with 8.6 hours pretreatment.

Atenolol

A double-blind crossover study against placebo demonstrated the efficacy of atenolol, 100 mg once daily.[13] Attacks were reduced to less than half the previous frequency in seven of the 20 patients. As with all β-blockers, the results were statistically significant but by no means dramatic. Merikangas and Merikangas[14] found that atenolol, 50–100 mg daily, could safely be combined with the monoamine oxidase (MAO) inhibitor phenelzine, 45–75 mg daily, in the management of migraine, leading to reduction in some of the side effects of phenelzine such as orthostatic hypotension.

Drugs That Act on 5-Hydroxytryptamine Mechanisms

Dihydroergotamine

Although oral dihydroergotamine (DHE) is poorly absorbed, it has been used as prophylactic medication. Bousser et al.[15] reported that DHE, 10 mg daily, administered together with acetylsalicylic acid, 80 mg daily, in a crossover trial with placebo diminished headache frequency over a 2-month period from 16.6 ± 9.9 to 11.5 ± 6.2, but the severity and duration of attacks did not change. No adverse effect was noted when sumatriptan (6 mg subcutaneously) was used to treat patients on DHE therapy.[16]

Pizotifen and Cyproheptadine

Pizotifen (pizotyline) is a benzocycloheptathiophene derivative, structurally similar to cyproheptadine and the tricyclic antidepressants. It has an elimination half-life of approximately 23 hours and can therefore be given as a single nocturnal dose. Pizotifen and cyproheptadine are 5-HT$_2$ and histamine$_1$ antagonists. They probably have a similar efficacy in the prevention of migraine and share the same side effects of drowsiness, increased appetite, and weight gain. Pizotifen has proven effective in controlled trials,[17] although less potent than methysergide. I am not aware of any double-blind trial of cyproheptadine, but an early open study of our own[18] followed 100 patients taking 12–24 mg daily for a period of 6 months and found that 15 became headache-free and 31 were substantially improved. This success rate of 46% compared with 64% for 150 patients treated with methysergide (2–6 mg daily) for 6 months and 20% of 50 patients given placebo medication for 1 month. A comparative trial, incorporating a placebo group, demonstrated that pizotifen, 0.5 mg three times daily, and naproxen sodium, 550 mg twice daily, were of equal value in prophylaxis[19] and that both were more effective than placebo. The number of headache days was reduced to about half with naproxen and to about two-thirds with pizotifen.

Methysergide

Methysergide (1-methyl-D-lysergic acid butanolamide) is an ergot derivative with an elimination half-life of approximately 3 hours. It breaks down to methylergometrine (methylergonovine), which is probably responsible for its sustained beneficial effect in the prophylaxis of migraine. Methysergide is a 5-HT$_2$ antagonist but also has agonist properties on 5-HT$_1$ receptors. It has been proven effective in the prevention of migraine in double-blind trials.[20–22] Graham reported that retroperitoneal fibrosis, pleural fibrosis, or cardiac valvular fibrosis had developed in about 100 patients of the estimated half-million who had been treated with methysergide at that time.[23] In 30 years of using methysergide extensively, I have known six patients with retroperitoneal fibrosis, three with pleural fibrosis, and one who developed a cardiac murmur while under observation. It must be borne in mind that other agents may cause fibrotic syndromes and that in some cases no cause may be apparent. Lewis et al.[24] reported a retrospective study of seven patients with retroperitoneal fibrosis from the London Hospital. None had ever taken methysergide, but four of the seven had taken excessive amounts of analgesics. Those cases that are associated with methysergide usually resolve completely once treatment is stopped.

The fibrotic complications of methysergide may well be the result of its 5-HT–like action. Graham commented on the similarity of the appearance at surgery for valvular fibrosis in methysergide-treated patients to that seen in carcinoid syndrome.[23] The administration of 5-HT to rats either decreases or increases granuloma formation, depending on the function of the adrenal gland.[25] Excessive fibrosis appears only if adrenal insufficiency is induced, which raises the question of whether there might be adrenal insufficiency in patients who develop fibrotic syndromes in response to 5-HT or methysergide. It is possible that any drug that relies upon a 5-HT–simulating action for the treatment of migraine has the potential for producing excessive fibrosis in susceptible persons. It is recommended that patients cease medication with methysergide for 1 month every 4–6 months to minimize the possibility of fibrotic complications.

Amitriptyline

Amitriptyline blocks the reuptake of 5-HT and noradrenaline at central synapses. It is effective in the prevention of migraine[7,26,27] independent of its antidepressant effect. Individual responses to amitriptyline vary greatly. Some patients are unable to tolerate as little as 10 mg given as a nocturnal dose because of intolerable drowsiness the next day, whereas others experience no side effects while taking 150 mg in divided doses or in a single nocturnal dose. Plasma levels on a given dosage vary widely (as much as tenfold) but a steady state is reached 7–14 days after a fixed dosage is achieved.[28] Apart from drowsiness and a "drugged feeling," weight gain and dryness of the mouth may be troublesome side effects. The addition of amitriptyline to propranolol does not improve the results of propranolol medication in migraine headache, but the combination is superior to either preparation alone in the management of headaches that combine the features of migraine and tension headache.[29]

Fluoxetine

Fluoxetine is a high-profile antidepressant that also blocks 5-HT reuptake. A small controlled trial against placebo, using doses varying from 20 mg every second day to 40 mg daily, showed a significant improvement in the fluoxetine group.[30] A larger trial involving 58 migraine patients given 20 mg daily[31] did not demonstrate any improvement compared with placebo, although another group with chronic daily headache showed some response. Side effects of fluoxetine included sleep disturbance, tremor, and abdominal pain.

Monoamine Oxidase Inhibitors

Because 5-HT levels are lowered in migraine, the use of a drug that maintains or increases 5-HT levels is a logical form of treatment. Anthony and Lance treated 25 patients, who had failed to respond to other forms of interval medication, with phenelzine (MAO-A inhibitor), 45 mg daily, for periods of up to 2 years.[32] The frequency of headache was reduced to less than half in 20 of the 25 patients. Although mean plasma 5-HT increased by about 50%, there was no correlation between the 5-HT level and the response of each individual patient. We have continued to use this form of treatment in patients resistant to other therapy. Patients are issued a notice stating that they must not consume cheese, meat extracts, red wines (or any alcoholic drink in excess), broad beans, pickled herring, chicken livers (pâté), or any tablets or injections other than those prescribed for their migraine, such as aspirin, codeine, or ergotamines. They are particularly warned against the use of nasal decongestants and bronchial dilators, pethidine (meperidine), morphine, reserpine, tranquilizers, sleeping tablets, blood pressure or weight-reducing tablets, or tablets for the control of diabetes.

Phenelzine has been used in conjunction with the β-blocker atenolol with the advantage that the side effect of postural hypotension is less frequent.[14] There appears to be no adverse effect from the use of sumatriptan to treat acute episodes in patients taking MAO inhibitors.[33] The MAO-B inhibitor selegiline, which prevents the breakdown of dopamine and phenylethylamine, is not helpful in the management of migraine.[34]

Miscellaneous

Calcium Channel–Blocking Agents

Despite initial enthusiastic reports concerning the benefit of calcium channel blockers in migraine, the subject remains controversial. The Migraine-Nimodipine European Study Group was unable to demonstrate any significant effect of nimodipine, 40 mg three times daily, over placebo in migraine without aura or in migraine with aura, although the researchers noted that a larger sample in the latter trial might have yielded a positive result.[35,36] Solomon summarized the results of three small controlled studies, which found verapamil more effective than placebo and reported that a dosage of 320 mg per day was more effective than 240 mg per day.[37] Constipation is the main side effect. Flunarizine is a calcium channel blocker with dopamine antagonist properties and a long half-life. Double-blind studies have demonstrated its efficacy in the dose of 10 mg per day.[38] Side effects include fatigue, depression, and the development of parkinsonian symptoms after prolonged use. Bassi et al.[39] found that a lower dose of 3 mg per day was as effective as 10 mg per day over a 4-month period. Al Deeb et al.[40] were not able to demonstrate any benefit of flunarizine, 10 mg daily, compared with placebo-treated controls over a 3-month period.

Anticonvulsants

The only anticonvulsant that has demonstrated efficacy against migraine in controlled trials is valproate. Hering and Kuritzky[41] found that migraine attacks were reduced to half the number and severity while patients were given 400 mg twice daily over a 2-month period. Jensen et al.[42] used a slow-release formulation of sodium valproate, 1,000–1,500 mg per day depending on blood levels, for comparison with placebo in a crossover design in which 12-week treatment periods were separated by 4-week washouts. Half the patients experienced a reduction of 50% or better on valproate compared with 18% on placebo. A similar result was reported by Mathew et al.: 48% of valproate-treated patients achieved a 50% or greater reduction in headache frequency, compared with 14% of those on placebo.[43] Mean headache frequency diminished from 6 to 3.5 each month, but the severity of each attack was unaltered.

Nonsteroidal Anti-Inflammatory Drugs

Masel et al. conducted a controlled crossover trial of aspirin, 325 mg twice daily, combined with dipyridamole, 25 mg three times daily, and found that the frequency and severity of migraine attacks were significantly reduced compared with the placebo period.[44] A crossover double-blind trial established that naproxen, 275 mg, two tablets given morning and night, gave significantly better results than placebo. Fifty-nine percent of patients on naproxen achieved freedom from severe headaches, compared with 19% on placebo.[45] Naproxen, 550 mg twice daily, was also found to be useful in menstrual migraine, but a significant difference from the placebo response occurred only after 3 months of treatment.[46] Gastrointestinal side effects limit the application of nonsteroidal anti-inflammatory drugs in the prophylaxis of migraine for many patients.

Feverfew

The herbal remedy feverfew, which inhibits the release of 5-HT from platelets, has enjoyed a vogue in the United Kingdom as a remedy for migraine. A double-blind study against placebo has confirmed that the daily consumption of one capsule of dried leaves was effective in reducing the number and severity of attacks.[47]

Histamine Antagonists

In a carefully controlled double-blind trial, we were unable to demonstrate any worthwhile effects of the histamine$_1$-blocking agent chlorpheniramine or the histamine$_2$-blocking agent cimetidine in preventing migraine.[48]

Clonidine

Clonidine is an α_2-adrenoceptor agonist that was proposed as a prophylactic agent for migraine. Initial optimistic reports were followed by a series of negative trials.

THE PRACTICAL APPLICATION OF PROPHYLACTIC THERAPY FOR FREQUENT MIGRAINE ATTACKS

Provided the patient is not overweight, pizotifen (not available in the United States) or cyproheptadine is worth trying first for migraine prevention. Tablets of pizotifen contain 0.5 mg, and the dose can be increased slowly from one to six at night if necessary, staying at a level that does not cause morning drowsiness. Alternatively, cyproheptadine 4 mg, one to two tablets at night, can be prescribed. Increase in appetite with resulting weight gain is a common side effect of both drugs. If a patient has not improved after 1 month on the optimum dose, my own policy is to change to a β-blocker such as propranolol (Inderal) after making sure the patient is not asthmatic. Some patients respond to as little as 10 mg twice daily of propranolol, but others require full β-blocking doses. For patients who do not respond to β-blockers, naproxen, 250–500 mg twice daily, can be tried.

When migraine is mixed with tension headache or recurs often, tricyclic antidepressants are useful even for those patients who are not depressed. Amitriptyline is probably the most effective, but it should be given at night and the dose increased slowly because many patients complain of morning drowsiness. The patient can start with a 10-mg tablet or half of a 25-mg tablet at night and increase to 75 mg or even 150 mg each night if the medication is well tolerated. Its use may be limited by dryness of the mouth or tremor as well as sedation. In such cases, dothiepin or imipramine can be employed instead.

Methysergide is a highly effective antimigrainous agent, but treatment must be started cautiously to minimize the incidence of side effects. Patients are well advised to cut a pill in half as a small test dose, because approximately 40% of patients experience side effects such as epigastric discomfort, muscle cramps, vasoconstrictive phenomena, or mood changes if the full dosage of one to two pills three times daily is taken immediately. Methysergide suppresses migraine completely in approximately 25% of patients and reduces the frequency of headaches by half or more in another 40% or 50%. If the patient's symptoms are substantially relieved, methysergide therapy is usually continued for 4–6 months and then reduced slowly and substituted by another prophylactic agent for a period of 1 month before being recommenced. The reason for this precaution is the rare complication of retroperitoneal or pleural fibrosis. Some patients choose to continue methysergide therapy uninterrupted because attempts at withdrawal lead to a severe and debilitating recrudescence of migraine. In such cases the patient should be aware of the possibility of fibrotic side effects and should report for a physical examination and a blood urea or creatinine estimation every 3 months; the patient must notify the medical adviser immediately should any symptoms appear. With these precautions, methysergide is a safe and useful form of migraine prophylaxis for many patients. It is uncertain whether methysergide reduces migraine by maintaining tonic constriction of large arteries or by acting on the central nervous system.

Some patients experience side effects, chiefly abdominal discomfort and muscle cramps, when methysergide treatment is first started, but these usually pass after some days or weeks. Less common side effects include insomnia, depression, a sensation of swelling in the face or throat, increase in the size of venules over the nose and cheeks, and weight gain.[21] Approximately 10% of patients are unable to tolerate methysergide because of persistent unpleasant symptoms or the appearance of peripheral vasoconstriction with pallor of the extremities, intermittent claudication or, rarely, angina pectoris. These symptoms disappear on ceasing medication or, if mild, may be overcome by the combination of a vasodilator drug with methysergide.[20] Peripheral vascular disease, coronary artery disease, hypertension, a history of thrombophlebitis or peptic ulcer, and pregnancy are all relative, but not absolute, contraindications to the use of methysergide. The reason for avoiding methysergide in the first four conditions is fairly clear, because arterial vasoconstriction is a recognized side effect. The administration of methysergide was found to double basal gastric secretion of hydrochloric acid in patients with peptic ulcer, and hence its use is best avoided in patients with this condition. There is no evidence to suggest that methysergide is harmful to mother or fetus, but it has been our own practice to suspend its use if pregnancy is planned or occurs unexpectedly.

For patients who have not responded to β-blockers, pizotifen (cyproheptadine), or methysergide or who have contraindications to their use, verapamil, flunarizine, and valproate are available as options. I have found flunarizine useful, particularly for patients with a prolonged aura or with hemiplegic migraine. Some 80% of patients with migraine who have proved to be resistant to other forms of therapy respond to phenelzine, 15 mg three times a day. A list of foods and drugs to be avoided while taking MAO inhibitors should be issued to each patient. Particular mention should be made of oral or inhaled nasal decongestant or bronchodilator agents, which commonly contain monoamines.

MIGRAINE IN CHILDREN

When migraine recurs frequently in children, interval therapy can be used as in adults, usually starting with pizotifen or cyproheptadine (if the child is not overweight) or propranolol (if there is no tendency to asthma). Once migraine is brought under control in children it goes into remission in about 60% of cases, though it may recur in later years in approximately 20%.

CONCLUSIONS

That such a variety of medications is employed in the treatment of migraine indicates that none is entirely effective. Nevertheless, most patients can obtain relief from a combination of behavioral management and drug therapy. For patients who do not respond satisfactorily to sumatriptan, ergotamine derivatives, or analgesics and whose frequency of attacks exceeds two per month, a thorough trial of prophylactic therapy is indicated with the aim of reducing the intensity or frequency of attacks or eliminating them completely.

REFERENCES

1. Steiner TJ, Catarci T, Hering R, et al. If migraine prophylaxis does not work, think about compliance. Cephalalgia 1994;14;463.
2. Tfelt-Hansen P. Therapy of migraine. Curr Opin Neurol Neurosurg 1989;2:212.
3. Bardwell A, Trott JA. Stroke in migraine as a consequence of propranolol. Headache 1987;27:381.
4. Weber RB, Reinmuth OM. The treatment of migraine with propranolol. Neurology 1971;21:404.
5. Pascual K, Polo JM, Berciano J. The dose of propranolol for migraine prophylaxis: Efficacy of low doses. Cephalalgia 1989;9:287.
6. Al-Qassab HK, Findley LJ. Comparison of propranolol LA 80 mg and propranolol LA 160 mg in migraine prophylaxis: A placebo-controlled study. Cephalalgia 1993;13:128.
7. Ziegler DK, Hurwitz A, Preskorn S, et al. Propranolol and amitriptyline in prophylaxis of migraine: Pharmacokinetic and therapeutic effects. Arch Neurol 1993;50:825.
8. Tfelt-Hansen P, Standnes B, Kangasniemi P, et al. Timolol vs propranolol vs placebo in common migraine prophylaxis: A double-blind multicenter trial. Acta Neurol Scand 1984;69:1.
9. Tfelt-Hansen P. Efficacy of β-blockers in migraine: A critical review. Cephalalgia 1986;6(Suppl 5):15.
10. Sudilovsky A, Elkind AH, Ryan RE, et al. Comparative efficacy of nadolol and propranolol in the management of migraine. Headache 1987;27:421.
11. Andersson PG, Dahl S, Hansen JH, et al. Prophylactic treatment of classical and non-classical migraine with metoprolol—a comparison with placebo. Cephalalgia 1983;3:207.
12. Kangasniemi P, Andersen AR, Andersson PG, et al. Classical migraine: Effective prophylaxis with metoprolol. Cephalalgia 1987;7:231.
13. Forssman B, Lindblad CJ, Zbornikova V. Atenolol for migraine prophylaxis. Headache 1983;23:188.

14. Merikangas KR, Merikangas JR. Combination monoamine oxidase inhibitor and β-blocker treatment of migraine with anxiety and depression. Biol Psychiatry 1995;37:1.
15. Bousser MG, Chick J, Fuseau E, et al. Combined low-dose acetylsalicylic acid and dihydroergotamine in migraine prophylaxis. Cephalalgia 1988;8:187.
16. Henry P, d'Allens H, French Migraine Network Bordeaux-Lyon-Grenoble. Subcutaneous sumatriptan in the acute treatment of migraine in patients using dihydroergotamine as prophylaxis. Headache 1993;33:432.
17. Speight TM, Avery GS. Pizotifen (BC105): A review of its pharmacological properties and its therapeutic efficacy in vascular headache. Drugs 1972;3:159.
18. Curran DA, Lance JW. Clinical trial of methysergide and other preparations in the management of migraine. J Neurol Neurosurg Psychiatry 1964;27:463.
19. Bellevance AJ, Meloche JP. A comparative study of naproxen sodium, pizotyline, and placebo in migraine prophylaxis. Headache 1990;30:710.
20. Lance JW, Fine RD, Curran DA. An evaluation of methysergide in the prevention of migraine and other vascular headaches. Med J Aust 1963;1:814.
21. Curran DA, Hinterberger H, Lance JW. Methysergide. Res Clin Stud Headache 1967;1:74.
22. Pedersen E, Moller CE. Methysergide in migraine prophylaxis. Clin Pharmacol Ther 1966;7:520.
23. Graham JR. Cardiac and pulmonary fibrosis during methysergide therapy for headache. Am J Med Sci 1967;254:23.
24. Lewis CT, Molland EA, Marshall VR, et al. Analgesic abuse, ureteric obstruction and retroperitoneal fibrosis. BMJ 1975;2:76.
25. Bianchine JR, Eade NR. The effect of 5-hydroxytryptamine on the cotton pellet local inflammatory response in the rat. J Exp Med 1967;125:501.
26. Gomersall JD, Stuart A. Amitriptyline in migraine prophylaxis: Changes in pattern of attacks during a controlled clinical trial. J Neurol Neurosurg Psychiatry 1973;36:684.
27. Couch JR, Ziegler DK, Hassanein R. Amitriptyline in the prophylaxis of migraine: Effectiveness and relationship of antimigraine and antidepressant drugs. Neurology 1976;26:121.
28. Ziegler VE, Clayton PJ, Biggs JT. A comparison study of amitriptyline and nortriptyline with plasma levels. Arch Gen Psychiatry 1977;34:706.
29. Mathew NT. Prophylaxis of migraine and mixed headache: A randomized controlled study. Headache 1981;21:105.
30. Adly C, Straumanis J, Chesson A. Fluoxetine prophylaxis of migraine. Headache 1992;32:101.
31. Saper JR, Silberstein SD, Lake AE, Winters ME. Double-blind trial of fluoxetine: Chronic daily headache and migraine. Headache 1994;34:497.
32. Anthony M, Lance JW. Monoamine oxidase inhibition in the treatment of migraine. Arch Neurol 1969;21:263.
33. Diamond S. The use of sumatriptan in patients on monoamine oxidase inhibitors. Neurology 1995;45:1039.
34. Kuritzky A, Zoldan Y, Melamed E. Selegiline, a MAO B inhibitor, is not effective in the prophylaxis of migraine without aura—an open study. Headache 1992;32:416.
35. Migraine-Nimodipine European Study Group (MINES). European multicenter trial of nimodipine in the prophylaxis of common migraine (migraine without aura). Headache 1989;29:633.
36. Migraine-Nimodipine European Study Group (MINES). European multicenter trial of nimodipine in the prophylaxis of classic migraine (migraine with aura). Headache 1989;29:639.
37. Solomon GD. Verapamil in migraine prophylaxis: A five-year review. Headache 1989;29:425.
38. Leone M, Grazzi L, La Mantia L, Bussone G. Flunarizine in migraine: A mini review. Headache 1991;31:388.
39. Bassi P, Brunati L, Rapuzzi B, et al. Low-dose flunarizine in the prophylaxis of migraine. Headache 1992;32:390.
40. Al Deeb SM, Biary N, Bahou Y, et al. Flunarizine in migraine: A double-blind placebo-controlled study (in a Saudi population). Headache 1992;32:461.
41. Hering R, Kuritzky A. Sodium valproate in the prophylactic treatment of migraine: A double-blind study versus placebo. Cephalalgia 1992;12:81.
42. Jensen R, Brinck T, Olesen J. Sodium valproate has a prophylactic effect in migraine without aura. Neurology 1994;44:647.
43. Mathew NT, Saper JR, Silberstein SD, et al. Migraine prophylaxis with divalproex. Arch Neurol 1995;52:281.
44. Masel BE, Chesson AL, Peters BH, et al. Platelet antagonists in migraine prophylaxis: A clinical trial using aspirin and dipyridamole. Headache 1980;20:13.
45. Welch KMA. Naproxen sodium in the treatment of migraine. Cephalalgia 1986;6(Suppl 4):85.

46. Sances G, Martignoni E, Fioroni L, et al. Naproxen sodium in menstrual migraine prophylaxis: A double-blind placebo-controlled study. Headache 1990;30:705.
47. Murphy JJ, Hepinstall S, Mitchell JRA. Randomized double-blind placebo-controlled trial of feverfew in migraine prevention. Lancet 1988;2:189.
48. Anthony M, Lord GDA, Lance JW. Controlled trials of cimetidine in migraine and cluster headache. Headache 1978;18:261.

10
Sex Hormones and Headache

Stephen D. Silberstein and George R. Merriam

Considerable evidence suggests a link between estrogen and progesterone, the female sex hormones, and migraine.[1-5] Although no gender difference is apparent in prepubertal children—migraine occurs equally in 4% of boys and girls[5,6]—it occurs more frequently in women (18%) than in men (6%). Migraine develops most frequently in the second decade, and the peak incidence occurs at menarche.[3,4]

Menstrually related migraine (MM) begins at menarche in 33% of affected women.[4] MM occurs at the time of menses in many migrainous women, and exclusively with menses (true menstrual migraine [TMM]) in some.[4] MM is not psychological; rather, the headache, like menstruation itself, appears to be the result of falling sex hormone levels.[1] Premenstrual migraine (PMM) may be part of the premenstrual syndrome (PMS), which is now included in the criteria for late luteal phase dysphoric disorder (LLPDD), a menstrually related mood disorder that may be associated with other somatic complaints, including nausea, backache, and breast swelling and tenderness. LLPDD recurs during the luteal phase of the menstrual cycle and usually, but not always, resolves with the onset of menstruation.[7] Migraine occurring during menstruation is usually not associated with LLPDD.

Migraine may worsen during the first trimester of pregnancy, and, although many women become headache-free during the last two trimesters, 25% have no change in their migraine.[8-10] MM typically improves with pregnancy, perhaps due to sustained high estrogen levels.[8-10] Hormonal replacement with estrogens can exacerbate migraine, and oral contraceptives (OCs) can change its character and frequency.[11,12] Migraine prevalence decreases with advancing age but may regress or worsen at the menopause.[5,13,14] Changes in the headache pattern with OC use and during menarche, menstruation, pregnancy, or menopause are related to changes in estrogen levels.[15] These phenomena suggest a relationship between migraine headaches and changes in sex hormone levels.[16]

This chapter covers the endocrinology of the menstrual cycle, neuropharmacology of estrogens and progestins, and approaches to the therapy of hormone-related headaches, particularly those headaches associated with the menstrual cycle, the menopause, and the use of OCs.

ENDOCRINOLOGY OF THE MENSTRUAL CYCLE

Cyclic ovarian function spans the time between puberty and menopause, which are transitional periods of increasing or decreasing ovarian activity over several years. The menstrual cycle, although a continuum, is usually represented as beginning on the first day of the menses and ending on the last day before the next menses. This arbitrary peripheral marker of steroid hormone withdrawal bridges smooth changes in hormone levels: follicular growth with rising estrogens is followed by ovulation and the organization and decline of the corpus luteum. By the next menses, growth of the next cohort of follicles has already begun.

Normal ovarian functioning requires the coordinated activity of the hypothalamus, which secretes gonadotropin-releasing hormone (GnRH); the pituitary, which secretes the glycoproteins luteinizing hormone (LH) and follicle-stimulating hormone (FSH); the ovary, which secretes estrogens and progesterone; and the endometrial lining of the uterus, which responds to estrogen and progesterone (Figure 10.1). Under the control of norepinephrine (NE), serotonin (5-HT), corticotropin-releasing hormone (CRH), the opioids, and other neurotransmitters, the hypothalamus secretes GnRH in a pulsatile manner, stimulating pituitary secretion of LH and FSH.[17] This in turn stimulates secretion of ovarian estrogen and progesterone, which feed back at the pituitary to modulate the relative amounts of LH and FSH and at the hypothalamus to regulate GnRH. NE stimulates GnRH secretion; opiates and CRH are inhibitory.[18] GnRH release also may be regulated directly by intraneuronal prostaglandin E_2 (PGE_2).[19]

GnRH secretion is pulsatile rather than continuous. This pulsatility is obligatory (continuous GnRH secretion does not stimulate the pituitary; it produces inhibition of pituitary and ovarian function)[17,20] and both the amplitude and the frequency of the pulses modulate the LH and FSH output. In the follicular phase of the cycle, pulses occur at intervals of 1–2 hours (Figure 10.2).[17,20,21] Changes in the pattern of episodic LH secretion during the menstrual cycle largely reflect the effects of progesterone on the hypothalamic pattern of secretion of GnRH and the effects of estrogens and progestins on the pituitary secretion of gonadotropins. In the luteal phase of the cycle, progesterone secretion by the corpus luteum progressively slows the frequency of episodic gonadotropin secretion, which nearly ceases just before menses.[22–24]

The target of the gonadotropins is the ovary, where FSH and LH stimulate follicular growth. Most become atretic and atrophy, but one or two mature with two layers of steroidogenic tissue: granulosa cells surrounded by theca cells. Ovulation carries away the oocyte and a cumulus of granulosa cells; the remaining theca and granulosa cells organize into a progesterone-secreting corpus luteum, which is active for about 2 weeks and then regresses.

The sex hormones are steroids synthesized in a sequence of enzymatic steps that rearrange the side groups on the steroid nucleus. Because of the rigidity of the linked rings of the steroid nucleus, minor chemical changes in these side groups can produce hormones that have distinctly different activity. Progesterone is a precursor of both male sex hormones (androgens) and female sex hormones (estrogens). As related compounds they retain some receptor cross-affinity. Progesterone has some androgenic properties; and some synthetic steroids and drugs, such as medroxyprogesterone and danazol, show mixed hormonal activity.

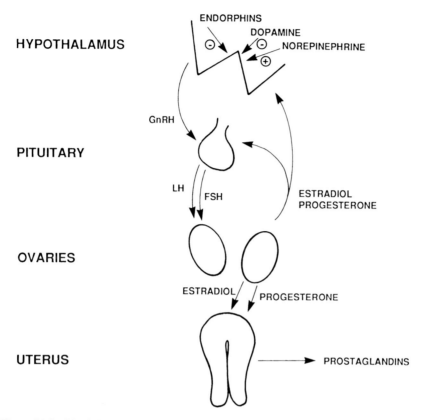

Figure 10.1 Physiology of the hypothalamic-pituitary-ovarian-uterine axis. Gonadotropin-releasing hormone (GnRH) stimulates pituitary secretion of luteinizing hormone (LH) and follicle-stimulating hormone (FSH). FSH and LH stimulate the ovary to secrete the sex steroids estrogen and progesterone, which feed back on the hypothalamus and pituitary to modulate GnRH and LH secretion. Estrogen and progesterone stimulate endometrial prostaglandin synthesis. (Reprinted with permission from SD Silberstein, G Merriam. Sex hormones and headache. J Pain Symptom Manage 1993;8:1.)

The two cell layers of the ovarian follicle divide the responsibility for steroidogenesis. The outer theca layer responds to LH and can carry out steroid synthesis from cholesterol to progesterone and androgens.[25–27] The inner granulosa layer responds to FSH and aromatizes androgens to estrogens. As the follicle develops, both cell groups proliferate. Many ovarian regulators, including growth factors, influence the theca cells to differentiate from fibroblasts of the ovarian stroma outside the follicular basement membrane.

Estrogen exerts negative feedback regulation on the pituitary; thus, as the follicle grows and estrogen levels increase, FSH initially decreases. At the middle of the cycle, however, there is a rapid reversal from inhibition to stimulation, and a large surge of LH secretion occurs. A small increase in progesterone plays a central role

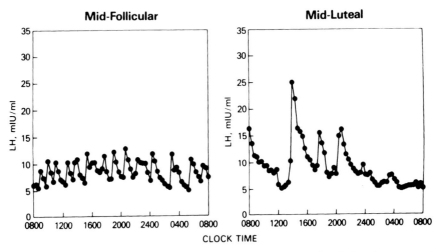

Figure 10.2   Patterns of episodic luteinizing hormone (LH) secretion during the menstrual cycle in women. During the follicular phase (left), LH secretion is of relatively high frequency and low amplitude. During the luteal phase (right), LH secretion is of lower frequency and higher amplitude (prior to cessation of secretion). (Reprinted with permission from SD Silberstein, G Merriam. Sex hormones and headache. J Pain Symptom Manage 1993;8:1.)

in this reversal, which in turn may reflect inhibition of the synthesis of estrogen due to product inhibition by the high levels of estrogen in the dominant follicle. Thus the increase in progesterone can serve as a signal that the follicle is ready to ovulate.[28,29]

High levels of LH at midcycle stimulate a further increase in progesterone, activating enzymes that digest the wall of the follicle. The oocyte and most of the granulosa cells float out. The crater of the ovulated follicle and the remaining granulosa organize as the corpus luteum, an evanescent gland that secretes progesterone for about 2 weeks and then regresses. Progesterone has two main target organs: the hypothalamus, where the GnRH pulse frequency is progressively reduced and where the temperature set point is increased by a half a degree Celsius, and the uterus, which responds to both estrogens and progestins. Estrogen stimulates growth of the endometrium; progesterone causes it to secrete mucus, specific proteins, and vasoactive substances. Progesterone withdrawal leads to arterial spasm and menses. The involved vasoactive substances include peptides and the prostaglandins.

In men, gonadotropin and steroid hormone levels are relatively stable over time, but in women the menstrual cycle requires a carefully coordinated sequence of changes. That sequence can be interrupted by subtle miscues that are not readily characterized as simply hypogonadism. Stressors such as weight change or exercise can result in amenorrhea in women, whereas changes of comparable magnitude in men may be clinically silent.[22]

The succession of hormones causes major changes in fluid balance, blood pressure, and uterine tone. The transitions between states may not be smooth. Estrogens cause fluid retention and have direct central nervous system (CNS) effects. Sex hormones bind to receptors in the area of the brain responsible for reproductive behavior and gonadotropin release.[30] They activate high-affinity intracellular receptors that undergo a process called nucleocytoplasmic shuttling, in which the receptors exit from the cell nucleus but are rapidly shuttled back in an energy-dependent process. The estrogen receptor (ER), when activated, is a transcription factor. In the absence of hormonal binding, the ER is an oligomeric complex containing the heatshock protein hsp 90. Following estrogen binding, the ER sheds the hsp 90, dimerizes, and binds with high affinity to estrogen-responsive genes (estrogen response elements). The result is transcription by means of two transcriptional activation functions (TAF-1 and TAF-2).[31] Steroids also modulate gene expression and the synthesis of new protein in the brain.

In addition, steroid hormones rapidly exert behavioral and electrophysiologic effects through nongenomic mechanisms by rapidly binding to neuronal membranes. Effector systems that transduce the signal of steroid-membrane interactions include neurotransmitter receptors, release mechanisms, and ion channels. Estradiol has rapid effects on membrane potentials in preoptic and septal neurons, and progesterone acts on dorsal midbrain neurons, presumably through receptor sites on neuronal membranes.[32] In rodents, estrogens increase the electrical activity of the neurons that foster female reproductive behavior and decrease the electrical activity of the preoptic neurons that disrupt feminine behavior. Progesterone initially facilitates and later inhibits sexual behavior.[33]

Estradiol changes the potassium permeability of postsynaptic medial amygdala neurons within minutes. Progestogen stimulates the release of dopamine from striatal tissue and of GnRH from hypothalamus tissue. Estrogens increase the number of progesterone and muscarinic receptors and modulate 5-HT_1, 5-HT_2, and beta-adrenergic receptors.[33] Long-term estrogen treatment decreases 5-HT_{1A} receptor sensitivity in the raphe presynaptically and enhances it postsynaptically in the hippocampus. These actions, in concert, increase serotonergic transmission.[34] Estrogen withdrawal increases the number of dopaminergic receptors.[35] Progesterone modulates the estrogen effects on the 5-HT_1 and 5-HT_2 receptors. Estrogens also affect the peripheral nervous system, increasing the size of the receptive fields of trigeminal mechanoreceptors in rats.[36]

Progesterone has other CNS effects. Some progesterone metabolites have potent interactions with the gamma-aminobutyric acid–responsive chloride channels in the brain.[37] Progesterone metabolites may modulate anxiety processes in susceptible individuals, perhaps by interacting with the endogenous benzodiazepine receptor ligands, which normally suppress anxiety.[38] This interaction may account in part for the mood changes of LLPDD. In self-scoring profiles,[39] women with LLPDD show a distinctive pattern: anxiety scores increase progressively during the late luteal phase, resolve rapidly with the onset of menstruation, and then remain stable until progesterone rises again. Depression scores are similarly affected by the phases of the menstrual cycle.

Many believe that the symptoms of PMS are related to changes in progesterone that occur during the late luteal phase of the menstrual cycle. However, most women with PMS who had their luteal phase truncated by the progestogen antagonist mifepristone (RU 486) continued to have PMS symptoms at the expected time despite hormonal conditions of the early follicular phase.[40] The cycle was maintained by giving human chorionic gonadotropin, which maintained high serum progesterone levels, but menstruation still occurred as a result of blocking the progesterone receptor with mifepristone. (Two women who received mifepristone did not have PMS symptoms when the menstrual cycle was reset, suggesting that in some women there is an obligatory relation between PMS and the endocrine events of the late luteal phase.) PMS symptoms may represent an autonomous cyclic disorder that is linked to, but can be dissociated from, the menstrual cycle. Alternatively, symptoms may be triggered by hormonal events before the late luteal phase, consistent with reports that suppression of ovulation results in a remission of PMS symptoms. PMS and premenstrual migraine may both result from a cyclic central disturbance of mood and pain perception.

MENSTRUAL MIGRAINE

Migraine can occur before, during, or after menstruation, or at the time of ovulation.[41,42] When migraine occurs before menstruation (PMM) there may also be features of PMS (LLPDD), including depression, anxiety, crying spells, difficulty in thinking, lethargy, backache, breast tenderness and swelling, and nausea.[4] Migraine that occurs during menstruation is often associated with dysmenorrhea[42] and is frequently refractory.[43] It is important to differentiate between the two conditions, because medications that may be useful in treating headache related to dysmenorrhea may not help headache associated with PMS.[1]

Based on clinical experience, the frequency of MM has been reported to be as high as 60–70%. Based on retrospective analysis, prevalence ranges from 26–60% in headache clinic patients. The prevalence is lower in patients seen in non–headache clinic settings. The relative frequency of MM depends on the means of ascertainment.[44]

In order to define the relationship between the frequency of migraine attacks and the menstrual cycle, MacGregor et al.[42] prospectively followed 55 women migraineurs who were attending a headache clinic. They defined TMM as attacks that occurred regularly on or between days –2 to +3 of the menstrual cycle and at no other time, and MM as attacks that occurred at all times during the cycle with an increased frequency during menstruation. Using these criteria, 7.2% of the patients studied had TMM (if –4 to +4 days was used as the interval, 10.9% had TMM). None had migraine with aura. Another 34.5% had increased attack frequency with MM; 32.7% did not. Increased severity or resistance to treatment occurring with MM was not analyzed.

Waters and O'Connor,[6] using a prospective diary assessment of 41 migraineurs and 14 nonmigraineurs, found that both migraine and nonmigraine headache were at least twice as frequent during menstruation as between menses, and that the highest incidence of migraine occurred during the first few days of menstruation.

Beckham et al.[45] monitored the headache activity and menstrual distress of 14 migraineurs. One patient (7.1%) had TMM and 10 (71.4%) had MM. Menstrual distress was highest during the premenstrual and menstrual phases, but headache activity was greatest in the premenstrual period.

In contrast to this is a 4-month diary study[44] of 79 women screened for migraine with aura in Washington County, MD, selected from a community survey of headache. The subjects completed daily diaries and recorded information regarding their menstrual cycle phase, time of headache, and occurrence and attack characteristics. Headache was classified into four categories (migraine with aura, migraine without aura, tension-type headache, and other headache types), and occurred on 30% of the study days. There was considerable variability between subjects, most of whom experienced at least three separate headache types. All headache types occurred more frequently during the first 3 days of the menstrual cycle, but this was statistically significant only for migraine without aura (66% higher). Headache frequency did not significantly increase in the premenstrual, postmenstrual, or ovulatory periods.

Keenan and Lindamer[46] preselected patients with PMS and followed them prospectively for both headache and PMS symptoms. When they compared these patients to a non-PMS control group, they found that severe (nonmigrainous) headaches were more common in the PMS group, were most severe during the late luteal phase, and peaked the day prior to menstruation. In contrast, women without PMS experienced a peak in severity only on the first day of menses. This difference in time course is also consistent with different mechanisms leading to headache in PMS.

Recall bias may account for the higher frequency of both PMM and MM in retrospective studies. When symptoms of PMS were collected both prospectively and retrospectively in the same group of women, 40% reported PMM retrospectively, but only 17% reported it with the diary.[47] Retrospectively, more (39.7% versus 35.6%) reported PMM. With the diary, migraine occurring after menstruation was more common (19.7% versus 17.4%).

Cupini et al.[48] looked at the relationship between the sex hormone milestones and migraine with aura and migraine without aura. They defined MM as attacks that occur from 2 days before to 3 days after menstruation, and TMM as attacks that occur *only* during that period. Consistent with previous reports, this study found both MM and TMM were common in migraine without aura. Migraine without aura was also found to be more frequently associated with menarche and the postpartum period than was migraine with aura, but not significantly so. These observations were retrospectively reported and thus more subject to bias. The menstrual migraine portion of the study, which was prospective and diary-based, was less subject to recall bias. Migraine that began with pregnancy or OC use was more likely to be migraine with aura. The researchers noted no difference between migraine with or without aura with menopause. This study suggests a difference in hormonal responsiveness between the two types of migraine. Migraine without aura is more likely to occur de novo or to be triggered by declining sex hormone levels (postpartum or at menarche), and migraine with aura is more likely to begin de novo with sustained high sex hormone levels (pregnancy, OC use).

Facchinetti et al.[49] prospectively studied women recruited from a PMS clinic who claimed that premenstrual discomfort, migraine, or both had interfered with their daily lives for at least the previous 2 years. In this population, 14 of 22 women with MM (migraine occurring between day −2 and day +3) and four of 12 women without MM had menstrual distress. Questionnaire scores (Menstrual Distress Questionnaire of Moos) were similar to those of women with PMS. Whether this relationship is a result of selection bias or of comorbidity is uncertain. PMS symptoms should not yet be part of the criteria for MM.

Most women have increased headache attacks at the time of menses. Women preselected on the basis of PMS have more headaches prior to the onset of menses, but most women have more headaches just before or with menstruation. Some women have migraine (usually without aura) only with menses. Menstrual migraine can be defined by looking at attacks regularly triggered by menstruation. Attacks occurring only with menstruation, even if infrequent, would be called TMM. Attacks occurring both at menstruation and at other times of the cycle could be called menstrually triggered migraine. A frequency indicator (e.g., frequent, ≥70%; common, 35–70%; and infrequent, ≤35%) would clarify the tightness of the association. The quality of the attacks, their response to treatment, and the hormonal changes in the patients could then be analyzed based on this association. Migraine attacks occurring –2 to –7 days before the onset of menses would be called premenstrual; those occurring from –1 to +4 days, menstrual. Proposed cutoffs are arbitrary and should be examined further.[50]

MM occurs at the time of greatest fluctuation in estrogen levels. Attempts to find consistent differences in ovarian hormone levels between women with MM and controls have not yielded consistent results. Some authors have reported higher estrogen and progestin levels in those with MM; others have not;[4,41,51,52] most find that testosterone, FSH, and LH levels are similar to those in controls. In the study by Beckham et al.,[45] headache activity correlated with high progesterone during the luteal phase. But progesterone is the marker for the luteal phase, so this correlation tells us nothing about any causal association between luteal headaches and progesterone.[50]

Somerville[53] reported that MM headache occurs during or after the simultaneous decrease of estrogens and progesterone. Estrogens given premenstrually delay the onset of migraine but not menstruation.[53] In contrast, progesterone administration delays menstruation but does not prevent migraine.[54] Somerville concluded that estrogen withdrawal may trigger migraine attacks in susceptible women.

Estrogen-withdrawal migraine requires several days of exposure to high levels of estrogen.[55] When Somerville used an erratic delivery system of long-acting estrogen implants to suppress migraine, his patients developed irregular bleeding and headaches associated with fluctuating estrogen levels.[56]

Pathogenesis of Menstrual Migraine

The fluctuation in estrogen levels produces many biochemical effects that may be relevant to the pathogenesis of MM. This section examines four of these: (1) prostaglandins and the uterus; (2) prolactin (PRL) release; (3) opioid regulation; and (4) melatonin secretion.

Prostaglandins and the Uterus

The prostaglandins, 20-carbon fatty acid derivatives of arachidonic acid, inhibit adrenergic transmission, sensitize nociceptors, and promote the development of neurogenic inflammation.[57,58] Prostaglandins modulate sympathetic activity.

Prostaglandins of the E series inhibit adrenergic transmission.[59] Nonsteroidal anti-inflammatory drugs (NSAIDs) block prostaglandin synthesis and enhance adrenergic transmission by increasing the amount of NE released.[60,61] Prostaglandins are synthesized in response to neuronal release of NE. The newly synthesized prostaglandins further inhibit NE release by a feedback mechanism.[60] Prostaglandins sensitize pain receptors[62] and increase neurogenic inflammation;[58] when injected they produce intense local pain, in part by lowering the threshold of nociceptors.[57] PGE_1 infusion produces migraine-like headaches and abdominal cramps;[63] prostacyclin infusion produces a dull, throbbing headache;[64] and PGF_2 infusion produces cramping, diarrhea, nausea, flushing, syncope, and inability to concentrate.

Antidromic sensory nerve stimulation results in the release of substance P, calcitonin gene-related peptide, and neurokinin A and produces vasodilation, leakage of plasma protein, and sterile inflammation.[58] The neurogenic inflammation may generate part of the painful sensation of headache. NSAIDs block prostaglandin synthesis and inhibit the development of neurogenic inflammation.[65] Ergotamine and sumatriptan, effective migraine abortives, prevent neurogenic inflammation by blocking transmission in unmyelinated C fibers.[66] Prostaglandins affect the CNS and may modulate the descending noradrenergic pain-control system.[67] Intrathecal PGE_2 decreases the pain threshold.[68] Prostaglandins block NE release in the CNS, antagonize electrical and morphine analgesia, and may regulate GnRH release.[19] This antagonism is blocked by intrathecal NSAIDs.[67]

Increased uterine contractions cause much of the pain of dysmenorrhea.[69] Prostaglandins, particularly PGF_2 and PGE_2, produced by the endometrium under the influence of estrogens and progesterone, intensify uterine contractions.[70,71] The endometrium and menstrual fluid of dysmenorrheic patients have been reported to contain increased concentrations of prostaglandins.[70,71] These increased prostaglandins are associated with menstrual headache.[70] PGF_2 plasma levels, which are normal throughout the menstrual cycle, significantly increase during a migraine attack.[72] Prostaglandin infusion produces menstrual symptoms, including dysmenorrhea and headache.[70] Plasma taken from menstruating women with severe dysmenorrhea and infused back to them when they were not menstruating reproduced dysmenorrhea and other symptoms of the menstrual syndrome, including headache.[72,73] Prostaglandins have a very short plasma half-life; therefore, a prostaglandin-generating factor, which enhances local prostaglandin production, may induce the menstrual syndrome,[72] including headache.

Grant[74] reported that women with migraine may have more endometrial arterial proliferation, and thus possibly an altered end-organ response to estrogen. Menstrual migraine may be a consequence of estrogen withdrawal that affects both the hypothalamus[19] and the uterus, mediated in part by increased prostaglandin and prostaglandin-generating factors.

Prolactin Release

PRL release is under tonic inhibitory control by the hypothalamus. Dopamine is the major PRL-inhibitory factor. Thyrotropin-releasing hormone (TRH), vasoactive intestinal peptide, and angiotensin also stimulate PRL, but their

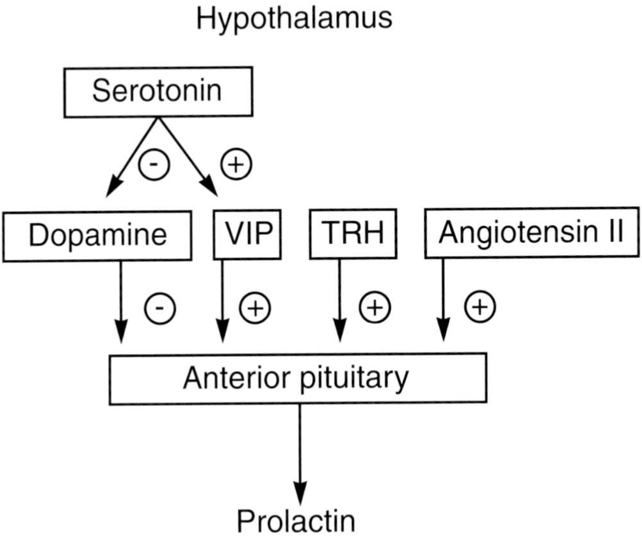

Hypothalamus

Figure 10.3   Neurotransmitter and neuropeptide modulation of prolactin (PRL) secretion. Dopamine inhibits PRL release. Thyrotropin-releasing hormone (TRH), vasoactive intestinal peptide (VIP), and angiotensin II promote PRL secretion. Serotonin increases PRL secretion by inhibiting dopamine and enhancing VIP release. (Reprinted with permission from SD Silberstein, G Merriam. Sex hormones and headache. J Pain Symptom Manage 1993;8:1.)

physiologic role is uncertain. Serotonin may increase PRL release by inhibiting dopamine and by stimulating TRH neurons.[75] Serotonin receptors themselves are modulated by estrogen and progesterone.[33] Acetylcholine, opiates, and estrogen act indirectly to enhance PRL release. PRL plasma levels are raised by estrogens, dopamine antagonists, and natural stimuli such as suckling and stress, and reduced by dopamine agonists.[75] In women migraineurs, PRL baseline levels are in the normal range in all phases of the menstrual cycle. However, the PRL response to exogenous TRH is enhanced during a migraine attack.[76,77] Enhanced PRL release by dopaminergic antagonists in women with MM occurs throughout the menstrual cycle and is maintained in post-menopausal migrainous women.[78,79] Inhibition of PRL release by L-dopa is less marked in migraineurs; therefore, dopaminergic receptor supersensitivity cannot account for these responses (Figure 10.3).[80]

TRH is both the releasing factor for thyroid-stimulating hormone (TSH) and one of the PRL-releasing factors.[75] Infusion of TRH during a migraine attack produces enhanced release of PRL but not of TSH.[77] Serotonin may modulate both PRL and TSH release; it may facilitate PRL release and inhibit TSH release. Possibly the enhancement of PRL release without enhancement of TSH release is an effect of increased hypothalamic serotonin. It may be speculated that these abnormalities are a by-product of central serotonin dysmodulation in MM.

Table 10.1   Opioids in headache, premenstrual syndrome, and menopause

| | Luteinizing hormone response to naloxone | | Cerebrospinal fluid beta endorphin levels |
	Midluteal phase	Late luteal phase	
Cluster headache	WNL	WNL	WNL
Menstrually related headache	WNL	↓	WNL
Menstrually related/unrelated migraine	↓	↓	↓
Premenstrual syndrome with or without migraine	WNL	↓	WNL
Chronic daily headache	↓	↓	↓
Menopause	NA*	NA*	↓

*No longer menstruating, decreased response at all times.
WNL = within normal limits; NA = not applicable.
Source: Reprinted with permission from SD Silberstein, G Merriam. Sex hormones and headache. J Pain Symptom Manage 1993;8:1.

Opioids

Opiate peptides tonically inhibit hypothalamic GnRH and thus pituitary LH secretion by acting on the mu-receptor in the arcuate nucleus of the hypothalamus (see Figure 10.1).[81] Naloxone, a mu-receptor antagonist, reverses this effect. The intensity of the inhibition depends on the phase of the menstrual cycle. Naloxone administration produces a significant increase in LH levels in the early luteal phase of the menstrual cycle.[82,83] But the LH response to naloxone is lost (1) in the late luteal phase in women with TMM, perhaps because of decreased functional hypothalamic opioid activity in MM;[84] (2) during PMS;[82] (3) earlier in the luteal phase with more severe and chronic headaches;[84] and (4) after menopause (Table 10.1). The response is restored by treatment with estrogens and progesterone.[85]

Most studies of hormonal profiles across the menstrual cycle have shown no difference between PMS patients and controls, consistent with the impression that PMS reflects an abnormal response to hormonal changes rather than a response to abnormal hormones.[86] However, one group has reported increased frequency and reduced amplitude of LH pulses during the late luteal phase in women with PMS; if this is so, it might reflect a dysfunction of hypothalamus GnRH release, possibly linked to a reduction of opioid inhibition.[87] Women with PMS and MM (occurring before the onset of menstruation) may lose the stimulatory response to clonidine-induced release of beta-endorphin and growth hormone (GH). This suggests a postsynaptic alpha$_2$-adrenoreceptor hyposensitivity—perhaps as a result of abnormal opioid content of the hypothalamus, because naloxone infusion can attenuate the GH response to clonidine in midluteal phase. Clonidine itself can alleviate symptoms of PMS.[88]

The pituitary is the primary source of plasma beta-endorphin; however, beta-endorphin synthesized in the brain acts locally as a neuromodulator[89] and is influenced by estrogens. Cerebrospinal fluid (CSF) beta-endorphin levels more accurately measure the central concentration of beta-endorphin than do plasma levels. CSF levels of beta-endorphin decrease with increasing chronicity and intensity of headache,[84] whereas plasma levels of beta-endorphin show no consistent change in migraine patients.[90]

A correlation has been reported between loss of naloxone responsiveness, decreased CSF beta-endorphin levels, and increasing severity of migraine.[84] The estrogen-sensitive changes in central opioid tone in women with menstrual migraine may relate to the genesis of their headaches.

Melatonin

Melatonin is synthesized from serotonin by two sequential enzymatic steps in the pineal gland, where tryptophan is first converted to serotonin (5-HT) by the sequential action of tryptophan hydroxylase and aromatic L-amino acid decarboxylase. 5-HT is then *N*-acetylated by the enzyme *N*-acetyl transferase and subsequently converted to melatonin by hydroxyindole-O-methyl transferase. The first enzyme, *N*-acetyl transferase, is rate limiting and under sympathetic control.[91]

Serum melatonin concentration shows a circadian pattern, with a high concentration at night and a very low concentration during the day. This pattern is under the influence of the sympathetic input to the pineal gland with primary control by NE released from sympathetic nerve endings. NE acts on beta-adrenergic receptors via cyclic AMP to activate *N*-acetyl transferase. The rhythm of the pineal gland is driven by the suprachiasmatic nucleus of the hypothalamus, which receives direct and indirect visual input.[91]

Melatonin concentration is elevated during darkness and suppressed by light. It has been implicated in synchronizing the endogenous cycles to the length of day. In humans, melatonin promotes sleep and entrains some biologic rhythms. In adults, the nocturnal increase in melatonin stimulates prolactin release. An abnormality in the circadian hypothalamic pacemaker could act both to trigger migraine and to decrease melatonin production.[91]

Brun et al.[92] compared nocturnal melatonin secretion in women with migraine without aura with that in healthy controls. To qualify as having MM, their patients had to have increased headache frequency and intensity at the time of menstruation and at least one attack per month during the study. Nocturnal urinary melatonin immunoactivity, a marker for nocturnal melatonin secretion, was decreased throughout the menstrual cycle in women with MM and did not increase in the luteal phase, whereas it increased significantly in the luteal phase in controls. Decreased melatonin immunoactivity could result from a phase delay in melatonin secretion or, more likely, from sympathetic hypofunction, which has been reported in migraine. Murialdo et al.[93] reported that nocturnal urinary melatonin immunoactivity was decreased in migraine without aura patients with menstrually triggered migraine (defined as migraine occurring 2 days before to 3 days after menses); however, they noted an increase in excretion during the luteal phase.

The difference between the two studies' results may be due to the fact that Brun used a less precise definition of menstrually related headache. Could the

Table 10.2   Preventive treatment of menstrual migraine

Perimenstrual use of standard drugs
Nonsteroidal anti-inflammatory drugs
Ergotamine and its derivatives
Magnesium
Hormonal therapy
    Estrogens (with or without androgens or progestin)
    Synthetic androgens (Danacrine)
    Antiestrogen (Tamoxifen)
    Dopamine agonists (Bromocriptine)
    Medical oophorectomy (gonadotropin-releasing hormone analogues)

Source: Reprinted with permission from SD Silberstein, G Merriam. Sex hormones and headache. J Pain Symptom Manage 1993;8:1.

headache have occurred premenstrually, during the luteal phase? It is recognized that melatonin secretion decreases during painful states (e.g., decreased melatonin secretion has been observed in cluster headache patients, in whom further decreases are associated with increased pain). A headache occurring during the premenstrual (luteal) phase could account for lower luteal melatonin excretion. However, McIntyre and Morse[94] could not find any difference in urinary immunoreactive 6-sulphatoxy melatonin levels between the early follicular and the late luteal phases of the menstrual cycle in healthy normal women or in patients with PMS. These findings do not support an involvement of melatonin in the development of PMS symptomatology or a role of melatonin in regulating ovulation in humans.

Treatment of Menstrual Migraine

The initial treatment of women who have migraine throughout their menstrual cycle should include general measures such as reassurance, identification and elimination of triggers, use of abortive and prophylactic medications and psychological modalities, and sleep hygiene (Table 10.2).[1]

Abortive therapy is used to decrease the duration and intensity of an individual attack and the associated symptoms of nausea and vomiting.[95] Preventive treatment should be considered when there are three or more attacks per month that are prolonged and unresponsive to abortive measures, or when abortive measures are contraindicated or produce significant side effects. Before preventive medication is initiated, analgesic or ergot overuse must be addressed.[95]

The goal of prophylactic therapy is to reduce the frequency, duration, and intensity of attacks. A 50% reduction without intolerable side effects is considered an acceptable outcome. If therapy is successful, dosages may be reduced after 4–6 months, with the ultimate aim of discontinuation. To ensure compliance, clinicians should educate patients concerning goals, dosages, benefits, and side effects of medication. Drug therapy should be started with low doses, which may be increased gradually based on response.[95] These measures may eliminate all headaches except those associated with menses.[96–98] MM typically occurs at the same time each month or in association with symptoms that herald its occurrence, allowing the timed use of medications.[1,2,97] Treatment of coexistent PMS may help control premenstrual headache.[99] Women who have migraine exclusively with their menses can be treated by the perimenstrual use of prophylactic medication (antidepressants, beta-blockers, calcium channel blockers, or methysergide).[1,2,95] Women already using prophylactic medication for nonmenstrual migraine can increase the dose of medication prior to their menses.

Nuclear magnetic resonance spectroscopy has shown magnesium deficiency in the cerebral cortex of migraineurs.[100] Ionized serum magnesium is low in some women who selectively respond to bolus intravenous magnesium.[101] A placebo-controlled double-blind study of 24 women with PMS and migraine has shown that oral magnesium (360 mg of magnesium pyrolidone carboxylic acid) decreases the severity of the PMS symptoms and the duration and intensity of MM occurring prior to the onset of menstruation.[102,103] Perhaps responders belong to the subset of women with low serum ionized magnesium.[101]

Popular but ineffective treatments include diuretics and vitamins. Diuretics help with fluid retention but not with MM.[16,104] The efficacy of pyridoxine to treat either PMS or MM has not been proven in double-blind studies.[105,106] In fact, high doses of pyridoxine have been reported to cause a sensory neuropathy.[107]

An attack of MM may be controlled by the use of NSAIDs, ergotamine, dihydroergotamine (DHE), or sumatriptan. Prostaglandin production may be enhanced in MM. The effectiveness of the NSAIDs[70,108] may be a result of their blocking prostaglandin synthesis by inhibiting the enzyme cyclooxygenase.[57] The meclofenamates, in addition, are prostaglandin receptor antagonists.[57] One NSAID, ketoprofen, inhibits the formation of leukotrienes by inhibiting 5-lipoxygenase.[57] NSAIDs in adequate doses can be used either abortively or prophylactically (beginning 1–2 days before the expected onset of headache and continuing for the duration of vulnerability).[109,110] If the first NSAID is ineffective, other classes of NSAIDs should be tried.

Ergotamine and DHE can be used prophylactically at the time of menses without significant risk of developing ergot dependence.[1,2,95,97] Ergotamine tartrate, at bedtime or twice a day, is an effective prophylactic agent.[2] Ergotamine in combination with belladonna and phenobarbital (Bellergal) may be useful in treating other perimenstrual symptoms in addition to headache.[110] Ergonovine maleate, an ergot derivative no longer available, provided a 65% improvement in severity and duration of headache when given perimenstrually.[111] Methylergonovine maleate is sometimes used in its place. DHE, currently available only in parenteral form, may be extremely effective in preventing and terminating MM.[112,113] In an open study, patients with MM responded equally as well to 1 mg of intramuscular DHE as did patients with nonmenstrual migraine.[114] Headache, nausea, and vomiting were all well controlled.

Sumatriptan is a selective 5-HT$_1$ agonist with specific activity at the 5-HT$_{1D}$ receptor site. A number of reviews of sumatriptan[115–117] have commented on subcutaneous sumatriptan's (6 mg) 86% efficacy and oral sumatriptan's (100 mg) 75% efficacy at 2 hours. By 24 hours, headache recurred in 35–40% of patients and was relieved with the same degree of efficacy by a second dose of sumatriptan. Subcutaneous sumatriptan is as effective for MM[118] as for nonmenstrually related migraine and, in addition, controls the nausea and vomiting associated with attacks.[117,119]

If severe MM cannot be controlled with NSAIDs, ergots, DHE, or sumatriptan, then analgesics in combination with narcotics,[95] high-dose corticosteroids, major tranquilizers (chlorpromazine, haloperidol, thiothixene), or a course of intravenous DHE can be tried.[113] If these therapies fail, a trial of hormonal therapy may be indicated. Successful hormonal therapy of MM has been reported with estrogens,[120] estrogen antagonists,[121] PRL-release inhibitors,[122] and estrogens in combination with progesterone or testosterone.[123] Progesterone is not effective in the treatment of headache or the symptoms of PMS,[122] despite many favorable anecdotal reports.[123,124]

The decrease in estrogen levels during the late luteal phase of the menstrual cycle is a trigger for migraine.[53,72] Estrogen replacement prior to menstruation has been used to prevent migraine.[56] In a double-blind crossover study, DeLignieres[120] used percutaneous estradiol gel perimenstrually with significant (30.8% versus 96.3%) headache reduction. In a double-blind trial of percutaneous estradiol gel, Dennerstein et al.[125] reported similar excellent results. Magos et al., in both an open study[126] and a double-blind study,[127] found estradiol implants (available investigationally in the United States) and cyclic progesterones to be effective in MM.

Somerville[56] attempted prophylaxis of menstrual migraine with estradiol implants. The implants did not produce stable plasma estrogen levels and caused severe menstrual disturbance, loss of periodicity of headaches, and unpredictable headache improvement. In contrast, the cutaneous gel[120] and the estradiol implant used by Magos et al.[127] provide stable blood estrogen levels. The estradiol cutaneous patch (Estraderm) provides a relatively stable plasma estrogen level over the time of application.[128–130] Levels are less stable with higher-dose patches. Serum estrogen levels rise within 4 hours of applying the transdermal patch and are proportional to the dose (patch Transdermal Therapeutic Systems [TTS] 25 ($\approx$ serum level of 23 pg per ml; TTS 50 $\approx$ 39 pg per ml; and TTS 100 $\approx$ 74 pg per ml).[131]

Pradalier et al.[132] found that using the TTS 25 patch from 4 days before to 4 days after menstruation was not as effective as using the TTS 100 patch. Dennerstein et al.[133] suggested that a serum estradiol level of 60–80 pg per ml is needed during the crucial week to prevent menstrual migraine. Pfaffenrath,[134] using TTS 50 patches, did not find a significant difference from placebo in a placebo-controlled double-blind trial. Similarly, Smits et al.[135] found minimal benefit of TTS 50 in a placebo-controlled trial, except for patients who had abnormal contingent negative variations and normal ES2. Women who received transdermal estradiol (two 100-mg patches) to suppress ovulation, supplemented by norethisterone, 5 mg on days 19 through 26 to ensure withdrawal bleeding, showed significant improvement in PMS symptoms at 6 months compared with those who received placebo.[136] During the first 3 months of the study there was a response to both placebo and active drug. The patches can be used both for contraception and treatment of PMS and MM in younger women for whom estrogens are not contraindicated or natural estrogens are preferred.

Combinations of estrogens and progestogens or progestogens alone in the form of OCs (discussed later in a separate section) may be a reasonable approach for some patients with intractable MM, particularly if it is associated with severe dysmenorrhea.[137] Anecdotally, the perimenstrual use of a synthetic oral estrogen (ethinyl estradiol, 0.05 mg) in combination with an androgen (methyl testosterone, 2 mg) was effective in 22 of 30 patients.[2]

Danazol (Danocrine),[121,138] an androgen derivative, suppresses the pituitary-ovarian axis by binding to androgen and progestogen receptors and by inhibiting ovarian steroidogenesis. It may be effective in the prophylaxis of menstrual migraine at a dose of 200–600 mg a day, starting before the expected onset of the headache and continuing through the menses.

Tamoxifen (Nolvadex),[139,140] an antiestrogen that binds to a cytosol estrogen receptor, may be effective in resistant MM. Its long-acting nuclear retention time results in estrogen antagonism by down-regulation of an estrogen receptor and inhibition of messenger RNA transcription. A dose of 5–15 mg per day for days 7–14 of the luteal cycle has provided significant relief of menstrual headache without side effects.

Bromocriptine (Parlodel),[141–144] a dopamine D2 receptor agonist, is an inhibitor of PRL release. A dose of 2.5–5.0 mg per day during the luteal phase of the menstrual cycle may decrease the premenstrual symptoms of breast engorgement, irritability, and headache. In an open trial,[145] 24 women with severe, disabling menstrual migraine (occurring within 3 days of menstruation) were treated with bromocriptine, 2.5 mg three times daily. Seventy-five percent of the women had at least a 25% reduction in headache compared with baseline. Overall headache frequency decreased by 72%. None of the patients had more than 10% increase in headache; three could not tolerate bromocriptine, and three did not benefit.

Neither hysterectomy nor oophorectomy has been proven to be effective in unselected cases in the treatment of migraine. However, medical ovariectomy using GnRH analogues to suppress ovulation are effective in refractory PMS.[17,146,147] In two placebo-controlled double-blind studies, GnRH was significantly better than placebo in controlling both behavioral and physical symptoms of PMS (headache, breast fullness and tenderness, bloating, and fatigue).[146,147] GnRH analogues may be effective in severe MM. Because GnRH analogues induce hypogonadism, with many of the same short-term and long-term side effects as menopause, treatment is usually limited to 6 months unless replacement estrogens are used.[17]

Adverse effects are related to profound hypoestrogenism and include hot flashes (91%), insomnia (55%), vaginal dryness (37%), and headache (39%). The onset of these symptoms clusters between 2 and 7 weeks after treatment is begun, when down-regulation of pituitary GnRH receptors is usually achieved.[148]

PMS sufferers who have had a hysterectomy without an oophorectomy continue to have cyclic mental and physical symptoms during the late luteal phase of the menstrual cycle, demonstrating that neither the presence of the uterus nor the occurrence of menstruation is necessary for the maintenance of PMS.[149]

Some physicians are again advocating the use of hysterectomy and oophorectomy in women with severe intractable PMS or MM who respond to medical ovariectomy.[150,151] There are no long-term follow-up or controlled studies to prove the effectiveness of this radical procedure. One retrospective study[150] reported oophorectomy in 14 women who responded to danazol suppression of ovulation. Postoperatively they were given conjugated estrogens without progestin. At 48-month follow-up, they were improved compared with their preoperative status. In another study,[151] 14 women with intractable PMS had total abdominal hysterectomy, bilateral salpingo-oophorectomy, and postoperative

Table 10.3   Menopausal symptoms

Early
  Hot flushes
    Associated with pulses of hypothalamic activity that lead to pulses of luteinizing
      hormone
    Atrophic vaginitis
  Psychological and somatic complaints
    Depression, anxiety, fatigue, dizziness, insomnia, altered libido, loss of concentration,
      headache
Late
  Dyspareunia, hirsutism, reduced breast size, dry skin, osteoporosis, arteriosclerotic
    cardiovascular disease

Source: Reprinted with permission from SD Silberstein, G Merriam. Sex hormones and headache. J Pain Symptom Manage 1993;8:1.

continuous estrogen replacement. At 6-month follow-up, none of the women had scores diagnostic of PMS.

The ability to gauge and interpret the effects of ovariectomy and hysterectomy on PMS and headache is contaminated by the postoperative use of daily estrogen. No study is placebo controlled, and women with PMS are very sensitive to placebo. The use of continuous estrogen alone could account for the positive results.[137] Until more conclusive data are available, we do not recommend oophorectomy for MM; instead, GnRH agonists should be used as a last resort, supplemented by estrogens (after 6 months), preferably in a patch or depo formulation. A sequential approach to the treatment of menstrual migraine is outlined in Table 10.2.

MIGRAINE IN MENOPAUSE

Normal menopause results from depletion of ovarian follicles that can be stimulated to ovulate. Sex steroid hormone levels are low and gonadotropin levels are elevated. The menopause is associated with both early and late symptoms (Table 10.3).[152,153] Hot flushes, representing a vasomotor change, correlate with bursts of activity in hypothalamic pacemaker neurons that lead to pulses of GnRH and thus LH.[154,155] Hormonal replacement with estrogens (estrogen replacement therapy), alone or in combination with progestins, is often used to treat symptoms and to prevent osteoporosis.[156,157] There is evidence that estrogen therapy decreases the risk of coronary artery disease and hip fracture, but long-term, unopposed estrogen therapy increases the risk of endometrial carcinoma.[158] The increase in endometrial cancer risk can probably be avoided by adding a progestin to the estrogen regimen for women who have a uterus, probably without reducing the beneficial effect on coronary artery disease risk.[156,159,160,161] The effect of estrogen replacement therapy on the risk of breast cancer is uncertain; studies continue to yield inconsistent results.[156] There appears to be no increased risk with short-term estrogen use, but the risk of breast cancer may increase slightly with long-term use. A mid-1995 review of 24 original articles and three meta-analyses

Table 10.4   Estrogen preparations

Conjugated steroidal estrogens
   Estrones
      Conjugated equine estrogens (Premarin, Estratab)
      From urine of pregnant mare (estrone sulfate, equilin sulfate, and 17-dihydroequilin)
         Oral (0.3, 0.625, 0.9, 1.25, 2.5 mg)
         Vaginal cream (0.00625%)
      Estropipate (Ogen)
         Oral (0.625, 1.25, 2.5 mg)
         Vaginal cream (0.15%)
   Estradiols
      Micronized 17-β-estradiol: Major natural estrogenic hormone
         Estrace
            Oral (1 or 2 mg)
            Vaginal cream (0.01%)
         Estraderm: Transdermal (0.05 or 0.1): Delivers 0.05 or 0.1 mg of estradiol per day
         Estrapel: Estradiol pellet (25 mg; investigational)
      Estradiol cypionate
         Depo-estradiol: Injection (1 or 5 mg/ml)
      Estradiol valerate
         Delestrogen, Estraval: Injection (10, 20, 40 mg/ml)
Nonconjugated steroidal estrogens
   17-ethinyl estradiol (Estinyl): Potent synthetic estrogen. Oral (0.02, 0.05, 0.5 mg)
   17-ethinyl estradiol-3-cyclopentoether (quinestrol; Estrovis). Oral (0.1 mg)
Synthetic estrogen analogues (nonsteroidal)
   Dienestrol (Ortho dienestrol cream, Estragard Cream): Vaginal cream (0.01%)

Source: Reprinted with permission from SD Silberstein, G Merriam. Sex hormones and headache. J Pain Symptom Manage 1993;8:1.

does not support an increased risk of breast cancer in women who ever used post-menopausal estrogens.[162]

The menopause presents a particular set of problems in women in whom estrogen replacement is indicated but leads to a worsening of migraine symptoms. The most commonly used estrogen, Premarin, is a mixture of estrogens including the equine estrogen equilin (Table 10.4).[130] Pure estrones, estradiols, and synthetic ethinyl estradiol are also available.[163] The lowest dose of estrogen that will effectively control symptoms should be used. Estrogens can be taken sequentially for 25 days per month with the addition of a progestational agent on days 16 through 25 to induce bleeding; alternatively, estrogens and progesterone can be taken continuously.[141] Estrogens are available orally or parenterally in the form of injection, vaginal cream, or transdermal patches.[130] Parenteral administration of estrogens produces fewer hepatic effects and a higher, more physiologic serum estradiol-to-estrone ratio than oral administration.[163,164] Experimental implants and transdermal patches provide stable blood estrogen levels;[155,156] however, estradiol pellets for implantation are available only on an investigational basis.[164] Adjunct hormones include progesterone[165] for prevention of endometrial cancer (not needed after hysterectomy) and androgens[166] for decreased libido and sexual responsiveness and perhaps for fatigue, depression, and headache.

Table 10.5 Treatment of estrogen replacement headache

Reduce estrogen dose
Change estrogen type from conjugated estrogen to pure estradiol to synthetic estrogen to
  pure estrone
Convert from interrupted to continuous dosing
Convert from oral to parenteral dosing
Add androgens

Source: Reprinted with permission from SD Silberstein, G Merriam. Sex hormones and headache. J Pain Symptom Manage 1993;8:1.

Although migraine prevalence decreases with advancing age,[5] migraine can either regress or worsen at menopause.[13] Neri et al.[14] investigated 556 consecutive postmenopausal women attending an outpatient clinic and found that headache was present in 13.7%. Most (82%) of the 13% who had headache had had headaches prior to the onset of menopause. Many (62%) had migraine without aura; the remainder had tension-type headaches. None of the women had migraine with aura or cluster headache. Women with prior migraine generally (two-thirds of the time) improved with physiologic menopause. In contrast, surgical menopause usually (two-thirds of the time) resulted in a worsening of migraine. Other studies have shown that hysterectomy or oophorectomy is not an effective treatment for migraine at any age,[167,168] despite recent suggestions to the contrary.[150,151] Estrogen replacement therapy can exacerbate migraine[11,169,170] or—alone[171] or with testosterone[172]—relieve it. This has been confirmed in one,[173] but not another,[174] double-blind study. The use of drugs for the treatment of migraine in menopausal women who do not need replacement estrogens should be guided by their cardiac and renal status.[141] Refractory cases may be treated with hormonal replacement.[133]

Headache management can be difficult in women who require estrogen replacement therapy for menopausal symptoms but develop headaches as a result of the therapy. Several empirical strategies may be used (Table 10.5). Reducing the dose of estrogen or changing the type of estrogen from a conjugated estrogen to pure estradiol, to synthetic ethinyl estradiol, or to a pure estrone may significantly reduce headache. Aylward et al.,[169] in a controlled double-blind crossover trial of menopausal women, found that oral estropipate decreased the frequency and intensity of headache, whereas ethinyl estradiol increased the headache. Changing from interrupted to continuous administration may be effective if the headaches are associated with estrogen withdrawal. Techniques may be combined. Kudrow[11] reported a 58% improvement in headache control with a reduced, continuous dose of estrogen. Parenteral estrogens, with or without adjunct hormones, can be effective. Greenblatt and Bruneteau[172] studied postmenopausal women with oral estrogen–induced headaches and found that their headaches could be improved by switching from oral to parenteral estrogens (estradiol) and adding androgens (testosterone). The estradiol cutaneous patch (Estraderm), which provides a physiologic ratio of estradiol to estrone and a steady-state concentration of estrogen, has been associated anecdotally with fewer headache side effects; however, this benefit has not been proven in any controlled study.[126,127,129]

MIGRAINE ASSOCIATED WITH ORAL CONTRACEPTIVE USE

Hormonal contraceptive steroids are available as oral preparations, subcutaneous implants, depo-injections, and vaginal preparations (in some countries).[175] The transdermal estrogen patch has been advocated for contraception by some.[130,136] The OCs most commonly used in the United States contain combinations of synthetic estrogen (ethinyl estradiol or mestranol) and synthetic progestin (derivatives of 9-norprogesterone) taken 21 days each month.[176,177] OCs interfere with the midcycle gonadotropin surge at both the hypothalamic and pituitary levels, thus preventing ovulation.[141] Another method of contraception uses a progestin alone, which inhibits the LH surge.[141] This progestin-only contraception would be expected to have fewer systemic side effects, but it is less effective and is associated with a high incidence of irregular bleeding.[175,178] The ethinyl estradiol content in combined OCs has progressively decreased; most now contain 35 mg or less. In an attempt to minimize the associated androgenic side effects, the type of synthetic progestin has been changed. The newest (desogestrel, gestodene, norgestimate) are less androgenic and have less effect on carbohydrate and lipid metabolism than prior progestins.[178] They appear to produce relatively minor effects on the coagulation system.[175] The new formulations of OCs, containing 35 mg of ethinyl estradiol and one of the new progestins, are comparable in efficacy to each other and to established agents.[175,178–182]

Controversy has persisted concerning OCs and the risk of stroke in migraineurs.[12] During the last two decades, at least 15 retrospective studies have looked at the influence of OCs on the risk of cerebral thromboembolic events. Most (11 of 15) were conducted during a period when high-dose estrogen pills were widely used. These data suggest that OCs containing more than 50 mg, 50 mg, and 30–40 mg of estrogen are associated with odds ratios for cerebral thromboembolic attacks of about 8–10, 2–4, and 1.5–2.5, respectively, whereas those containing only a progestin are not associated with any increased risk. Smoking was associated with an odds ratio of 1.5–1.6, independent of age and use or nonuse of OCs.[183] The Collaborative Group for the Study of Stroke in Young Women did not confirm reports that migraine may increase the risk of stroke in women using OCs.[184] Migraine itself may be a risk factor for stroke.

The older combined OCs can induce, change, or alleviate headache.[12] OCs can trigger the first migraine attack, most often in women with a family history of migraine.[11,12,185] Existing migraine may be exacerbated, and headaches may occur on the days off the OC.[12,13,185,186] The headaches may become more severe and frequent and may be associated with neurologic symptoms.[185–187] In most women, however, the headache pattern does not change, and some women may have a distinct improvement in their headaches.[188,189]

New onset of migraine usually occurs in the early cycles of OC use, but it can occur after prolonged OC use.[185] Stopping the OC may not bring immediate headache relief; there may be a delay of 6 months to 1 year, or no improvement.[13,187]

Studies from neurologic or migraine clinics show increased incidence and severity of migraine in users of the older OCs (Table 10.6).[186,187,190] Although headaches frequently occur on the days off the OC, Whitty[13] found that many women had relief with certain OCs, and Ryan[185] found that 12 of 40 of his patients improved. Studies from contraceptive clinics and general practitioners (Table 10.7) have shown results more favorable toward OCs. Larsson-Cohen and Lundberg,[189] Diddle,[191] Ramchurian et al.,[192] Kappius and Goolkasian,[137] and others[193–195] reported either improvement or

Table 10.6   Oral contraceptives and headaches: neurologic and migraine clinics

Study	Year	Country	Type	No. studied	Effect of contraceptive
Whitty et al.[188]	1966	United Kingdom	Retrospective	50	Decreased attack frequency in many women. Remaining migraine attacks increased in severity in days off OC
Phillips[186]	1968	United Kingdom	Retrospective	41	21 patients reported new migraine on OC. 78% of migraine patients had increased severity and frequency of headache on OC
Carroll[190]	1971	United Kingdom	Retrospective	290	Increased frequency or intensity of migraine in 49%
Kudrow[11]	1975	United States	Retrospective	60	Increased migraine frequency in OC users versus nonusers Stopping OC decreased migraine frequency in 70% of patients
Dalton[187]	1976	United Kingdom	Retrospective	886	Increased migraine frequency in 34% of OC users and 60% of ex-OC users. New migraine in 5%. Stopping OC decreased migraine in 39% of ex-OC users
Ryan[185]	1978	United States	Prospective, 4 mo	40	40 migraine patients treated with OC: 12 better, 28 worse

OC = oral contraceptive.

Source: Reprinted with permission from SD Silberstein, G Merriam. Sex hormones and headache. J Pain Symptom Manage 1993;8:1.

no worsening of migraine in OC users. The headaches that occurred appeared to cluster around the menses. Aznar-Ramos et al.[196] gave placebo to 147 women who believed they were getting an OC and found a headache incidence of 15.6%. A study from the Philippines[197] of 1,800 women using three different low-dose estrogen OCs reported headache incidence between 5.2% and 8.0%, significantly below that reported with placebo. Four double-blind placebo-controlled studies[198–201] showed no difference in headache incidence between OC and placebo. Both groups had a decreasing incidence of headache with continued observation. Some uncontrolled studies show an increase in headache frequency in women using OCs.[202–205]

A new OC containing 35 mg of the new, third-generation progestin, Norgestimate (Ortho-Cyclen), was associated with a low incidence of headaches over three cycle intervals (5% after the third cycle, 3% after the sixth cycle) in an open prospective study.[180] A review of studies for the new combined OC containing 150 mg of desogestrel and 30 mg of ethinyl estradiol found headache incidence to be low (approximately 5% at the sixth cycle).[206]

Contraception with progestins alone is a hormonal alternative to the use of the combined OCs. Progestins have no effect on blood clotting or platelet aggregation and are

Table 10.7   Oral contraceptives and headaches: contraceptive clinics and general practitioners

Study	Year	Country	Type	No. studied	Effects of contraceptive
Nilsson et al.[202]	1967	Sweden	R	281	Increased headache symptoms, 20.2% of OC users. Decreased headache symptoms, 14.7% of OC users
Nilsson and Solwell[198]	1967	Sweden	P, 12 mo; DB CO	159	Headache incidence: 50% during treatment with placebo and OC
Grant[203]	1968	United Kingdom	P, 12 mo	532	Headache incidence: 17% pretreatment, 29% on OC
Aznar-Ramos et al.[196]	1969	Mexico	P, 12 mo; placebo only	147	Headache incidence: 15.6% on placebo
Cullberg et al.[204]	1969	Sweden	P, 6 mo	99	New headache in 2% of OC users
Diddle et al.[191]	1969	United States	P	10,889	Headache incidence: 8% of controls, 3.2% of OC users. New headaches in 0.8% of OC users
Herzberg and Coppers[193]	1970	United Kingdom	P, 11 mo; IUD controls	163	Headache incidence (moderate to severe): 5 wk: 4% on OC, 0% on IUD; 11 mo: 2% on OC, 0% on IUD
Larsson-Cohn and Lundberg[189]	1970	Sweden	P, 12 mo	1,676	New migraine in 10% of OC users. Migaine patients: 36% improved, 18% worsened on OCs
Herzberg et al.[194]	1971	United Kingdom	P, 12 mo; IUD controls	272	Headache incidence: 5 mo, OC = IUD; 10 mo, OC > IUD
Goldzieher et al.[199]	1971	United States	P, 6 mo; DB placebo CO	398	Headache incidence decreased 68% with both placebo and OC
Silbergeld et al.[200]	1971	United States	P, 4 mo; DB placebo CO	8	No increase in headache with OC
Cullberg[201]	1972	Sweden	P, 2 mo; DB placebo CO	332	No difference in headache frequency between OC and placebo
Desrosiers[205]	1973	Canada	P	125	Headache incidence: 27.4% pretreatment; 36.8% on OC
Royal College General Practitioners[195]	1974	United Kingdom	P, 48 mo	46,000	No evidence that headache is a pharmacologic side effect of OC use

Study	Year	Country	Type	No. studied	Effects of contraceptive
Ramchurian et al.[192]	1980	United States	P, 96 mo	16,638	No evidence of increased frequency of migraine or tension headache in OC users
Kappius and Goolkasian[137]	1987	United States	P, 2 mo	78	Headache on OCs less severe, less frequent, clustered around menses
Ramos et al.[197]	1989	The Philippines	P, 12 mo	1,800	Headache incidence on OC: 0–3 mo, 6%; 10–12 mo, 2%; 2.7% stopped OC because of headache

R = retrospective; P = prospective; OC = oral contraceptive; DB = double blind; CO = crossover; IUD = intrauterine device.

Source: Reprinted with permission from SD Silberstein, G Merriam. Sex hormones and headache. J Pain Symptom Manage 1993;8:1.

the contraceptive of choice for hypertensive women.[175] Norplant, a system of subdermal implants that release a steady dose of levonorgestrel (a progestin), is an effective contraceptive that lasts 5 years. The primary side effects are irregular menstrual bleeding and headaches. Headache, which was the primary reason cited for removal other than menstrual disturbance, occurs in approximately 5–20% of patients. The cumulative headache rate was 6.4 per 100 by the end of the second year.[207] In one study, headache was a complaint of 4% of women at 3 months compared with 2% of women using a copper IUD.[208] A new system, Norplant II, using two implanted rods instead of five, is being tested.[209] Recently, Depo-Provera (medroxyprogesterone acetate suspension), a long-acting parenteral progestin, has been approved as a contraceptive agent. The exact frequency of headache with its use is uncertain.

OCs may generate new headaches or aggravate or ameliorate preexisting headaches. This variability is also noted with pregnancy and menopause and may be a consequence of a variation in intrinsic neuronal response to estrogen. Women with intractable menstrual migraine or a history of headache relief with OCs may be candidates for a trial of OC. They must be followed for headache aggravation or the development of neurologic symptoms. Progestins can be used for contraception when estrogens have caused increased headaches or are otherwise contraindicated.

CONCLUSION

The normal female life cycle is associated with a number of hormonal milestones: menarche, pregnancy, contraceptive use, menopause, and the use of replacement sex hormones. Menarche marks the onset of menses and cyclic changes in hormone levels. Pregnancy is associated with rising noncyclic levels of sex hormones, and menopause with declining noncyclic levels. Hormonal contraceptive use during the reproductive years and hormone replacement in menopause are therapeutic hormonal interventions that alter the levels and cycling of sex hormones. These events and interventions may cause a change in the prevalence or intensity of headache.

The menstrual cycle is the result of a carefully orchestrated sequence of interactions between the hypothalamus, pituitary, ovary, and endometrium, in which the sex hormones act as modulators and effectors at each level. Estrogen and progestins have potent effects on central serotonergic and opioid neurons, modulating both neuronal activity and receptor density. The primary trigger of MM appears to be the withdrawal of estrogen rather than the maintenance of sustained high or low estrogen levels. However, changes in the sustained estrogen levels with pregnancy (increased) and menopause (decreased) also appear to affect headaches.

Headaches that occur with PMS appear to be centrally generated, involving the inherent rhythm of CNS neurons, perhaps including the serotonergic pain-modulating systems. Headaches associated with OC use or menopausal hormonal replacement therapy may be related, in part, to periodic discontinuation of oral sex hormone preparations. The treatment of migraine associated with changes in sex hormone levels is frequently difficult, and the condition is often refractory. Based on what is known of the pathophysiology of migraine, we have attempted to provide a logical approach to the treatment of headaches that are associated with menses, menopause, and OCs using abortive and preventive medications and hormonal manipulations.

REFERENCES

1. Silberstein SD, Merriam GR. Estrogens, progestins, and headache. Neurology 1991;41:786.
2. Raskin NH. Headache (2nd ed). New York: Churchill Livingstone, 1988.
3. Selby G, Lance JW. Observations on 500 cases of migraine and allied vascular headache. J Neurol Neurosurg Psychiatry 1960;23:23.
4. Epstein MT, Hockaday JM, Hockaday TDR. Migraine and reproductive hormones throughout the menstrual cycle. Lancet 1975;1:543.
5. Goldstein M, Chen TC. The Epidemiology of Disabling Headache. In M Critchley (ed), Advances in Neurology (Vol. 33). New York: Raven, 1982;377.
6. Waters WE, O'Connor PJ. Epidemiology of headache and migraine in women. J Neurol Neurosurg Psychiatry 1971;34:148.
7. American Psychiatric Association. Diagnostic and Statistical Manual of Mental Disorders (4th ed). Washington, DC: American Psychiatric Association, 1994.
8. Somerville BW. A study of migraine in pregnancy. Neurology 1972;22:824.
9. Lance JW, Anthony M. Some clinical aspects of migraine. Arch Neurol 1966;15:356.
10. Ratinahirana H, Darbois Y, Bousser MG. Migraine and pregnancy: A prospective study in 703 women after delivery. Neurology 1990;40:437.
11. Kudrow L. The relationship of headache frequency to hormone use in migraine. Headache 1975;15:36.
12. Bickerstaff ER. Neurological Complications of Oral Contraceptives. Oxford: Clarendon, 1975.
13. Whitty CWM, Hockaday JM. Migraine: A follow-up study of 92 patients. Br Med J Clin Res 1968;1:735.
14. Neri I, Granella F, Nappi R, Manzoni GC, et al. Characteristics of headache at menopause: A clinico-epidemiologic study. Maturitas 1993;17:31.
15. Welch KMA, Darnley D, Simkins RT. The role of estrogen in migraine: A review. Cephalalgia 1984;4:227.
16. Lundberg PO. Endocrine Headaches. In FC Rose (ed), Handbook of Clinical Neurology, Vol 48. New York: Elsevier, 1986;431.
17. Conn PM, Crowley WF. Gonadotropin-releasing hormone and its analogues. N Engl J Med 1991;324:93.

18. Fink G, Stanley HF, Watts AG. Central Nervous Control of Sex and Gonadotropin Release: Peptide and Nonpeptide Transmitter Interactions. In D Krieger, M Brownstein, J Martin (eds), Brain Peptides. New York: Wiley, 1983;413.

19. Behrman HR, Caldwell BV. Prostaglandins, Thromboxanes, and Leukotrienes. In SCC Yen, RB Jaffe (eds), Reproductive Endocrinology: Physiology, Pathophysiology, and Clinical Management. Philadelphia: Saunders, 1986.

20. Dierschke DJ, Bhattacharya AN, Atkinson LE, Knobil E. Circhoral oscillations of plasma LH in the ovariectomized rhesus monkey. Endocrinology 1970;87:850.

21. Belchetz P, Plant TM, Nakai Y, Keogh EJ, et al. Hypophysial responses to continuous and intermittent delivery of hypothalamic gonadotropin-releasing hormone. Science 1978;202:631.

22. Merriam GR, Brody SA, Collins RL, Evans WS, et al. Episodic Gonadotropin Secretion in Normal and Hyperprolactinemic Men and Women. In C Dotti (ed), Gonadotropins and Prolactin. Milan: Dotti, 1984;61.

23. Filicori M, Butler JP, Crowley WF Jr. Neuroendocrine regulation of the corpus luteum in the human: Evidence for pulsatile progesterone secretion. J Clin Invest 1984;73:1639.

24. Backstrom CT, McNeilly AS, Leask RM, Baird DT. Pulsatile secretion of LH, FSH, prolactin, oestradiol, and progesterone during the human menstrual cycle. Clin Endocrinol 1982;17:29.

25. McNatty PK, Makris A, DeGrazia C, Osathanondh R, et al. Effects of luteinizing hormone on steroidogenesis by thecal tissue from human ovarian follicles in vitro. Steroids 1980;36:53.

26. Ryan KJ, Petro Z. Steroid biosynthesis by human ovarian granulosa and theca cells. J Clin Endocrinol Metab 1966;26:46.

27. Ryan KJ, Petro Z, Kaiser J. Steroid formation by isolated and recombined ovarian granulosa and thecal cells. J Clin Endocrinol Metab 1968;28:355.

28. Batista MC, Cartledge TP, Zellmer A, Merriam GR, et al. The antiprogesterone RU 486 delays ovulation in spontaneous and GnRH-induced menstrual cycles [Abstract 1634]. Endocrine Society 71st Annual Meeting, Seattle, Washington, 1989;431.

29. Laborde N, Carril M, Cheviakoff A, et al. The secretion of progesterone during the periovulatory period in women with certified ovulations. J Clin Endocrinol Metab 1976;43:1157.

30. Pfaff DW, McEwen BS. Actions of estrogens and progestins on nerve cells. Science 1983;219:808.

31. Parker MG. Structure and function of the oestrogen receptor. J Neuroendocrinol 1993;5:223.

32. Schumacher M. Rapid membrane effects of steroid hormones: An emerging concept in neuroendocrinology. Trends Neurosci 1990;13:359.

33. Biegon A, Reches A, Snyder L, McEwen BS. Serotonergic and noradrenergic receptors in the rat brain: Modulation by chronic exposure to ovarian hormones. Life Sci 1983;32:2015.

34. Clarke WP, Goldfarb J. Estrogen enhances a 5-HT$_{1A}$ response in hippocampal slices from female rats. Eur J Pharmacol 1989;160:195.

35. Gordon JH, Diamond BI. Antagonism of dopamine supersensitivity by estrogen: Neurochemical studies in an animal model of tardive dyskinesia. Biol Psychiatry 1981;16:365.

36. Bereiter DA, Stanford LR, Barker DJ. Hormone-induced enlargement of receptive fields in trigeminal mechanoreceptive neurons. II: Possible mechanisms. Brain Res 1980;184:411.

37. Baunea A, Hajibeigi A, Trant JM, Mason JI. Expression of steroid-metabolizing enzymes by brain cells in culture: A model for developmental regulation of the progesterone 5X-reductase pathway. Endocrinology 1990;127:500.

38. Harris NL, Majewska MD, Harrington JW, Barker JL. Structure-activity relationships for steroid interaction with the gamma-aminobutyric acid receptor complex. J Pharmacol Exp Ther 1987;241:346.

39. Rubinow DR, Roy-Byrne P, Hoban MC, Gold PW, et al. Prospective assessment of menstrually related mood disorders. Am J Psychiatry 1984;141:686.

40. Schmidt PJ, Nieman LK, Grover GN, Muller KL, et al. Lack of effect of induced menses on symptoms in women with premenstrual syndrome. N Engl J Med 1991;324:1174.

41. Nattero G. Menstrual Headache. In M Critchley (ed), Advances in Neurology (Vol 33). New York: Raven, 1982;215.

42. MacGregor EA, Chia H, Vohrah RC, Wilkinson M. Migraine and menstruation: A pilot study. Cephalalgia 1990;10:305.

43. Solbach P, Sargent J, Coyne L. Menstrual migraine headache: Results of a controlled, experimental, outcome study of nondrug treatments. Headache 1984;24:75.

44. Johannes CB, Linet MS, Stewart WF, Celentano DD, et al. Relationship of headache to phase of the menstrual cycle among young women: A daily diary study. Neurology 1995;45:1076.

45. Beckham JC, Krug LM, Penzien DB, et al. The relationship of ovarian steroids, headache activity, and menstrual distress: A pilot study with female migraineurs. Headache 1992;32:292.

46. Keenan PA, Lindamer LA. Nonmigraine headache across the menstrual cycle in women with and without premenstrual syndrome. Cephalalgia 1992;12:356.
47. Woods NF, Most A, Dery GK. Estimating perimenstrual distress: A comparison of two methods. Res Nurs Health 1982;34:263.
48. Cupini LM, Matteis M, Troisi E, Calabresi P, et al. Sex-hormone–related events in migrainous females: A clinical comparative study between migraine with aura and migraine without aura. Cephalalgia 1995;15:140.
49. Facchinetti F, Neri I, Martignoni E, Fioroni L, et al. The association of menstrual migraine with the premenstrual syndrome. Cephalalgia 1993;13:422.
50. Silberstein SD. Menstrual migraine (editorial). Headache 1992;32:312.
51. Davies PTG, Eccles NK, Steiner TJ, Leathard HL, et al. Plasma oestrogen, progesterone and sex-hormone binding globulin levels in the pathogenesis of migraine. Cephalalgia 1989;9:143.
52. Facchinetti F, Sances G, Volpe A, et al. Hypothalamus pituitary-ovarian axis in menstrual migraine: Effects of dihydroergotamine retard prophylactic treatment. Cephalalgia 1983;1:159.
53. Somerville BW. The role of estradiol withdrawal in the etiology of menstrual migraine. Neurology 1972;22:355.
54. Somerville BW. The role of progesterone in menstrual migraine. Neurology 1971;21:853.
55. Somerville BW. Estrogen-withdrawal migraine. I: Duration of exposure required and attempted prophylaxis by premenstrual estrogen administration. Neurology 1975;25:239.
56. Somerville BW. Estrogen-withdrawal migraine. II: Attempted prophylaxis by continuous estradiol administration. Neurology 1975;25:245.
57. Moncada S, Flower RJ, Vane JR. Prostaglandins, Prostacyclin, Thromboxane A2, and Leukotrienes. In AG Gilman, LS Goodman, TW Rall, F Murad (eds), The Pharmacological Basis of Therapeutics. New York: Macmillan, 1985.
58. Moskowitz MA. The neurobiology of vascular head pain. Ann Neurol 1984;16:157.
59. Brody MJ, Kadowitz PJ. Prostaglandins as modulators of the autonomic nervous system. Fed Proc 1974;33:48.
60. Samuelsson B, Wennmalm A. Increased nerve stimulation induced release of noradrenaline from the rabbit heart after inhibition of prostaglandin synthesis. Acta Physiol Scand 1971;83:163.
61. Stjarne L. Prostaglandin- versus adrenoceptor-mediated control of sympathetic neurotransmitter secretion in guinea-pig isolated vas deferens. Eur J Pharmacol 1973;22:233.
62. Levine J, Taiwo YO, Collins SD, Tam JK. Noradrenaline hyper algesia is mediated through interaction with sympathetic postganglionic neurone terminals rather than activation of primary afferent nociceptors. Nature 1986;323:158.
63. Carlson LA, Ekelund LG, Oro L. Clinical and metabolic effects of different doses of prostaglandin E1 in man. Acta Med Scand 1968;183:423.
64. Peatfield RC, Gawel MJ, Rose FC. The effect of infused prostacyclin in migraine and cluster headache. Headache 1981;21:190.
65. Buzzi MG, Sakas DE, Moskowitz MA. Indomethacin and acetylsalicylic acid block neurogenic plasma protein extravasation in rat dura mater. Eur J Pharmacol 1989;165:251.
66. Saito K, Markowitz S, Moskowitz MA. Ergot alkaloids specifically block the development of neurogenic inflammation within the dura mater induced by chemical or electrical stimulation. Ann Neurol 1988;24:732.
67. Taiwo YO, Levine JD. Prostaglandins inhibit endogenous pain control mechanisms by blocking transmission at spinal noradrenergic synapses. J Neurosci 1988;8:1346.
68. Ferreira SH, Lorenzetti BB, Correa FMA. Blockade of central and peripheral generation of prostaglandins explains the antialgic effect of aspirin-like drugs. Pol J Pharmacol Pharm 1978;30:133.
69. Akerlund M. Pathophysiology of dysmenorrhea. Acta Obstet Gynecol Scand 1979;87:27.
70. Chan WY. Prostaglandins and nonsteroidal anti-inflammatory drugs in dysmenorrhea. Annu Rev Pharmacol Toxicol 1983;23:131.
71. Pickles VR. Prostaglandins and dysmenorrhea. Acta Obstet Gynecol Scand 1979;87:7.
72. Nattero G, Allais G, DeLorenzo C, et al. Relevance of prostaglandins in true menstrual migraine. Headache 1989;29:232.
73. Irwin J, Morse E, Riddick D. Dysmenorrhea induced by autologous transfusion. Obstet Gynecol 1981;58:286.
74. Grant ECG. Relation of arterioles in the endometrium to headache from oral contraceptives. Lancet 1965;1:1143.
75. Yen SSC. Prolactin in Human Reproduction. In SSC Yen, RB Jaffe (eds), Reproductive Endocrinology, Physiology, Pathophysiology, and Clinical Management. Philadelphia: Saunders, 1986.

76. Papakostas Y, Daras M, Markianos M, Stefanis C. Increased prolactin response to thyrotropin-releasing hormone during migraine attacks. J Neurol Neurosurg Psychiatry 1987;50:927.

77. Murialdo G, Martignoni E, DeMaria A, et al. Changes in the dopaminergic control of prolactin secretion and in ovarian steroids in migraine. Cephalalgia 1986;6:43.

78. Awaki E, Takeshima T, Takahashi K. A neuroendocrinological study in female migraineurs: Prolactin and thyroid-stimulating hormone responses. Cephalalgia 1989;9:187.

79. Klimek A. Growth Hormone and Prolactin Release in Migraine Patients. In V Pfaffenrath, P-O Lundberg, O Sjaastad (eds), Updating in Headache. New York: Springer, 1983;241.

80. Nattero G, Corno M, Savi L, Isaia GC, et al. Prolactin and migraine: Effect of L-dopa on plasma prolactin levels in migraineurs and normals. Headache 1986;26:9.

81. Yen SSC. Neuroendocrine Control of Hypophyseal Function. In SSC Yen, RB Jaffe (eds), Reproductive Endocrinology, Physiology, Pathophysiology, and Clinical Management. Philadelphia: Saunders, 1986.

82. Dyer RG, Bicknell RJ. Brain Opioid Systems in Reproduction. New York: Oxford University Press, 1989.

83. DeCree C. Endogenous opioid peptides in the control of the normal menstrual cycle and their possible role in athletic menstrual irregularities. Obstet Gynecol Surv 1989;44:720.

84. Nappi G, Martignoni E. Significance of Hormonal Changes in Primary Headache Disorders. In J Elesen, L Edvinsson (eds), Basic Mechanisms of Headache. New York: Elsevier, 1988;277.

85. Genazzani AR, Petraglia F, Volpe A, Facchinetti F. Estrogen changes as a critical factor in modulation of central opioid tonus: Possible correlations with postmenopausal migraine. Cephalalgia 1985;2:211.

86. Rubinow DR, Hoban MC, Grover GN, Anderson R, et al. Changes in plasma hormones across the menstrual cycle in patients with menstrually related mood disorders and controls. Am J Obstet Gynecol 1988;158:5.

87. Facchinetti F, Genazzani AD, Martignoni E, Fioroni L, et al. Neuroendocrine correlates of premenstrual syndrome: Changes in the pulsatile pattern of plasma LH. Psychoneuroendocrinology 1990;15:269.

88. Facchinetti F, Martignoni E, Nappi G, Fioroni L, et al. Premenstrual failure of α-adrenergic stimulation on hypothalamus–pituitary responses in menstrual migraine. Psychosom Med 1989;51:550.

89. Polinsky RJ, Brown RT, Lee GK, et al. β-Endorphin, ACTH, and catecholamine responses in chronic autonomic failure. Ann Neurol 1987;21:573.

90. Bach FW, Jensen K, Blegvad N, Fenger M, et al. β-Endorphin and ACTH in plasma during attacks of common and classic migraine. Cephalalgia 1985;5:177.

91. Brown GM. Melatonin in psychiatric and sleep disorders: Therapeutic implications. CNS Drugs 1995;3:210.

92. Brun J, Claustrat B, Saddier P, Chazol G. Nocturnal melatonin excretion is decreased in patients with migraine without aura attacks associated with menses. Cephalalgia 1995;15:136.

93. Murialdo G, Fonzi S, Costelli P, Solinas GP, et al. Urinary melatonin excretion throughout the ovarian cycle in menstrually related migraine. Cephalalgia 1994;14:205.

94. McIntyre IM, Morse C. Urinary 6-sulphatoxy melatonin levels within the menstrual cycle and in patients with premenstrual syndrome. Psychoneuroendocrinology 1990;15:233.

95. Silberstein SD, Saper J. Migraine: Diagnosis and Treatment. In D Dalessio, SD Silberstein (eds), Wolff's Headache and Other Head Pain (6th ed). New York: Oxford University Press, 1993;96.

96. Digre KB, Damasio H. Menstrual migraine: Differential diagnosis, evaluation, and treatment. Clin Obstet Gynecol 1987;30:417.

97. Edelson RN. Menstrual migraine and other hormonal aspects of migraine. Headache 1985;25:376.

98. Silberstein SD, Lipton RB. Overview of diagnosis and treatment of migraine. Neurology 1994;44:6.

99. DeMonico SO, Brown CS, Ling FW. Premenstrual syndrome. Obstet Gynecol 1994;6:499.

100. Ramadan NM, Halvorson H, Vande-Linde A, Levine SR, et al. Low brain magnesium in migraine. Headache 1989;29:416.

101. Mauskop A, Altura BT, Cracco RQ, Altura BM. Intravenous magnesium sulfate relieves acute migraine in patients with low serum ionized magnesium levels [Abstract]. Neurology 1995;45:A379.

102. Facchinetti F, Montorsi S, Borella P, Sances G, et al. Magnesium Prevention of Premenstrual Migraine: A Placebo-Controlled Study. In FC Rose (ed), New Advances in Headache Research (2nd ed). London: Smith-Gordon, 1991.

103. Facchinetti F, Borella P, Sances G, Fioroni L, et al. Oral magnesium successfully relieves premenstrual mood changes. Obstet Gynecol 1991;78:177.

104. Reid RL, Yen SSC. Premenstrual syndrome. Am J Obstet Gynecol 1981;139:85.

105. Williams MJ, Harris RI, Dean BC. Controlled trial of pyridoxine in the premenstrual syndrome. J Int Med Res 1985;1:174.

106. Hagen I, Nesheim B, Tuntland T. No effect of vitamin B-6 against premenstrual tension: A controlled clinical study. Acta Obstet Gynecol Scand 1985;64:667.
107. Schaumburg H, Kaplan J, Windebank A, Vick N, et al. Sensory neuropathy from pyridoxine abuse. N Engl J Med 1983;309:445.
108. Vardi J, Rabey JM, Streifler M. Prostaglandins and Their Synthesis Inhibitors in Migraine. In SMM Karin (ed), Practical Applications of Prostaglandins and Their Synthesis Inhibitors. Baltimore: University Park Press, 1979;139.
109. Sargent J, Solbach P, Damasio H, et al. A comparison of naproxen sodium to propranolol hydrochloride and a placebo control for the prophylaxis of migraine headache. Headache 1985;25:320.
110. Robinson K, Huntington KM, Wallace MG. Treatment of the premenstrual syndrome. Br J Obstet Gynaecol 1977;84:784.
111. Gallagher, RM. Menstrual migraine and intermittent ergonovine therapy. Headache 1989;29:366.
112. D'Alessandro R, Gamberini G, Lozito A, Sacquegna T. Menstrual migraine: Intermittent prophylaxis with a timed-release pharmacological formulation of dihydroergotamine. Cephalalgia 1983;15:158.
113. Silberstein SD, Schulman EA, McFadden-Hopkins M. Repetitive intravenous DHE in the treatment of refractory headache. Headache 1990;30:334.
114. Winner P, Sheftel F, Sadowsky C, Dalessio D, et al. A profile of menstrual migraine sufferers. Cephalalgia 1993;13:242.
115. Ferrari MD, Saxena PR. Clinical and experimental effects of sumatriptan in humans. Trends Pharmacol Sci 1993;14:129.
116. Bateman DN. Sumatriptan. Lancet 1993;341:221.
117. Tfelt-Hansen P. Sumatriptan for the treatment of migraine attacks: A review of controlled clinical trials. Cephalalgia 1993;13:238.
118. Solbach MP, Waymer RS. Treatment of menstruation-associated migraine headache with subcutaneous sumatriptan. Obstet Gynecol 1993;82:769.
119. Sheftel F, Silberstein SD, Rapoport A. Pharmacological treatment of chronic headache. Drug Therapy 1992;22:47.
120. DeLignieres B, Vincens M, Mauvais-Jarvis P, Mas JL, et al. Prevention of menstrual migraine by percutaneous oestradiol. Br Med J Clin Res 1986;293:1540.
121. Calton GJ, Burnett JW. Danazol and migraine. N Engl J Med 1984;310:721.
122. Freeman E, Rickels K, Sondheimer SJ, Polansky M. Ineffectiveness of progesterone suppository treatment for premenstrual syndrome. JAMA 1990;264:349.
123. Dalton K. Progesterone suppositories and pessaries in the treatment of menstrual migraine. Headache 1973;13:151.
124. Bancroft J, Backstrom T. Premenstrual syndrome. Clin Endocrinol 1985;22:313.
125. Dennerstein L, Morse C, Burrows G, Oats J, et al. Menstrual migraine: A double-blind trial of percutaneous estradiol. Gynecol Endocrinol 1988;2:113.
126. Magos AL, Zilkha KJ, Studd JWW. Treatment of menstrual migraine by oestradiol implants. J Neurol Neurosurg Psychiatry 1983;46:1044.
127. Magos AL, Brincat M, Studd JWW. Treatment of the premenstrual syndrome by subcutaneous oestradiol implants and cyclical oral norethisterone: Placebo-controlled study. Br Med J Clin Res 1986;292:1629.
128. Transdermal estrogen. Med Lett Drugs Ther 1986;28:119.
129. Judd H. Efficacy of transdermal estradiol. Obstet Gynecol 1987;156:1326.
130. Stumpf PG. Pharmacokinetics of estrogen. Obstet Gynecol 1990;75:9.
131. Schwartz J, Freeman R, Frishman W. Clinical pharmacology of estrogens: Cardiovascular actions and cardioprotective benefits of replacement therapy in postmenopausal women. J Clin Pharmacol 1995;35:1.
132. Pradalier A, Vincent D, Beaulieu PH, Baudesson G, et al. Correlation between Oestradiol Plasma Level and Therapeutic Effect on Menstrual Migraine. In FC Rose (ed), New Advances in Headache Research (4th ed). London: Smith-Gordon, 1994;129.
133. Dennerstein L, Laby B, Burrows GD, Hyman GJ. Headache and sex hormone therapy. Headache 1978;18:146.
134. Pfaffenrath V. Efficacy and safety of percutaneous estradiol vs. placebo in menstrual migraine [Abstract]. Cephalalgia 1993;13:168.
135. Smits MG, VanDerMeer YG, Pfeil JP, Rijnierse JJ, et al. Perimenstrual migraine: Effect of estraderm TTS and the value of contingent negative variation and exteroceptive temporalis muscle suppression test. Headache 1993;34:103.
136. Watson NR, Studd JWW, Savvas M, Garnett T, et al. Treatment of severe premenstrual syndrome with oestradiol patches and cyclical oral norethisterone. Lancet 1989;2:730.

137. Kappius REK, Goolkasian P. Group and menstrual phase effect in reported headaches among college students. Headache 1987;27:491.
138. Sarno AP, Miller EJ, Lundblad EG. Premenstrual syndrome: beneficial effects of periodic, low-dose danazol. Obstet Gynecol 1987;70:33.
139. Powles, TJ. Prevention of migrainous headaches by tamoxifen. Lancet 1986;2:1344.
140. O'Dea PK, Davis EH. Tamoxifen in the treatment of menstrual migraine. Neurology 1990;40:1470.
141. Wentz AC. Management of the Menopause. In HW Jones, AC Wentz, LS Burnett (eds), Novak's Textbook of Gynecology (11th ed). Baltimore: Williams & Wilkins, 1985;397.
142. Andersch B, Hahn L, Wendestam C, Ohman R, et al. Treatment of premenstrual syndrome with bromocriptine. Acta Endocrinol 1978;88:165.
143. Ylostalo P, Kauppila A, Puolakka J, Ronnberg L, et al. Bromocriptine and norethisterone in the treatment of premenstrual syndrome. Obstet Gynecol 1982;58:292.
144. Andersen AN, Larsen JF, Steenstrup OR, Svendstrup B, et al. Effect of bromocriptine on the premenstrual syndrome: A double-blind clinical trial. Br J Obstet Gynaecol 1977;84:370.
145. Herzog AG. Continuous bromocriptine therapy in menstrual migraine [abstract]. Neurology 1995;45:A465.
146. Muse N, Cetel NS, Futterman LA, Yen SSC. The premenstrual syndrome: Effects of "medical ovariectomy." N Engl J Med 1984;311:1345.
147. Hammarbäck S, Bäckström T. Induced anovulation as treatment of premenstrual tension syndrome. A double-blind cross-over study with GnRH-agonist versus placebo. Acta Obstet Gynecol Scand 1988;67:159.
148. Friedman AJ, Juneau-Norcross M, Rein MS. Adverse effects of leuprolide acetate depot treatment. Fertil Steril 1993;59:448.
149. Bäckström CT, Boyle H, Baird DT. Persistence of symptoms of premenstrual tension in hysterectomized women. Br J Obstet Gynaecol 1981;88:530.
150. Casson P, Hahn PM, Van Vugt DA, Reid RL. Lasting response to ovariectomy in severe intractable premenstrual syndrome. Obstet Gynecol 1990;162:99.
151. Casper RF, Hearn MT. The effect of hysterectomy and bilateral oophorectomy in women with severe premenstrual syndrome. Am J Obstet Gynecol 1990;162:105.
152. Utian WH. Overview on menopause. Am J Obstet Gynecol 1987;156:1280.
153. Utian WH. The fate of the untreated menopause. Obstet Gynecol Clin North Am 1987;14:1.
154. Rebar RW, Spitzer IB. The physiology and measurement of hot flushes. Am J Obstet Gynecol 1987;156:1284.
155. Ravnikar V. Physiology and treatment of hot flushes. Obstet Gynecol 1990;75:3S.
156. Shoemaker ES, Forney JP, MacDonald PC. Estrogen treatment of postmenopausal women. JAMA 1977;238:1524.
157. LaRosa JC. Has HRT come of age? Lancet 1995;345:76.
158. Grady D, Rubin SM, Petitti DB, Fox CS, et al. Hormone therapy to prevent disease and prolong life in postmenopausal women. Ann Intern Med 1992;117:1016.
159. Martin KA, Freeman MW. Postmenopausal hormone-replacement therapy. N Engl J Med 1993;328:1115.
160. Nablusi AA, Folsom AR, White A, Patsch W, et al. Association of hormone-replacement therapy with various cardiovascular risk factors in postmenopausal women. N Engl J Med 1993;328:1069.
161. Grady D, Gebretsadik T, Kerlikrowske K, Ernster V, et al. Hormone replacement therapy and endometrial cancer risk: A meta-analysis. Obstet Gynecol 1995;85:304.
162. Henrich JB. The postmenopausal estrogen–breast cancer controversy. JAMA 1992;268:1900.
163. Cedars MI, Judd HL. Nonoral routes of estrogen administration. Obstet Gynecol Clin North Am 1987;14:269.
164. Studd J, Magos A. Hormone pellet implantation for the menopause and premenstrual syndrome. Obstet Gynecol Clin North Am 1987;14:229.
165. Whitehead MI, Hillard TC, Crook D. The role and use of progestogens. Obstet Gynecol 1990;75:59S.
166. Greenblatt RB. The use of androgens in the menopause and other gynecic disorders. Obstet Gynecol Clin North Am 1987;14:251.
167. Utian WH. Oestrogen, headache, and oral contraceptives. S Afr Med J 1974;48:2105.
168. Alvarez WC. Can one cure migraine in women by inducing menopause? Report on forty-two cases. Mayo Clin Proc 1940;15:380.
169. Aylward M, Holly F, Parker RJ. An evaluation of clinical response to piperazine oestrone sulphate ("Harmogen") in menopausal patients. Curr Med Res Opin 1974;2:417.
170. Kaiser HJ, Meienberg O. Deterioration or onset of migraine under oestrogen replacement therapy in the menopause. J Neurol 1993;240:195.

171. Martin PL, Burnier AM, Segre EJ, Huix FJ. Graded sequential therapy in the menopause: A double-blind study. Am J Obstet Gynecol 1971;111:178.
172. Greenblatt RB, Bruneteau DW. Menopausal headache: Psychogenic or metabolic? J Am Geriatr Soc 1974;283:186.
173. Campbell S. Double-Blind Psychometric Studies on the Effects of Natural Estrogens on Postmenopausal Women. In S Campbell (ed), The Management of the Menopause and Postmenopausal Years. Baltimore: University Park Press, 1975;149.
174. Coope J. Double-Blind Crossover Study of Estrogen Replacement Therapy. In S Campbell (ed), The Management of the Menopause and Postmenopausal Years. Baltimore: University Park Press, 1975;149.
175. Baird DT, Glasier AF. Hormonal contraception. N Engl J Med 1993;328:1543.
176. Wentz AC. Contraception and Family Planning. In HW Jones, AC Wentz, LS Burnett (eds), Novak's Textbook of Gynecology (11th ed). Baltimore: Williams & Wilkins, 1985;204.
177. Derman R. Oral contraceptives: A reassessment. Obstet Gynecol Surv 1989;44:662.
178. Speroff L, DeCherney A, and the Advisory Board for the New Progestins. Evaluation of a new generation of oral contraceptives. Obstet Gynecol 1993;81:1034.
179. Corson SL. Contraceptive efficacy of a monophasic oral contraceptive containing desogestrel. Am J Obstet Gynecol 1993;168:1017.
180. Huber J. Clinical experience with a new norgestimate-containing oral contraceptive. Int J Fertil 1992;32:47.
181. Dunson TR, McLaurin VL, Israngkura B, Leelapattana B, et al. A comparative study of two low-dose combined oral contraceptives: Results from a multicenter trial. Contraception 1993;48:109.
182. Shoupe D. Effects of desogestrel on carbohydrate metabolism. Am J Obstet Gynecol 1993;168:1041.
183. Lidegaard Ø. Oral contraception and risk of a cerebral thromboembolic attack: Results of a case-control study. Br Med J Clin Res 1993;306:956.
184. Collaborative Group for the Study of Stroke in Young Women. Oral contraceptives and stroke in young women. JAMA 1975;231:718.
185. Ryan RE. A controlled study of the effect of oral contraceptives on migraine. Headache 1978;17:250.
186. Phillips BM. Oral contraceptive drugs and migraine. Br Med J Clin Res 1968;2:99.
187. Dalton K. Migraine and oral contraceptives. Headache 1976;15:247.
188. Whitty CWM, Hockaday JM, Whitty MM. The effect of oral contraceptives on migraine. Lancet 1966;1:856.
189. Larsson-Cohn U, Lundberg PO. Headache and treatment with oral contraceptives. Acta Neurol Scand 1970;46:267.
190. Carroll JD. Migraine and Oral Contraception. In Proceedings of the International Headache Symposium. Basel: Sandoz, 1971;45.
191. Diddle AW, Gardner WH, Williamson PJ. Oral contraceptive medications and headache. Am J Obstet Gynecol 1969;105:507.
192. Ramchurian S, Pellegrin FA, Ray RM, Hsu JP. The Walnut Creek contraceptive drug study. J Reprod Med 1980;25:346.
193. Herzberg B, Coppen A. Changes in psychological symptoms in women taking oral contraceptives. Br J Psychiatry 1970;116:161.
194. Herzberg BN, Draper KC, Johnson AL, Nicol GC. Oral contraceptives, depression, and libido. Br Med J Clin Res 1971;3:495.
195. Oral Contraceptives and Health: An Interim Report from the Oral Contraception Study of the Royal College of General Practitioners. London: Whitefriars, 1974.
196. Aznar-Ramos R, Giner-Velazquez J, Lara-Ricalde R, Martinez-Manautou J. Incidence of side effects with contraceptive placebo. Am J Obstet Gynecol 1969;105:1144.
197. Ramos R, Apelo R, Osteria T, Vilar E. A comparative analysis of three different dose combinations of oral contraceptives. Contraception 1989;39:165.
198. Nilsson L, Solvell L. Clinical studies on oral contraceptives: A randomized, double-blind, cross-over study of 4 different preparations (Anovlar mite, Lyndiol mite, Ovulen, and Volidan). Acta Obstet Gynecol Scand 1967;46:3.
199. Goldzieher JW, Moses LE, Averkin E, Scheel C, et al. A placebo-controlled double-blind cross-over investigation of the side effects attributed to oral contraceptives. Fertil Steril 1971;22:609.
200. Silbergeld S, Brast N, Noble EP. The menstrual cycle: A double-blind study of symptoms, mood and behavior, and biochemical variables using enovid and placebo. Psychosom Med 1971;33:411.
201. Cullberg J. Mood changes and menstrual symptoms with different gestagen/estrogen combinations: A double-blind comparison with a placebo. Acta Psychiatr Scand 1972;236:259.
202. Nilsson A, Jacobson L, Ingemanson C-A. Side effects of an oral contraceptive with particular attention to mental symptoms and sexual adaptation. Acta Obstet Gynecol Scand 1967;46:537.

203. Grant ECG. Relation between headaches from oral contraceptives and development of endometrial arterioles. Br Med J Clin Res 1968;3:402.
204. Cullberg J, Celli MG, Jonsson CO. Mental and sexual adjustment before and after six months use of an oral contraceptive. Acta Psychiatr Scand 1969;45:259.
205. Desrosiers JJJ. Headaches related to contraceptive therapy and their control. Headache 1973;13:117.
206. Fotherby K. Twelve years of clinical experience with an oral contraceptive containing 30 µg ethinyloestradiol and 150 µg desogestrel. Contraception 1995;51:3.
207. Lopez G, Rodriguez A, Rengifo J, Sivin I. Two-year prospective study in Colombia of Norplant implants. Obstet Gynecol 1985;68:204.
208. Shaaban MM, Salah M, Zarzour A, Abdullah SA. A prospective study of Norplant implants and the Tcu 380Ag IUD in Assiut, Egypt. Stud Fam Plann 1983;14:163.
209. Buckshee K, Chatterjee P, Dhall GI, Hazra MN, et al. Phase III clinical trials with Norplant II (two covered rods): Report on five years of use. Contraception 1993;48:120.

TWO

PRIMARY NONMIGRAINOUS HEADACHES

11
Tension-Type Headache

Jean Schoenen and Wei Wang

Tension-type headache (TTH) has in the past been an ill-defined syndrome, and it probably still is heterogeneous. The headaches formerly described as "muscular contraction," "psychogenic," "psychomyogenic," "tension," "stress," "essential," and "nonmigrainous" are now classified in this group. The term *tension-type headache* has been chosen by the Classification Committee of the International Headache Society (IHS),[1] in order to offer a new heading that underlines the uncertain pathogenesis but nonetheless indicates that some kind of mental or muscular tension may play a causative role. Whereas previous definitions have been imprecise and nonoperational, the IHS classification has provided operational diagnostic criteria.

Although TTH is the most common form of headache, it receives much less attention from health authorities, clinical researchers, or industrial pharmacologists than does migraine. This situation may be due to the fact that most subjects with TTH never consult a doctor and treat themselves, if necessary, with over-the-counter analgesic drugs. However, TTH also occurs in frequent and severe forms and as such constitutes a major health problem with an enormous socioeconomic impact.

The exact causes of TTH are still unknown. There are no ancillary investigations that are diagnostic for this form of headache; the disease definition relies exclusively on symptomatology, which is not as distinct in TTH as in migraine. Despite the meager scientific foundations regarding both mechanisms and treatments of TTH and the lack of a major therapeutic breakthrough in recent years, it is possible to manage TTH patients with some success.

CLASSIFICATION AND DIAGNOSTIC FEATURES

The term *tension-type headache* has been chosen in order to offer a new category heading that underlines the uncertainties about the precise pathogenesis but

Table 11.1   Episodic tension-type headache (code 2.1): diagnostic criteria

A.   At least 10 previous headache episodes fulfilling criteria B–D listed below. Number of days with such headache < 180/year (<15/month)
B.   Headache lasting from 30 minutes to 7 days
C.   At least two of the following pain characteristics:
   1.   Pressing/tightening (nonpulsating) quality
   2.   Mild or moderate intensity (may inhibit, but does not prohibit activities)
   3.   Bilateral location
   4.   No aggravation by walking stairs or similar routine physical activity
D.   Both of the following:
   1.   No nausea or vomiting (anorexia may occur)
   2.   Photophobia and phonophobia are absent, or one but not the other is present
E.   At least one of the following:
   1.   History and physical and neurologic examinations do not suggest one of the disorders listed in groups 5–11*
   2.   History and/or physical and/or neurologic examinations do suggest such disorder, but it is ruled out by appropriate investigations
   3.   Such disorder is present, but tension-type headache attacks do not occur for the first time in close temporal relation to the disorder

*Disorders listed in groups 5–11 refer to the headache associated with (1) head trauma, (2) vascular disorders, (3) nonvascular intracranial disorder, (4) substance use or withdrawal, (5) noncephalic infection, (6) metabolic disorder, or (7) cranium, neck, eyes, ears, nose, sinuses, teeth, mouth, or other facial or cranial structures.

nonetheless indicates that some kind of mental or muscular tension may play a causative role. In the IHS classification,[1] TTH has been classified to the level of the four-digit code (see also Chapter 12).

Definition

TTHs are recurrent episodes of headache lasting minutes to weeks. The pain is typically pressing or tightening in quality, of mild or moderate intensity, and bilateral in location, and does not worsen with routine physical activity. Nausea is usually absent, but photophobia or phonophobia may be present (Table 11.1).

Second-Digit Level

At the two-digit level, TTH is subdivided into episodic (code 2.1, ETTH) and chronic (code 2.2, CTTH) forms. The principal difference between these two forms is the frequency of headache episodes. With episodes occurring up to 15 days per month (180 days per year) the patient qualifies for ETTH; above that limit the patient is classified in the CTTH group. This subdivision may appear arbitrary because clinical features are similar in both types of TTHs. The chronic type may be accompanied by nausea as an isolated associated symptom, but the main reason to distinguish the two forms is the difference in management strategies.

Table 11.2   Classification of tension-type headache

International Headache Society code	International Classification of Diseases-10 NA code
2. Tension-type headache	G44.29
2.1. Episodic tension-type headache	
2.1.1. Episodic tension-type headache associated with disorder of pericranial muscles	G44.20
2.1.2. Episodic tension-type headache unassociated with disorder of pericranial muscles	G44.21
2.2. Chronic tension-type headache	
2.2.1. Chronic tension-type headache associated with disorder of pericranial muscles	G44.22
2.2.2. Chronic tension-type headache unassociated with disorder of pericranial muscles	G44.23
2.3. Headache of the tension type not fulfilling above criteria	G44.28

Third-Digit Level

The three-digit code level (Table 11.2) subdivides TTH into a form with a disorder of pericranial muscles (codes 2.1.1 and 2.2.1) and a form without such a disorder (codes 2.1.2 and 2.2.2). Pericranial muscle disorder is supposed to be present when pericranial muscles are excessively tender as indicated by manual palpation or pressure algometer measurements, or when increased electromyographic (EMG) levels can be recorded in pericranial muscles at rest or during physiologic tests. There is at present no scientific basis for a such a subdivision. Increased pericranial tenderness is found in most TTH patients in clinical samples[2,3] and in population-based studies,[4] but it can also be detected in other pain disorders such as fibromyalgia or low back pain[5,6] as well as in migraine.[2] Although pericranial tenderness and pericranial muscle activity vary greatly between patients, there is at present no conclusive evidence that patients with higher levels differ from those with normal findings in clinical presentation, pathogenesis of pain, or response to therapy.[3]

Fourth-Digit Level

In contrast to migraine, TTH is subdivided up to the four-digit code, which is supposed to indicate the most likely causative factors (Table 11.3). This subdivision has little clinical utility. It has no indisputable scientific basis and should be considered only for research purposes. For instance, simple concurrence of oromandibular dysfunction and headache is frequent, but could be due to chance because both disorders are extremely prevalent. An extensive population-based study[7] performed on 735 adults representative of the total Danish population has shown that the prevalence of oromandibular dysfunction does not differ between subjects with frequent TTH, migraineurs, and headache-free persons. A causal relationship between oromandibular dysfunction and TTH, therefore, seems to be absent or weak, and only a minor positive relation with increased frequency of TTH was found.

Table 11.3   Subdivision of tension-type headache according to the most likely causative factor(s)

0	No identifiable causative factor
1	More than one of the causative factors 2–9
2	Oromandibular dysfunction
3	Psychosocial stress
4	Anxiety
5	Depression
6	Headache as delusion or an idea (psychogenic headache)
7	Muscular stress
8	Drug overuse for tension-type headache
9	One of the disorders causing secondary headaches

Note: Fourth digit code 6 for tension-type headache could correspond to delusional disorder (297.1) or hypochondriasis (300.7) in the *Diagnostic and Statistical Manual of Mental Disorders* (4th ed) classification.

The possible psychological and psychiatric causative factors are defined according to the *Diagnostic and Statistical Manual*, 4th edition (DSM-IV-R), criteria. Psychosocial stress may be causative, but in the Danish population-based study,[8] stress and mental tension were the most frequent precipitating factors, not only in TTH but also in migraine. Some of the psychosocial and personality factors that have been suspected as causal may in fact be results of specific coping strategies for recurrent pain rather than primary causative factors. Most patients suffering from TTH have no overt depression, despite increased scores on scales indicating a depressive mood.[9] According to studies of genetic epidemiology, depression and anxiety disorders are associated with migraine but not with TTH.[10]

Muscular stress and strain are considered to be prominent causes of TTH, especially of the episodic form. Whether the pain is directly related to the initial muscular stress or to defective central pain perception is not yet clear (see the later section on pathophysiology). TTH is also associated with menstrual periods: Menstruation is cited as a precipitating factor by 38% of 102 women with TTH.[8] Drug overuse is a complication of TTH rather than a cause of it. Headache related to drug overuse or misuse is classified in a separate section of the IHS classification.

CLINICAL FEATURES

Clinical Heterogeneity

The clinical pattern of TTH is different in general practice compared with specialized headache clinics. The latter deal chiefly with the chronic form of the disorder and with patients in whom the clinical picture is modified by aggravating factors such as drug overuse. In a survey performed in our headache clinic of 596

Table 11.4 Clinical diagnoses in 596 outpatients of the University of Liège Headache Clinic, January to June 1992

	Number	*Percentage*
Migraine	186	31
Without aura	166	28
With aura	20	3
Tension-type headache	137	23
Drug abuse headache	60	10
Initially migraine	25	4
Initially tension-type headache	28	5
Initially not defined	7	1
Cluster headache	38	6
"Cervicogenic" headache*	60	9
Others	160	27

*In many cases the syndrome of "cervicogenic" headache may be a cervicotrigeminal pain pattern of tension-type headache. Diagnostic criteria for cervicogenic headache from OTA Sjaastad, V Frederisksen, V Pfaffenrath. Cervicogenic headache: Diagnostic criteria. Headache 1990;30:725.

patients over 6 months, no patient consulted for ETTH, 23% of patients had CTTH, and 5% had drug-abuse headache with initial TTH (Table 11.4). Most TTH sufferers in the general population have only occasional headache episodes and have never consulted a doctor.[11] Because of the high prevalence of TTH and its variable temporal profile, it was proposed to define 14 headache days per year as the lower limit; below that, subjects may be regarded as, practically speaking, headache-free.[7] The duration of each episode of TTH is also variable: A median value of 12 hours, with extreme values of 30 minutes and 72 hours, has been reported.[12] The median number of headache days per month in the chronic form may be as high as 30.[13] If headache frequency is greater than 15–20 days per month, it often becomes a daily and constant headache. However, most patients overreport the frequency of their TTH during the initial clinical interview, as compared with the prospective headache diary.[14]

Pain

In concordance with the IHS diagnostic criteria, the pain is mild or moderate in 99% of ETTH sufferers in the general population.[15] Its intensity increases with frequency.[11] Most patients with TTH report that their headache does not interfere with daily activities[13]; 42% report inhibition and 11% report prohibition of normal activities.

The pain of TTH is usually described as dull, aching, pressure-like, constricting, or giving a sense of fullness in the head. Patients may describe their pain as like wearing a tight hat, wearing a tight band around the head, or bearing a heavy burden on the head.[16] In the majority of patients, physical activity has no influence on headache intensity (i.e., in 71% of TTH patients, compared with 2% of migraineurs in the Danish population-based study).[15] Aggravation of pain by routine physical activity is therefore one of the best criteria with which to distinguish between migraine and TTH—better than unilaterality or pulsating quality of pain.

Bilateral location of pain is the rule in TTH. In a recent study from a specialized headache clinic, 89% of patients reported bilateral location.[17] Location of pain, however, varies considerably within and between patients. Contrary to the previous National Institutes of Health Ad Hoc Committee classification,[18] which postulates that the headache is usually posterior, occipital location (25%) was less frequent than frontal/temporal pain (66%) in a large clinical study.[13]

Associated Symptoms

Whereas the pain intensity is graded in the IHS classification, the accompanying symptoms are listed only as present or absent. Although most patients have no associated symptoms, some patients may report slight photophobia or phonophobia or nausea. Grading the accompanying symptoms may improve the differentiation of migraine from TTH, and has been suggested for a revised version of IHS criteria.[15]

Lack of sleep is frequently reported as a precipitating factor for headache.[8] Headache of the tension type occurs in 39% of healthy volunteers after sleep deprivation.[19] In the general population, subjects with TTH have a significantly higher number of sleeping problems compared with migraineurs and the rest of the normal population.[8,20] The precise relationship between CTTH and the fibromyalgia syndrome is not clear, but in the latter, disturbances of sleep patterns (alpha-delta sleep) are frequent.[21] The sleep apnea syndrome may also be associated with headache that mimics TTH.[20]

Time Course

Classically, TTH is reported to start sometime during the day and to increase slowly during the second part of the day, in contrast to migraine, which may be severe on early morning awakening. Many patients with CTTH, however, awake with headache or notice it shortly after rising. The headache usually lasts the whole day and is little influenced by daily activities. In clinical studies, no specific diurnal variation of the pain is found.[13,17]

Clinical Examination

As is true of other so-called functional headaches, the diagnosis of TTH requires exclusion of other organic disorders and therefore a meticulous general and neurologic examination. If even subtle abnormalities are noticed, a diagnostic evaluation should be made using appropriate investigations and with the advice of relevant specialists. The physical examination should include manual palpation of pericranial and neck muscles in order to identify tender and trigger points. A method for cranial palpation and calculation of a total tenderness score has been described.[2] The temporomandibular joints should be examined. Reciprocal clicking of the temporomandibular joint or pain with maximum jaw opening and pain on palpation have been proposed as sensitive clinical signs for oro-mandibular dysfunction.[22]

Prognosis

The prognosis and clinical course of TTH are variable. Subjects with frequent ETTH are probably at increased risk of developing CTTH over a period of many years.[13] The question of whether subjects with more severe TTH are at increased risk for developing migraine, or whether subjects with migraine are more likely to develop more severe and frequent TTH, is still controversial. A recent study suggests that migraineurs are more prone to TTH.[23] The continuum theory, implying that migraine and TTH are part of the same syndrome and that associated symptoms are consequences of severe pain,[24] has not been proven. On the contrary, results of recent epidemiologic studies favor the existence of separate clinical entities.[11,25] Various factors can influence headache frequency and transform ETTH into CTTH; among these the most frequent is overuse of analgesics or ergotamine (or both).[26] Another factor important for the onset of primary headaches and for their persistence is psychosocial stress. There is some evidence that chronic recurrent headache is associated with high reported frequency and severity of minor life events and so-called daily hassles.[9,27] This association is more pronounced in TTH than in migraine.

DIFFERENTIAL DIAGNOSIS

Although the pain characteristics listed in the IHS classification (see Table 11.1) are encountered in the majority of patients, it must be kept in mind that in the general population 17.5% of patients may have a pulsating headache, 10% unilateral pain, 27.7% aggravation by routine physical activity, 18.2% anorexia, 4.2% nausea, and 10.6% photophobia.[15] Two problems therefore arise in diagnosing TTH. On the one hand, TTH, although the most frequent, is also the least distinct of all headache types, because its clinical diagnosis is based chiefly on negative features, i.e., on the absence of symptoms that characterize other idiopathic or symptomatic headaches (such as unilaterality, pulsatility, aggravation by physical activity, associated symptoms, etc.). On the other hand, a significant minority of patients may present with symptoms that are found in other headache types. The lack of specificity as well as the uncommon features may make the clinician, and thus the patient, hesitant about the correct diagnosis and may explain why paraclinical investigations to exclude organic disease are (and probably should be) more frequently performed in TTH than in other types of headaches such as migraine. Many of the various headache types listed under the major headings of the IHS classification[1] may mimic TTH at some stage in their clinical course. The following are some illustrative examples.

It is usually not difficult to distinguish symptomatic headache due to sinus or eye disease from TTH. Chronic sinusitis cannot be accepted as a cause of headache on the basis of simple radiologic thickening of sinus mucosae. At least intermittent radiologic or clinical signs of ongoing sinus disease must be present.

Similarly, radiologic evidence of cervical spondylosis is rarely a satisfactory explanation for a headache, because it can be found with equal prevalence in aged-matched headache-free subjects.[28]

Changes in intracranial pressure are a well-known cause of headache. Although spontaneous or symptomatic intracranial hypotension (code 7.2) is most often distinguishable from other headache types by its accentuation in the erect position (so-called orthostatic headache), intracranial hypertension may produce a headache that can mimic migraine or TTH. In brain tumors, obviously of major concern to patients and clinicians, the headache overlies the tumor in a minority of patients but is usually generalized.[29] The syndrome of idiopathic intracranial hypertension, also known as pseudotumor cerebri or benign intracranial hypertension (code 7.1.1), may mimic TTH. The following characteristic features can guide the diagnosis: predominant occurrence among young obese women (93%), the most severe headache ever (93%), pulsatile character (83%), nausea (57%), vomiting (30%), orbital pain (43%), transient visual obscuration (71%), diplopia (38%), and visual loss (31%).[30] Papilledema without neurologic abnormalities except for a possible empty sella is pathognomonic for this condition, but it may be lacking in a small subgroup of patients. As mentioned before, the most frequent cause of chronic daily headache in clinical practice is abuse of analgesics or ergotamine (major heading 8.2 in the IHS classification[1]). Recognizing this condition is of crucial importance, because drug withdrawal is a prerequisite for therapeutic success.

ETTH (code 2.1) can be difficult to distinguish from migraine without aura (code 1.1) in patients with atypical, but not necessarily uncommon, clinical features. The importance of this distinction is underlined by the fact that TTH and migraine coexist in many patients.[11]

There is no straightforward diagnostic test for TTH. Pericranial tenderness, which is frequent in TTH and increases with recency, presence, or intensity of headache,[4] can also be found in other primary as well as symptomatic headaches, e.g., in intracerebral lesions such as tumor or hemorrhage. Pericranial EMG levels may be within the normal range in the majority of patients with TTH when recordings are performed at rest and in one muscle. The proportion of abnormal findings increases with multiple recording sites and under stressful conditions.[3] There is no correlation between pericranial tenderness and EMG levels, and patients with abnormal EMG levels or increased tenderness do not differ clinically from those without such abnormalities.[31] The second exteroceptive suppression of temporalis muscle activity (ES2), an inhibitory brain stem reflex, is shortened or abolished in most patients with CTTH.[32] Its diagnostic sensitivity and specificity are highest when comparing CTTH and migraine,[33] but obviously this differential diagnosis is seldom a problem in clinical practice.

EPIDEMIOLOGY

In surveys of the general population in the United States and Western Europe, a considerable variation in the prevalence of TTH has been reported, ranging from 30–80%. Few studies have been performed in other parts of the world. A study among Nigerian university students showed a prevalence of muscle contraction

Table 11.5 The Danish population-based study of headache

Number of respondents	740
Age	25–64 years
Prevalence	
Lifetime	All, 79%; male, 69%; female, 88%
1 year	All, 74%; male, 63%; female, 86%
Point	All, 12%; male, 9%; female, 16%
Frequency	
≤ 1/month	59%
> 1/month	37%
≥ 15/month	3%
Disability	
Daily activities inhibited	59%

Source: Data summarized from BK Rasmussen, R Jensen, J Olesen. A population-based analysis of the diagnostic criteria of the International Headache Society. Cephalalgia 1991;11:129.

headache of 42%,[34] and a study of an urban population in Zimbabwe arrived at a figure of 10%, but subjects with rare episodes were not included.[35] In an Ethiopian rural community the 1-year prevalence of CTTH was 1.7%.[36] In an Israeli study covering Jewish immigrants, the prevalence of nonmigrainous headaches was found to be 65% in men and 66% in women.[37] Differences in diagnostic criteria, methodology, and cultural background are responsible for the variations. In the Danish population-based study using IHS diagnostic criteria,[15] lifetime prevalence of TTH was 79% (Table 11.5).

As mentioned previously, TTH varies widely in frequency and severity, from rare, brief episodes of discomfort to frequent, long-lasting, or even continuous disabling headaches. At the two extremes of disability, 59% of Danish subjects had TTH 1 day per month or less and 3%, more than 15 days per month, i.e., the chronic form.[15] The 1-year prevalence of frequent TTH (more than one per month) is estimated at 20–30%.

TTH seems to be more prevalent in women than in men, and in both sexes the prevalence tends to decline with age. In clinical studies, gender differences are even more pronounced,[38] but this may be due to the fact that women are more likely to seek care for their headaches than men. Other possible explanations for the female preponderance are physiologic differences, such as lowering of pain thresholds in women, and the influence of female hormones. The latter, however, seems to be of less importance for TTH than for migraine, although menstruation may be a precipitating factor in both conditions. Prevalence of TTH does not differ significantly with socioeconomic background.[39,40] Among TTH sufferers in the Danish population, only 16% had at some time consulted a doctor because of their headaches.[40]

PATHOPHYSIOLOGY

From the clinical heterogeneity of TTH one may infer that pathophysiologic mechanisms are multiple. Traditionally, muscular factors have been

Table 11.6 Biochemical studies in tension-type headache

Plasma 5-HT	Decreased[50,51]
	Normal[52,53]
	Increased (during headache)[47,54]
Platelet 5-HT	Increased[46,55]
Met-enkephalin	Increased in plasma[48]
	Increased in plasma and CSF[49]
β-endorphin	Decreased in plasma and CSF[56]
	Normal in plasma and CSF[57]
Dynorphin	Decreased in CSF[49]

CSF = cerebrospinal fluid.

thought to play an important role, as illustrated by the previously used term "muscle contraction headache." Other former denominations, "psychogenic headache" or "stress headache," suggest that psychological factors play a dominant role. The controversy regarding peripheral versus central pathogenic aspects is ongoing. It may be a false debate: Both peripheral and central factors could be at work, interacting and varying in importance between patients, TTH subtypes, or even during the course of the disorder. The following is a synthesis of available data arguing in favor of one or the other pathophysiologic mechanisms.

Peripheral Aspects

Experimental ischemic exercise of temporal muscles may cause pain. Blood-flow studies, however, have ruled out the possibility that TTH is caused by ischemia of the temporal muscles.[41] Cerebral blood flow has been found normal in TTH, but in transcranial Doppler studies, increased flow velocities have been reported in ETTH compared with CTTH or control subjects' flow velocities.[42–44]

The results of biochemical studies performed in TTH have been synthesized by Ferrari.[45] The results are in part contradictory because of varying methodologies. Several recent biochemical studies tend to indicate nonetheless that serotonin[46,47] and met-enkephalin[48,49] disposition may be high in TTH, in contrast to migraine (Table 11.6).

Evidence both for and against a myofascial origin of pain has accumulated over recent years (Table 11.7). EMG levels in pericranial muscles may be on average increased in TTH, but there is no correlation between EMG activity and headache severity. In a clinical sample of CTTH patients, pressure pain thresholds (PPTs) were found on average to be lowered at pericranial sites. In a population-based study,[4] however, PPTs were normal over the temporal region. Palpation tenderness is increased in patients, more so during an actual headache. In ETTH, cephalic PPTs are usually normal.[4,58–60] Studies of extracephalic pain thresholds are scarce. In one study,[59] a more rapid increase of pain in fingers was found in ETTH patients compared with healthy volunteers; in another study,[3] PPTs were decreased over the Achilles tendon in CTTH (Figure 11.1). During isometric con-

Table 11.7   Evidence for and against a myofascial origin of pain in tension-type headache

For	*Against*
Pericranial electromyographic activity	
Increased in 50% of studies[64]	Normal in 50% of studies[64]
Increased on average in CTTH[65,66]	Significantly increased in less than 34% of CTTH patients[65,66]
Increased on average in ETTH[60]	Significantly increased in only 11% of ETTH patients[67]
Stress-induced increase superior in TTH[67]	Stress-induced increase similar in TTH and controls[69]
	Not correlated with headache intensity[66,69,70,71]
Experimental tooth clenching produces headache[72]	May be secondary to the pain as in patients with low back pain[73,74]
Pericranial pain sensitivity	
Increased palpation tenderness is correlated with headache frequency and intensity[7,59]	Increased palpation tenderness also found in migraineurs[59]
	Increased palpation tenderness not correlated with intensity, frequency, or chronicity[75]
	Increased palpation tenderness rarely over frontal or temporal region[7]
Decreased PPT on average in CTTH[3,66]	PPT normal over temple[7]
	PPT significantly decreased in 50% or less of CTTH[3,31,60]
	PPT not correlated with headache severity[3,31,60]
Qualitative difference of pericranial myofascial tenderness (linear stimulus-respective function)[76]	Pain sensitivity increased also at extracephalic sites[3,59,77,78]

CTTH = chronic tension-type headache; ETTH = episodic tension-type headache; TTH = tension-type headache; PPT = pressure pain threshold.

traction, PPTs tend to decrease over the temporal muscle in TTH patients (Jensen et al., submitted) whereas they increase markedly over the quadriceps muscle in healthy controls.[61] In addition to sensitization of peripheral nociceptors, central disnociception may therefore play a role in the increased pericranial tenderness of TTH patients.

Central Nervous System Aspects

Electroencephalogram and evoked potentials are normal in TTH.[62] Contingent negative variation, an event-related potential, was normal in most studies, but one study found a reduced amplitude.[63]

Many psychological abnormalities have been associated with TTH (Table 11.8) as mentioned in the discussion on the four-digit level of the classification

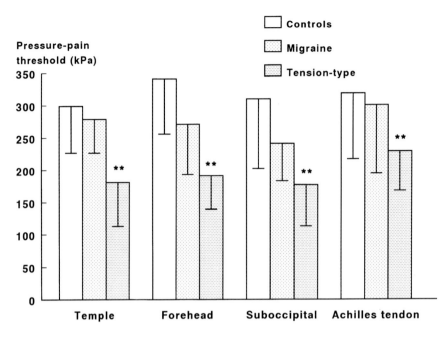

Figure 11.1   Pressure pain thresholds (mean ± standard error of the mean) in healthy controls, migraine patients, and tension-type headache patients. ** *P* < 0.05 versus controls.

Table 11.8   Psychological factors associated with tension-type headache

Anger, stress[80–82]
Depressive tendency (not overt depression)[9,83–85]
Increased daily hassles[27]
"Psychobiological disregulation" [86,87]
External locus of control[88]

code. It remains to be determined whether these psychological abnormalities are related to TTH etiology or just consequences of the headache.[78]

In recent years, much attention has been paid to an inhibitory reflex of jaw-closing muscles, called exteroceptive suppression or silent period. The second exteroceptive suppression of temporalis muscle (ES2) is shortened or abolished in CTTH patients (Table 11.9). Although not confirmed in two recent studies, this observation is of pathophysiologic interest.[75,98] ES2 duration reflects excitability of inhibitory brain stem interneurons, which receive afferent inputs from several brain stem centers and limbic structures, in particular from serotonergic raphe nuclei (Figure 11.2). The following data suggest that the descending con-

Table 11.9   Temporalis ES2 duration in various headache types

Headache type	ES2 duration
Chronic tension-type headache	Reduced or abolished[62,89–94]
Episodic tension-type headache	Normal[58,91,94]
Migraine between attacks	Normal[62,89–94]
Migraine during attacks	Normal[95]
Headache with daily analgesic or ergotamine abuse	Decreased, but individual values are scattered[31]
Post–lumbar puncture headache	Normal[95,96]
Cluster headache	Normal[97]
Meningitis	Normal[95]
Symptomatic headache	Normal[85]

trol, and not the inhibitory interneurons themselves, may be abnormal in TTH: Inhibition of ES2 by a preceding peripheral stimulus is greatly enhanced; habituation of ES2 at high-frequency stimulation is normal in CTTH but increased in ETTH; direct suppression of temporalis activity by exteroceptive stimuli at the upper limbs is normal.[94,99,100]

A Model for the Pathogenesis of Tension-Type Headache

Considering the heterogeneity of available pathophysiologic data in TTH, a comprehensive model was recently proposed as a working hypothesis.[101] According to this concept, TTH may be the result of an interaction between changes in the descending control of nociceptive brain stem neurons and interrelated peripheral changes, such as myofascial pain sensitivity and strain in pericranial muscles (Figure 11.3). An acute episode of ETTH may occur in most individuals otherwise perfectly normal. It can be brought on by physical stress, usually combined with psychological stress, or by nonergonomic working positions. In such cases, increased nociception from strained muscles may be the primary cause of the attack, possibly favored by a central temporary change in pain control due to stress. Emotional mechanisms may indeed increase muscle tension via the limbic system of muscle control and at the same time reduce tone in the endogenous antinociceptive system. With more frequent episodes of headache, central changes may become increasingly important. Long-term potentiation of nociceptive neurons and decreased activity in the antinociceptive system could cause CTTH. This process is probably the most important mechanism in frequent ETTH and in CTTH.

The importance of peripheral and central factors, however, may vary between patients and over time in the same patient. The complex interrelation between various pathophysiologic aspects of TTH may explain why the disorder is so difficult to treat. It certainly suggests that various therapeutic approaches should be used, in sequence or in combination, and that in the future determining the relative importance of peripheral and central mechanisms might be of some utility in determining therapeutic strategy.

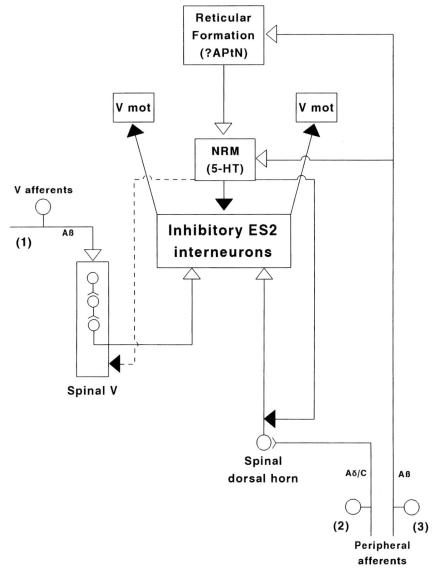

Figure 11.2　Illustration of some of the neuronal circuits modulating excitability of medullary inhibitory interneurons, which mediate exteroceptive suppression of temporalis/masseter muscle activity. (1) ES2 after labial stimulation is due to activation of an interneuronal net in the spinal trigeminal nucleus via Aß (and Aδ, C) fibers. ES2 is reduced in tension-type headache because of increased inhibition of inhibitory ES2 interneurons by descending (5-HT) pathways. (2) Temporalis "ES2" after peripheral upper limb stimulation is normal in tension-type headache. (3) Inhibition of labial ES2 by a nonpainful peripheral stimulus is markedly enhanced in tension-type headache, probably because of increased activity in descending pathways. (APtN = anterior pretectal nucleus; V mot = trigeminal motor nucleus; NRM = nucleus raphe magnus; open triangle = excitation; closed triangle = inhibition.)

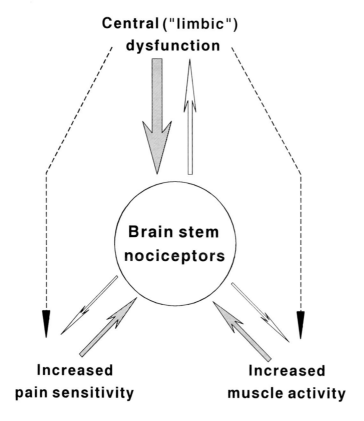

Figure 11.3   Illustration of the concept that tension-type headache is the result of an interaction between changes of the descending control of nociceptive brain stem neurons and interrelated peripheral changes, i.e., myofascial pain sensitivity and strain in pericranial muscles. (Reprinted with permission from J Olesen, J Schoenen [eds], Tension-type Headache: Classification, Mechanisms, and Treatment. New York: Raven, 1993;127–130.)

THERAPIES

A variety of treatment modalities are used in TTH. Only some of them have been proven effective in good quality, controlled clinical trials. Designing and performing such trials is more difficult for TTH than for migraine, for a number of reasons. TTH has a highly variable attack and disease course; the headache is lower in intensity, and aggravating factors such as those listed at the four-digit code level may play a confounding role. Most patients with ETTH treat themselves with over-the-counter drugs without consulting a physician. At the other end of the spectrum, CTTH is much more difficult to treat than migraine, because of the lower intensity of the pain and possibly because of other physiologic and psychological factors. The placebo effect may be superior in TTH, exceeding 30% in many studies.[102]

A subcommittee of the IHS recently proposed guidelines for clinical drug trials in TTH[103]; these guidelines are recommended as a standard against which the reader can assess the scientific value of published treatment trials.

As in the case of migraine, therapies for TTH can be schematically subdivided into short-term, abortive (mainly pharmacologic) treatments of the individual headache attack and long-term, prophylactic (pharmacologic or nonpharmacologic) treatments that may prevent headache.

Abortive Pharmacotherapy

Many controlled studies of simple analgesics and nonsteroidal anti-inflammatory drugs (NSAIDs) have been performed in TTH, using the headache attack as a model for acute pain. From these studies (for review see reference 104), one may conclude that NSAIDs are the drugs of first choice. Ibuprofen, 400 or 800 mg, is significantly more effective than placebo, and even a low 200-mg dose is more effective than aspirin.[105] Significant effects of ibuprofen on the headache can be detected within 15–30 minutes. Naproxen sodium, 550 mg, provided superior analgesia compared with placebo or acetaminophen. Other NSAIDs such as ketoprofen, ketorolac, and indomethacin are also effective but are less well studied. Because of the overall lower prevalence of gastrointestinal side effects,[106] ibuprofen (800 mg) is probably the first choice, followed by naproxen sodium (825 mg). Several studies have shown that aspirin (650 mg, or better, 1,000 mg) is superior to placebo and comparable with 650 mg (or better, 1,000 mg) of acetaminophen; the gastric side-effect profile of the latter is, however, much better.

In some patients, a combination of analgesics with caffeine, sedatives, or tranquilizers may be more effective than simple analgesics or NSAIDs, but in many cases this impression comes from too low a dosage of the latter. Whenever possible, combination analgesics for TTH should be avoided because of the risk of dependency, abuse, and chronification of the headache. There is at present no scientific basis for the use of muscle relaxants, such as the mephenesin-like compounds, baclofen, diazepam, tizanidine, cyclobenzaprine, or dantrolene sodium, in the treatment of TTH.

Prophylactic Pharmacotherapy

The tricyclic antidepressants are the most widely used first-line therapeutic agents for CTTH. Surprisingly, few controlled studies have been performed and not all of them have found an efficacy superior to placebo (Table 11.10). The drawbacks of these studies are small patient numbers, inadequate efficacy parameters, or short duration. Only a few of them can be considered adequate according to the IHS guidelines.[103] One major problem that arises with trials showing statistical differences between placebo and tricyclics is how to evaluate whether the observed effect is clinically relevant. In one study, for instance,[114] a reduction in average daily headache duration was selected as the primary efficacy parameter. Amitriptyline reduced daily headache duration by an average of 3.2 hours, from 11.1 hours per day to 7.9 hours per day. This effect was significantly dif-

Table 11.10   Controlled studies on prophylactic pharmacotherapy for tension-type headache

Study and drugs tested	No. of subjects	Results	Significance
Lance and Curran[107]	27	> 50% improved	$P < 0.01$
Amitriptyline (75 mg/day)		56%	
Placebo		11%	
Diamond and Baltes[108]		Decreased headache intensity	$P < 0.05$
Placebo	29	33%	
Amitriptyline, 10 mg (up to six/day)	28	54%	
Amitriptyline, 25 mg (up to six/day)	28	38%	
Morland et al.[109]	23	Headache days decreased 15% by doxepin compared with placebo	$P < 0.05$
Doxepin			
Placebo			
Fogelholm and Murros[110]	30	Headache intensity diminished by 25% and headache-free days increased by 40% on maprotiline	$P < 0.001$
Maprotiline (75 mg/day)			
Placebo			
Langemark et al.[111]		% intensity improvement (day 43):	Nonsignificant
Placebo	36	49%	
Clomipramine	28	57%	
Mianserine	28	54%	
Pfaffenrath et al.[112]		50% reduction in duration × frequency and in intensity	Nonsignificant
Placebo	64	21.9%	
Amitriptyline (50–75 mg/day)	67	22.4%	
Amitriptylinoxide (60–90 mg/day)	66	30.3%	
Göbel et al.[113]		Change in mean daily duration	$P \leq 0.001$
Placebo	29	–0.28 hours	
Amitriptyline (75 mg/day)	24	–3.2 hours	

ferent from placebo, but the clinical significance of such a reduction is questionable. Nonetheless, in clinical practice the tricyclic antidepressants remain the most useful prophylactic drugs for CTTH or frequent ETTH. Amitriptyline is the most frequently used. Clomipramine may be slightly superior but has more side effects. Other antidepressants, such as doxepin, maprotiline, or mianserine can be used as a second choice.

The initial dosage of tricyclics should be low: 10–25 mg of amitriptyline or clomipramine at bedtime. Many patients will be satisfied by such a low dose. The average dose of amitriptyline in CTTH, however, is 75–100 mg per day.[102] If a patient is insufficiently improved on this dose, a trial of higher doses of amitriptyline or clomipramine is warranted. If the headache is improved by at least 80% after 4 months, it is reasonable to attempt discontinuation of the medication. Decreasing the daily dose by 20–25% every 2–3 days may avoid rebound headache. The recent generation of antidepressants that selectively block the reuptake of serotonin (e.g., fluoxetine) may be effective in TTH prophylaxis (see Chapter 4). In clinical practice, they seem to be less efficient than the tricyclics, but they may be useful in certain subgroups of patients. There is at present no way to identify this subgroup of patients. In obese patients, selective serotonin reuptake inhibitors may be preferred to tricyclics as first-line drug treatment.

The mechanism of action of antidepressants in CTTH remains to be determined. Their effect on the headache may be partly independent of their antidepressant effect. Tricyclics have a variety of pharmacologic actions. Serotonin increase by inhibition of its reuptake, endorphin release, and inhibition of *N*-methyl-D-aspartate receptors that play a role in pain transmission may all be relevant for the pathophysiology of TTH.

Nonpharmacologic Treatments

Psychological and Behavioral Techniques

There is solid scientific support for the usefulness of relaxation and EMG biofeedback therapies in the management of TTH (see Chapter 3). Across studies, relaxation training, EMG biofeedback training, and their combination have all yielded a near 50% reduction in headache activity. Improvements are similar for each treatment modality but significantly greater than those observed in untreated patients or in patients with false or noncontingent biofeedback (Table 11.11).[115] Nonetheless, these treatments do not seem to be interchangeable; for example, some patients who fail to respond to relaxation training may benefit from subsequent EMG biofeedback training.

Cognitive-behavioral interventions, such as stress management programs, alone can effectively reduce TTH activity, but they seem to be most useful when added to biofeedback or relaxation therapies in patients with higher levels of daily hassles. Limited-contact treatment, based on the patient's guidance at home by audiotapes and written materials and requiring only three or four monthly clinical sessions, may be a cost-effective alternative to fully therapist-administered treatment in many patients. Still, behavioral therapies are time-consuming for patients and therapists. Although there is no infallible means of predicting treatment outcome, a number of factors have been identified that may have some predictive value. In one study,[116] relaxation producing at least 50% reduction of EMG activity at the fourth session was predictive of an excellent outcome. Excessive analgesic or ergotamine use limits the therapeutic benefits. Patients with continuous headache are less responsive to relaxation or biofeedback therapies, and patients with elevated scores on psychological tests that assess depression or psychiatric disturbance have done poorly with behavioral treatment in some studies.[114] Behavioral treatment may produce

Table 11.11   Global efficacy of biobehavioral therapies for tension-type headache

	Electromyo- graphic biofeedback	Relaxation	Relaxation and biofeedback	Noncontingent biofeedback	Controls (moni- toring)
Improvement range (%)	13–87	17–94	29–88	–14–40	–28–12

Source: Data summarized from KA Holroyd. Tension-Type Headache, Cluster Headache, and Miscellaneous Headaches: Psychological and Behavioral Techniques. In J Olesen, P Tfelt-Hansen, KMA Welch (eds), The Headaches. New York: Raven, 1993;515.

improvement more slowly than pharmacologic treatment, but the improvement is maintained for long periods, up to several years without monthly burst sessions or contact with the therapist.

Other Nonpharmacologic Treatments

Physical therapy techniques employed in the treatment of TTH include positioning, ergonomic instruction, massage, transcutaneous electrical nerve stimulation, heat or cold application, and manipulations. None of these techniques has been proven to be effective in the long-term. Physical treatment such as massage may be useful for acute episodes of TTH.

Oromandibular treatment may be helpful in selected TTH patients (see Chapter 3). Unfortunately, most studies claiming efficacy of treatments such as occlusal splints, therapeutic exercises for masticatory muscles, or occlusal adjustment are uncontrolled. In one single trial comparing occlusal equilibration with placebo equilibration in 56 TTH patients, headache frequency was reduced in 80% and intensity in 47% of patients in the active group compared with 50% and 16%, respectively, in the placebo group.[117] In another study[118] headache frequency decreased in 56% of patients treated with occlusal stabilization splints compared with 32% in patients receiving neurologic treatments. Considering the large number of headache-free subjects who display signs and symptoms of oromandibular dysfunction,[7] caution should be taken not to advocate irreversible dental treatments in TTH. A minority of selected patients may, however, benefit from oromandibular treatment.

Conclusion

There is little scientific evidence to guide the selection of treatment modalities in TTH. The best treatment is often found by trial and error. Because the success rates with the different therapeutic strategies, both pharmacologic and nonpharmacologic, appear very similar, it is of little surprise that dental treatment will be prescribed if the patient sees a dentist, that of behavior therapy if the patient sees a psychologist, and pharmacologic treatment if he or she consults a neurologist.

This situation is unfortunate because the multifactorial etiopathogenesis of TTH suggests that therapy should be tailored individually to each patient and that a combination of different therapeutic methods, such as pharmacologic and nonpharmacologic treatments, may yield better results than either treatment by itself. To prove this superior efficacy of combination therapies, multidisciplinary collaborations and large-scale comparative trials will be required.

REFERENCES

1. International Headache Society. Classification and diagnostic criteria for headache disorders, cranial neuralgias, and facial pain. Cephalalgia 1988;8(Suppl 7):1.
2. Langemark M, Olesen J. Pericranial tenderness in chronic tension-type headache: A blind controlled study. Cephalalgia 1987;7:249.
3. Schoenen J, Bottin D, Hardy F, Gérard P. Cephalic and extracephalic pressure pain thresholds in chronic tension-type headache. Pain 1991;47:145.
4. Jensen R, Rasmussen BK, Pedersen B, Olesen J. Cephalic muscle tenderness and pressure pain threshold in headache. Pain 1993;52:193.
5. Yunus M, Masi AT, Calabro JJ, et al. Primary fibromyalgia (fibrositis): Clinical study of 50 patients with matched controls. Semin Arthritis Rheum 1981;11:151.
6. Tunks E, Crook J, Norman G, Kalaher S. Tender points in fibromyalgia. Pain 1988;34:11.
7. Jensen R, Rasmussen BK, Pedersen B, et al. Oromandibular disorders in a general population. J Craniomandib Disord Facial Oral Pain 1993;7:175.
8. Rasmussen BK. Migraine and tension-type headache in a general population: Precipitating factors, female hormones, sleep patterns, and relation to lifestyle. Pain 1993;53:65.
9. Dawans A, Schoenen J, Timsit M, Timsit-Berthier M. Comparative Study of Psychopathological Features and Temporalis Second Exteroceptive Silent Period in Chronic Tension-Type Headache: Is 5-HT the Common Denominator? In J Olesen, PR Saxena (eds), 5-Hydroxytryptamine Mechanisms in Primary Headaches, Vol 2. New York: Raven, 1992;220.
10. Merikangas KR, Stevens DE, Angst J. Headache and personality: Results of a community sample of young adults. J Psychiatr Res 1993;27:187.
11. Rasmussen BK, Jensen R, Schroll M, Olesen J. Interrelations between migraine and tension-type headache in the general population. Arch Neurol 1992;49:914.
12. Iversen HK, Langemark M, Andersson PG, et al. Clinical characteristics of migraine and episodic tension-type headache in relation to old and new diagnostic criteria. Headache 1990;30:514.
13. Langemark M, Olesen J, Poulsen DL, Bech P. Clinical characterization of patients with chronic tension headache. Headache 1988;28:590.
14. Russel MB, Rasmussen BK, Brennum J, et al. Presentation of a new instrument: The diagnostic headache diary. Cephalalgia 1992;12:369.
15. Rasmussen BK, Jensen R, Olesen J. A population-based analysis of the diagnostic criteria of the International Headache Society. Cephalalgia 1991;11:129.
16. Kudrow L. Muscle Contraction Headache. In F Clifford-Rose (ed), Handbook of Clinical Neurology, Vol 48, Headache. Amsterdam: Elsevier, 1986;343.
17. Solomon S, Lipton RB, Newman LO. Evaluation of chronic daily headache: Comparison to criteria for chronic tension-type headache. Cephalalgia 1992;12:365.
18. Ad Hoc Committee on the Classification of Headache. Classification of headache. JAMA 1962;179:717.
19. Blau JN. Sleep deprivation headache. Cephalalgia 1990;10:157.
20. Paiva T, Batista A, Martins P, Martins A. The relationship between headaches and sleep disturbances. Headache 1995;35:590.
21. Moldofsky H, Scarisbrick P, England R, Smythe H. Musculoskeletal symptoms and REM sleep disturbance in patients with "fibrositis syndrome" and healthy subjects. Psychosom Med 1975;37:341.
22. Schiffman E, Haley D, Baker C, Lindgren B. Diagnostic criteria for screening headache patients for temporomandibular disorders. Headache 1995;35:121.
23. Ulrich, V, Russell MB, Jenson R, Olesen J. Tension-type headache among migraineurs. An epidemiological survey of the general population. Pain 1996, in press.

24. Featherstone HJ. Migraine and muscle contraction headaches: A continuum. Headache 1985;25:194.
25. Celentano DD, Steward WF, Linet MS. The relationship of headache symptoms with severity and duration of attacks. J Clin Epidemiol 1990;43:983.
26. Schoenen J, Lenarduzzi P, Sianard-Gainko J. Chronic Daily Headaches Associated with Analgesics and/or Ergotamine Abuse: A Clinical Survey of 434 Consecutive Out-patients. In F Clifford-Rose (ed), New Advances in Headache Research. London: Smith-Gordon, 1989;255.
27. DeBenedittis G, Lorenzetti A. Minor stressful life events (daily hassles) in chronic primary headache: Relationship with MMPI personality patterns. Headache 1992;22:140.
28. Wöber-Bingöl C, Wöber C, Zeiler K, et al. Tension headache and cervical spine-plain X-ray findings. Cephalalgia 1992;12:152.
29. Silberstein SD, Marcelis J. Headache associated with changes in intracranial pressure. Headache 1992;32:84.
30. Wall M. The headache profile of idiopathic intracranial hypertension. Cephalalgia 1990;10:331.
31. Schoenen J, Gérard P, De Pasqua V, Sionard-Gainko J. Multiple clinical and paraclinical analyses of chronic tension-type headache associated or unassociated with disorders of pericranial muscles. Cephalalgia 1991;11:135.
32. Schoenen J. Exteroceptive suppression of temporalis muscle activity in patients with chronic headache and in normal volunteers: Methodology, clinical and pathophysiological relevance. Headache 1993;33:3.
33. Wang W, De Pasqua V, Gérard P, Schoenen J. Specificity and sensitivity of temporalis ES2 measurements in the diagnosis of chronic primary headaches. Headache 1995;25:85.
34. Ogunyemi AO. Prevalence of headache among Nigerian university students. Headache 1984;24:127.
35. Levy LM. An epidemiological study of headache in an urban population in Zimbabwe. Headache 1983;23:2.
36. Tekle Haimanot R, Seraw B, Forsgren L, et al. Migraine, chronic tension-type headache, and cluster headache in an Ethiopian rural community. Cephalalgia 1995;15:482.
37. Abramson JH, Hopp C, Epstein LM. Migraine and nonmigrainous headaches: A community survey in Jerusalem. J Epidemiol Community Health 1980;34:188.
38. Friedman AP, von Storch TJC, Merritt TDR. Migraine and tension headaches: A clinical study of two thousand cases. Neurology 1954;4:773.
39. Waters WE. Migraine: Intelligence, social class, and familial prevalence. BMJ 1971;2:77.
40. Rasmussen BK. Migraine and tension-type headache in a general population: Psychosocial factors. Int J Epidemiol 1992;21:1138.
41. Langemark M, Jensen K, Olesen J. Temporal muscle blood flow in chronic tension-type headache. Arch Neurol 1990;47:654.
42. Reinecke M, Konen T, Langohr HD. Autonomic Cerebrovascular Reactivity and Exteroceptive Suppression of Temporalis Muscle Activity in Migraine and Tension-Type Headaches. In F Clifford-Rose (ed), New Advances in Headache Research. London: Smith-Gordon, 1991;115.
43. Wallasch TM. Transcranial Doppler ultrasonic features in episodic tension-type headache. Cephalalgia 1992;12:293.
44. Wallasch TM. Transcranial Doppler Ultrasonic Findings in Episodic and Chronic Tension-Type Headache. In J Olesen, J Schoenen (eds), Tension-Type Headache: Classification, Mechanisms, and Treatment. New York: Raven, 1993;127.
45. Ferrari MD. Tension-Type Headache, Cluster Headache, and Miscellaneous Headaches: Biochemistry. In J Olesen, P Tfelt-Hansen, KMA Welch (eds), The Headaches. New York: Raven, 1993;455.
46. D'Andrea G, Hasselmark L, Alecci M, et al. Increased platelet serotonin content and hypersecretion from dense granules in vitro in tension-type headache. Cephalalgia 1993;13:349.
47. Jensen R, Hindberg I. Plasma serotonin increase during episodes of tension-type headache. Cephalalgia 1994;14:219.
48. Ferrari MD, Odink J, Frölich M, et al. Methionine-enkephalin in migraine and tension headache: Differences between classic migraine, common migraine, and tension headache, and changes during attacks. Headache 1990;30:160.
49. Langemark M, Bach FW, Ekman R, Olesen J. Increased CSF levels of met-enkephalin immunoreactivity in patients with chronic tension-type headache [Abstract]. Pain 1995;63:103.
50. Rolf LH, Wiele G. 5-Hydroxytryptamine in platelets of patients with muscle contraction headache. Headache 1981;21:10.
51. Anthony M, Lance JW. Platelet serotonin in patients with chronic tension headache. J Neurol Neurosurg Psychiatry 1989;52:182.
52. Shukla R, Shanker K, Nag D, et al. Serotonin in tension headache. J Neurol Neurosurg Psychiatry 1987;50:1682.

53. Ferrari MD, Odink J, Tapparelli C, et al. Serotonin metabolism in migraine. Neurology 1989;39:1239.
54. Castillo J, Martinez F, Leira R, et al. Plasma monoamines in tension-type headache. Headache 1994;34:531.
55. Leira R, Castillo J, Martinez F, et al. Platelet-rich plasma serotonin levels in tension-type headache and depression. Cephalalgia 1993;13:346.
56. Nappi G, Facchinetti F, Martignoni E, et al. Plasma and CSF endorphin levels in primary and symptomatic headaches. Headache 1985;25:141.
57. Bach FW, Langemark M, Secher NH, Olesen J. Plasma and cerebrospinal fluid β-endorphin during chronic tension-type headache. Pain 1992;51:163.
58. Bovim G. Cervicogenic headache, migraine, and tension-type headache: Pressure pain thresholds measurements. Pain 1992;51:169.
59. Drummond PD. Scalp tenderness and sensitivity to pain in migraine and tension headache. Headache 1987;27:45.
60. Göbel H, Weigle L, Kropp P, Soyka D. Pain sensitivity and pain reactivity of pericranial muscles in migraine and tension-type headache. Cephalalgia 1992;12:142.
61. Kosek E, Ekholm J. Modulation of pressure pain thresholds during and following isometric contraction. Pain 1995;61:481.
62. Schoenen J. Clinical neurophysiology studies in headache: A review of data and pathophysiological hints. Funct Neurol 1992;7:191.
63. Wallasch TM, Kropp P, Weinschütz T, König B. Contingent Negative Variation in Tension-Type Headache. In J Olesen, J Schoenen (eds), Tension-Type Headache: Classification, Mechanisms, and Treatment. New York: Raven, 1993;173.
64. Pikoff H. Is the muscular model of headache viable? A review of conflicting data. Headache 1984;24:186.
65. Schoenen J, Gérard P, De Pasqua V, Juprelle M. EMG activity in pericranial muscles during postural variation and mental activity in healthy volunteers and patients with chronic tension-type headache. Headache 1991;31:321.
66. Sandrini G, Antonaci F, Pucci E, et al. Comparative study with EMG, pressure algometry, and manual palpation in tension-type headache and migraine. Cephalalgia 1994;14:451.
67. Hatch JP, Prihoda TJ, Moore PJ, et al. A naturalistic study of the relationships among electromyographic activity, psychological stress, and pain in ambulatory tension-type headache patients and headache-free controls. Psychosom Med 1991;53:576.
68. Traue HC, Bischoff C, Zeng H. Sozialer Stress, Muskelspannung und Spaerasgakopfachmerz. Z F Klin Psychol 1986:15:57.
69. Rugh JD, Hatch JP, Moore PJ. The effects of psychological stress on electromyographic activity and negative effect in ambulatory tension-type headache patients. Headache 1990;30:216.
70. Clark GT, Sakai S, Merrill R, et al. Cross-correlation between stress, pain, physical activity, and temporalis muscle EMG in tension-type headache. Cephalalgia 1995;15:511.
71. Jensen R. Mechanisms of spontaneous tension-type headache: An analysis of tenderness, pain thresholds and EMG. Pain 1995;64:251.
72. Jensen R, Olesen J. Initiating mechanisms of experimentally induced tension-type headache. Cephalalgia 1996;16:175.
73. Arena JG, Sherman RA, Bruno GM, Young TR. Electromyographic recordings of low back pain subjects and non-pain controls in six different positions: Effect of pain levels. Pain 1991;45:23.
74. Lund JP, Donga R, Widmer CG, Stohler CS. The pain-adaptation model: A discussion of the relationship between chronic musculoskeletal pain and motor activity. Can J Physiol Pharmacol 1991;69:683.
75. Lipchick GL, Holroyd KA, France CR, et al. Central and peripheral mechanisms in chronic tension-type headache. Pain 1996;64:467.
76. Bendtsen L, Jensen R, Olesen J. Qualitatively altered nociception in chronic myofascial pain. Pain 1996;65:259.
77. Langemark M, Bach FW, Jensen TS, Olesen J. Decreased nociceptive flexion reflex threshold in chronic tension-type headache. Arch Neurol 1993;50:1061.
78. Bendtsen L, Jensen R, Olesen J. Decreased pain detection and tolerance thresholds in chronic tension-type headache. Arch Neurol 1996;53:373.
79. Andrasik F, Passchier J. Tension-Type Headache, Cluster Headache, and Miscellaneous Headaches: Psychological Aspects. In J Olesen, P Tfelt-Hansen, KMA Welch (eds), The Headaches. New York: Raven, 1993;489.
80. Dalkvist J, Ekbom K, Waldenlind E. Headache and mood: A time-series analysis of self-ratings. Cephalalgia 1984;4:45.

81. Donias SH, Peioglou-Harmoussi S, Georgiadis G, Manos N. Differential emotional precipitation of migraine and tension-type headache attacks. Cephalalgia 1991;11:47.
82. Hatch JP, Schoenfeld LS, Boukros NM, et al. Anger and hostility in tension-type headache. Headache 1991;31:302.
83. Kudrow L, Sutkus BJ. MMPI pattern specificity in primary headache disorders. Headache 1979;19:18.
84. Diamond S. Depression and Headache: A Pharmacological Perspective. In CS Adler, SM Packard (eds), Psychiatric Aspects of Headache. Baltimore: Williams & Wilkins, 1987;259.
85. Francis-Jones NF. Cognitive, behavioural, and emotional responses to stressful events: A study of their relationship to headache severity. Cephalalgia 1989;9:248.
86. Schwartz GE. Psychosomatic Disorder and Biofeedback: A Psychobiological Model of Disregulation. In JD Maser, MEP Seligman (eds), Psychopathology: Experimental Models. San Francisco: Freeman, 1977.
87. Hovanitz CA, Wander MR. Tension headache: Disregulation at some levels of stress. J Behav Med 1986;13:539.
88. Andrasik F, Holroyd KA. Physiological and self-report comparisons between tension headache sufferers and nonheadache controls. J Behav Assess 1980;2:135.
89. Schoenen J, Jamart B, Gérard P, et al. Exteroceptive suppression of temporalis muscle activity in chronic headache. Neurology 1987;37:1834.
90. Wallasch TM, Reinecke M, Langohr HD. Exterozeptive Suppression der Temporalismuskelaktivität bei Kopfschmerzen: Seitenvergleich der Dauer der ipsi- und kontralateralen Suppressionsperioden. Nervenheilkunde 1990;9:58.
91. Wallasch TM, Reinecke M, Langohr HD. EMG analysis of the late exteroceptive suppression period of temporal muscle activity in episodic and chronic tension-type headache. Cephalalgia 1991;11:109.
92. Göbel H. Schmerzmessung. Methodisch-theoretische Grundlagen. Experimentelle und Klinische anwendungen. Habilitationschrift. Medizinische Fakultät der Christian-Albrechts-Univerversität zu Kiel, 1990.
93. Nakashima K, Takahashi K. Exteroceptive suppression of the masseter, temporalis, and trapezium muscles produced by mental nerve stimulation in patients with chronic headaches. Cephalalgia 1991;11:23.
94. Wang W, Schoenen J. Reduction of temporalis ES2 by peripheral electrical stimulation in migraine and tension-type headaches. Pain 1994;59:327.
95. Paulus W, Raubüchl O, Straube A, Schoenen J. Exteroceptive suppression of temporalis muscle activity in various types of headache. Headache 1992;32:41.
96. Wallasch TM, Niemann U, Strenge H. The "temporalis inhibitory reflex" in post-lumbar puncture headache [Abstract]. Funct Neurol 1992;5:725.
97. Schoenen J. Exteroceptive Silent Periods of Temporalis Muscle in Headache. In D Van Steenberghe, A De Laat (eds), Electromyography of Jaw Reflexes in Man. Leuven, Belgium: University Press, 1989;357.
98. Bendtsen L, Jensen R, Brennan J, et al. Exteroceptive suppression of temporal muscle activity in normal and chronic tension type headache and not related to actual headache data. Cephalalgia 1986;76:257.
99. Wang W, Schoenen J. Habituation of temporalis ES2 in healthy volunteers, migraine and tension-type headache patients [Abstract]. Proceedings of the EHF 2nd International Conference, Liège, Belgium, 1994;32a.
100. Wang W, Schoenen J. Suppression of temporalis EMG by upper limb stimulations: Results in healthy volunteers, migraine and tension-type headache patients [Abstract]. Proceedings of the EHF 2nd International Conference, Liège, Belgium, 1994;33a.
101. Olesen J, Schoenen J. Tension-Type Headache, Cluster Headache, and Miscellaneous Headaches: Synthesis. In J Olesen, P Tfelt-Hansen, KMA Welch (eds), The Headaches. New York: Raven, 1993;493.
102. Couch JR, Micieli G. Tension-Type Headache, Cluster Headache, and Miscellaneous Headaches: Prophylactic Pharmacotherapy. In J Olesen, P Tfelt-Hansen, KMA Welch (eds), The Headaches. New York: Raven, 1993;537.
103. International Headache Society Committee on Clinical Trials. Guidelines for trials of drug treatments in tension-type headache. Cephalalgia 1995;15:165.
104. Mathew NT. Tension-Type Headache, Cluster Headache, and Miscellaneous Headaches: Acute Pharmacotherapy. In J Olesen, P Tfelt-Hansen, KMA Welch (eds), The Headaches. New York: Raven, 1993;531.
105. Nebe J, Heier M, Diener HC. Low-dose ibuprofen in self-medication of mild to moderate headache: A comparison with acetylsalicylic acid and placebo. Cephalalgia 1995;15:531.

106. Ryan RE. Motrin: A new agent for symptomatic treatment of muscle contraction headache. Headache 1977;16:280.
107. Lance JW, Curran DA. Treatment of chronic tension headache. Lancet 1964;1:1236.
108. Diamond S, Baltes BJ. Chronic tension headache treated with amitriptyline: A double-blind study. Headache 1971;11:110.
109. Morland TJ, Storli OV, Mogstad TE. Doxepin in the prophylactic treatment of mixed "vascular" and tension headache. Headache 1979;19:382.
110. Fogelholm R, Murros K. Maprotiline in chronic tension headache: A double-blind cross-over study. Headache 1985;25:273.
111. Langemark M, Loldrup D, Bech P, Olesen J. Clomipramine and mianserin in the treatment of chronic tension headache: A double-blind, controlled study. Headache 1990;30:118.
112. Pfaffenrath V, Hummelsberger J, Pöllmann W, et al. MMPI personality profiles in patients with primary headache syndromes. Cephalalgia 1991;11:215.
113. Göbel H, Hamouz V, Hansen C, et al. Effect of Amitriptyline Prophylaxis on Headache Symptoms and Neurophysiological Parameters in Tension-Type Headache. In J Olesen, J Schoenen (eds), Tension-Type Headache: Classification, Mechanisms, and Treatment. New York: Raven, 1993;275.
114. Holroyd KA. Tension-Type Headache, Cluster Headache, and Miscellaneous Headaches: Psychological and Behavioral Techniques. In J Olesen, P Tfelt-Hansen, KMA Welch (eds), The Headaches. New York: Raven, 1993;515.
115. Holroyd KA, Penzien DB. Client variables and behavioral treatment of recurrent tension headaches: A meta-analytic review. J Behav Med 1986;9:515.
116. Schoenen J, Pholien P, Maertens de Noordhout A. EMG biofeedback in tension-type headache: Is the 4th session predictive of outcome? Cephalalgia 1985;5:132.
117. Forsell H, Kirveskari P, Kangasniemi P. Changes in headache after treatment of mandibular dysfunction. Cephalalgia 1985;5:229.
118. Schokker RP, Hansson TL, Ansink BJ. The results of treatment of the masticatory system of chronic headache patients. J Craniomandib Disord Facial Oral Pain 1990;4:126.

12
Chronic Daily Headache

Stephen D. Silberstein and Richard B. Lipton

There is no consensus on the classification of very frequent primary headache disorders or on the appropriate use of the term chronic daily headache (CDH). Some authors use it to refer to transformed migraine (TM), a distinct clinical syndrome described in the next section of this chapter. Others use it for any headache disorder that occurs on a daily or near daily basis, regardless of etiology. Although the International Headache Society (IHS) has done much to provide a uniform nomenclature system for headache, it has not yet fully addressed the classification of very frequent primary headache disorders. In this chapter, we use the term CDH to refer to the broad group of frequent (more than 15 days per month) primary headaches, including those associated with medication overuse.

When a patient presents with frequent headaches that are not related to a structural or systemic illness, the physician faces a substantial diagnostic and therapeutic challenge. Although only 0.5% of the population have severe headaches on a daily basis,[1] and only 3% meet IHS criteria for chronic tension-type headache (CTTH),[2] these groups account for the majority of consultations in headache subspecialty practices.[3] Often, such patients are overusing medication, which may play a role in initiating or sustaining the pattern of frequent headaches. Anxiety, depression, and other psychological disturbances may accompany CDH and require treatment.[3]

Several studies have shown that patients with CDH are difficult to classify using the IHS system as currently framed.[4-7] When they can be classified, many individuals with CDH are placed in the CTTH group. If there are superimposed attacks of severe headache, a second IHS diagnosis of migraine is often assigned. Several lines of evidence (outlined below) suggest that patients with CDH evolving from migraine have a form of migraine. Therefore, it seems inappropriate to classify their headaches as a form of tension-type headache (TTH).[3]

Several groups have proposed revisions to the IHS criteria to better encompass the CDH disorders.[3,4,7-9] Even in the absence of uniform terminology, clinicians must develop a systematic approach to these difficult patients. Once secondary headache has been excluded, we recommend dividing frequent headache suffer-

Table 12.1   Headache classification for chronic daily headache

Daily or near daily headache lasting > 4 hours/day for > 15 days/month
- 1.8   Transformed migraine (TM)
    - 1.8.1 with medication overuse
    - 1.8.2 without medication overuse
- 2.2   Chronic tension-type headache (CTTH)
    - 2.2.1 with medication overuse
    - 2.2.2 without medication overuse
- 4.7   New daily persistent headache (NDPH)
    - 4.7.1 with medication overuse
    - 4.7.2 without medication overuse
- 4.8   Hemicrania continua (HC)
    - 4.8.1 with medication overuse
    - 4.8.2 without medication overuse

ers into two groups based on headache duration. When headache duration is less than 4 hours, the differential diagnosis includes cluster headache, chronic paroxysmal hemicrania, idiopathic stabbing headache, hypnic headache, and other miscellaneous headache disorders beyond the scope of this chapter.[10] When the headaches are of longer duration (> 4 hours) the major primary disorders to consider are TM, hemicrania continua (HC), chronic tension-type headache (CTTH), and new daily persistent headache (NDPH) (Table 12.1).[3]

Several authors have examined the relative frequency of some of these conditions in CDH patients. For example, Sandrini et al.[9] classified 90 consecutive outpatients with CDH who attended a clinic in Italy. Most had CDH evolving from migraine (75%), whereas 16.7% had CDH that had begun de novo, and 7.7% had CDH that had evolved from episodic tension-type headache (ETTH). They differentiated two subsets of patients with CDH evolving from migraine. TM referred to those patients who had distinct bouts of migraine that evolved into CDH with the disappearance of typical migraine attacks. Migraine with interparoxysmal headache was defined as recurrent bouts of migraine with a constant, low-severity headache between attacks. These two conditions are most likely different manifestations of the same process.

Silberstein et al.[11] studied 300 patients who were admitted to an inpatient unit with chronic refractory headache. Most patients (216) had CDH associated with medication overuse. A subset of these patients (50) who overused medication were followed for 2 years.[12] Most had TM (74%), some had NDPH (24%), and only 2% had CTTH with a diagnosis of prior ETTH. Most patients (80%) reverted to episodic headache following detoxification, suggesting that both TM and NDPH associated with medication overuse are perpetuated by drug overuse. This conclusion will be validated only after long-term follow-up.

In this chapter, we discuss the classification and treatment of CDH, grouped into the four categories outlined previously. At present, the IHS provides criteria for only one of those disorders. We have proposed revisions to the IHS system and offered criteria for TM, HC, CTTH, and NDPH.[3] We recognize that our proposal is not universally accepted and that other rational systems using alternative terminology exist (see Chapter 6). Ultimately, the Classification Committee of the IHS will have to establish uniform terminology through an international consensus process. We present our framework to facilitate clinical diagnosis and research. We also discuss the role of medication overuse in the development and treatment of CDH disorders, as well as their mechanisms and treatment.

CATEGORIES OF CHRONIC DAILY HEADACHE

Transformed Migraine

Many studies have described the process and associated features of transformed migraine.[3,13–16] Patients with TM often have a history of episodic migraine, typically beginning in their teens or twenties.[3,13] The majority of patients with this disorder are women, 90% of whom have a history of migraine without aura. The headaches grow more frequent over months to years, and the associated symptoms of photophobia, phonophobia, and nausea become less severe and less frequent than in typical migraine.[13–16] Patients often develop a pattern of daily or almost daily headaches that resemble CTTH. That is, the pain is often mild to moderate and not associated with photophobia, phonophobia, or gastrointestinal symptoms. Other features of migraine, including aggravation by menstruation and other trigger factors, as well as unilaterality and gastrointestinal symptoms, may persist. Attacks of full-blown migraine superimposed on a background of less severe headaches occur in many patients. Ninan Mathew coined the term TM to refer to this process.

Most patients with TM overuse symptomatic medication.[13–16] Stopping the overused medication frequently results in distinct headache improvement. Many patients have significant long-term improvement after detoxification. Eighty percent of patients with TM have depression.[13,16] The depression often lifts when the pattern of medication overuse and daily headache is interrupted. Although TM is well recognized as a clinical entity, widely accepted formal diagnostic criteria are lacking. We have proposed revisions to the IHS criteria that would include TM as a form of migraine. In our initial proposal[3] (referred to hereafter as 1994 criteria), the diagnosis of TM depended on a past history of migraine as defined by IHS criteria and a process of transformation leading to headaches that last more than 4 hours a day and occur at least 15 days per month. The period of transformation is characterized by increasing headache frequency and decreasing prominence of associated migrainous features. We elected not to require particular characteristics for the daily or near daily headaches, in part because these headaches are pleomorphic. Patients with TM often continue to have episodic superimposed bouts of full-blown migraine. Some patients find that their migraine headaches disappear completely.[9,17] For this reason, we did not originally include the continuing occurrence of superimposed migraine attacks as part of our definition.

We tested our 1994 criteria for TM in 150 consecutive patients who presented to a headache subspecialty clinic with more than 15 headaches per month.[8] We tested the comprehensiveness of the IHS system with the addition of our revisions. That is, we wanted to be able to assign a clinically useful diagnosis to every patient with CDH. Despite our revisions, we still could not classify 29% of

Table 12.2   1995 criteria for transformed migraine

1.8   Transformed migraine
    A.   Daily or almost daily (> 15 days/month) head pain for > 1 month
    B.   Average headache duration of > 4 hours/day (if untreated)
    C.   At least one of the following:
        1.   History of episodic migraine meeting any IHS criteria 1.1–1.6
        2.   History of increasing headache frequency with decreasing severity of migrainous features over at least 3 months
        3.   Headache at some time meets IHS criteria for migraine 1.1–1.6 other than duration
    D.   Does not meet criteria for new daily persistent headache (4.7) or hemicrania continua (4.8)
    E.   At least one of the following:
        1.   There is no suggestion of one of the disorders listed in groups 5–11*
        2.   Such a disorder is suggested, but it is ruled out by appropriate investigations
        3.   Such a disorder is present, but first migraine attacks do not occur in close temporal relation to the disorder

*Disorders listed in groups 5–11 refer to International Headache Society diagnostic groups.
IHS = International Headache Society.
Source: SD Silberstein, RB Lipton, M Sliwinski. Classification of daily and near daily headaches: field trial of revised IHS criteria. Neurology 1996;47:871.

patients. We reviewed our classification failures and found that 41% of the unclassified patients were not able to provide an accurate history of prior headaches, and 55% could not describe a period of escalation, often because consultation occurred many years after the daily or near daily headaches developed.[8] Because most of these patients had a clinical diagnosis of TM, we reasoned that our criteria, as originally proposed, were too restrictive.

Based on these data, we developed our "1995 criteria" for TM[17a] (Table 12.2). We argued that the requirements of diagnosable migraine in the past and a history of escalation over 3 months imposed undue burdens given the limitations of patient recall. Although we believed that links to migraine were important, we wanted to provide alternative criteria to reduce the proportion of patients who could not be classified. We therefore provided three *alternative* diagnostic links to migraine: (1) prior history of IHS-defined migraine, or (2) a clear period of escalating headache frequency with decreasing severity of migrainous features (both were required in the 1994 criteria), or (3) current superimposed attacks of headaches that meet the IHS criteria for migraine except for duration.

A consequence of this less restrictive definition was that some patients met the criteria for more than one disorder, for example, both TM and CTTH. When this problem was encountered in the classification of psychiatric diseases the solution was to develop hierarchical rules. That is, if a patient meets the criteria for two disorders, a hierarchical rule establishes which diagnosis should be used. In our 1995 criteria the diagnosis of TM precludes a diagnosis of either episodic migraine (IHS 1.1–1.7) or CTTH. A limitation of this hierarchical rule is that some patients with episodic migraine and independent CTTH will be misclassified as TM. We predict this should be a rare event. With these revisions, we were able to classify virtually all of our CDH patients. The number of patients with TM increased dramatically. Using our revisions, essentially every patient not classi-

Table 12.3 Proposed criteria for hemicrania continua

4.8 Hemicrania continua[a]
   A. Headache present for at least 1 month
   B. Strictly unilateral headache
   C. Absolute response to indomethacin
   D. Pain has all three of the following characteristics present:
      1. Continuous but fluctuating
      2. Moderate severity, at least some of the time
      3. Lack of precipitating mechanisms
   E. May have associated stabbing headaches
   F. At least one of the following:
      1. There is no suggestion of one of the disorders listed in groups 5–11[b]
      2. Such a disorder is suggested, but it is ruled out by appropriate investigations
      3. Such a disorder is present, but first headache attacks do not occur in close temporal relation to the disorder

[a]Hemicrania continua is usually nonremitting, but rare cases of remission have been reported.
[b]Disorders listed in groups 5–11 refer to International Headache Society diagnostic groups.

fied as TM or CTTH met the criteria for NDPH or HC. Thus, the objective of comprehensiveness was met. Reliability and validity still need to be studied.

Migraine transformation most often develops in the setting of medication overuse, but transformation may occur without overuse.[18] Using the IHS criteria, a firm diagnosis of "headache induced by substance use or exposure" requires that the headaches remit after the overused medication is discontinued. This criterion is difficult to apply reliably, and diagnosis is impossible until the overused medication is discontinued. As an alternative, we provide definitions for medication overuse based on a review of published reports and clinical experience (in a separate section later in the chapter).[3] This is intended to supplement, but not replace, the more restrictive but useful construct of the IHS classification of headache induced by substance use or exposure.

Hemicrania Continua

Hemicrania continua is a rare, indomethacin-responsive headache disorder characterized by a continuous, moderately severe, unilateral headache that varies in intensity, waxing and waning without disappearing completely.[19] In the rarest of patients, it may alternate sides.[20] HC is frequently associated with jabs and jolts (idiopathic stabbing headache). Exacerbations of pain are often associated with autonomic disturbances such as ptosis, miosis, tearing, and sweating. HC is not triggered by neck movements, but tender spots in the neck may be present (Table 12.3). Some patients may have photophobia, phonophobia, and nausea.

Although the disorder almost invariably has a prompt and enduring response to indomethacin, the requirement of a therapeutic response as a diagnostic criterion is problematic. It effectively excludes the diagnosis of HC in patients never treated with indomethacin (perhaps because another agent helped) and in patients who failed to respond to indomethacin. Treatment response is generally

Table 12.4   Proposed criteria for new daily persistent headache

4.7   New Daily Persistent Headache
A. Average headache frequency > 15 days/month for > 1 month
B. Average headache duration > 4 hours/day (if untreated). Frequently constant without medication but may fluctuate
C. No history of tension-type headache or migraine that increases in frequency and decreases in severity in association with the onset of NDPH (over 3 months)
D. Acute onset (developing over < 3 days) of constant unremitting headache
E. Headache is constant in location? (Needs to be tested)
F. Does not meet criteria for hemicrania continua (4.8)
G. At least one of the following:
1. There is no suggestion of one of the disorders listed in groups 5–11*
2. Such a disorder is suggested, but it is ruled out by appropriate investigations
3. Such a disorder is present, but first headache attacks do not occur in close temporal relation to the disorder

*Disorders listed in groups 5–11 refer to International Headache Society diagnostic groups.

not part of IHS case definitions of headache disorders. Although a good therapeutic response to indomethacin adds confidence that HC is present, the significance of a lack of response is less clear. Despite these reservations, our draft criteria include indomethacin response as a diagnostic feature. When the IHS criteria are revised, the Classification Committee may elect to include it as a confirmatory feature.

HC exists in both continuous and remitting forms. In the continuous form, headaches occur on a daily, continuous basis, sometimes for years. Many patients with this disorder overuse acute medication; it must be differentiated from TM. In the remitting form, periods of daily headache alternate with pain-free remissions. Both forms meet the criteria in Table 12.3. HC takes precedence over the diagnosis of other types of primary CDH.

New Daily Persistent Headache

NDPH (Table 12.4) is characterized by the relatively abrupt onset of an unremitting CDH: a patient develops a headache that does not go away.[21] NDPH is likely to be a heterogeneous disorder. Some cases may reflect a postviral syndrome.[21] The development of daily headache is abrupt, occurring over less than 3 days. In fact, some patients remember the exact day or time the headache started. Patients with NDPH are generally younger than those with TM.[21]

We elected not to classify NDPH as a type of de novo CTTH, for it is not clear whether this condition is etiologically related to TTH. Because NDPH and CTTH have similar characteristics, the disorders are distinguished by the absence or presence of a past history of headache. NDPH requires the absence of a history of evolution from migraine or ETTH. Excluding all patients with a history of ETTH is problematic, because almost 70% of men and 90% of women have had a TTH in the past. We allow a diagnosis of NDPH in patients with migraine or ETTH if those disorders do not increase in frequency to give rise to NDPH.

Table 12.5   Proposed criteria for chronic tension-type headache

2.2   Chronic tension-type headache
    A.   Average headache frequency more than 15 days/month (180 days/year) with average duration of 4 hours/day (if untreated) for 6 months fulfilling criteria B–D listed below
    B.   At least two of the following pain characteristics:
        1.   Pressing/tightening quality
        2.   Mild or moderate severity (may inhibit, but does not prohibit, activities)
        3.   Bilateral location
        4.   No aggravation by walking stairs or similar routine physical activity
    C.   History of episodic tension-type headache in the past
    D.   History of evolutive headaches that gradually increased in frequency over at least a 3-month period [a]
    E.   Both of the following:
        1.   No vomiting
        2.   No more than one of nausea, photophobia, or phonophobia
    F.   At least one of the following:
        1.   There is no suggestion of one of the disorders listed in groups 5–11 [b]
        2.   Such a disorder is suggested, but it is ruled out by appropriate investigations
        3.   Such a disorder is present, but first headache attacks do not occur in close temporal relation to the disorder

[a]May be difficult to document or may not be applicable.
[b]Disorders listed in groups 5–11 refer to International Headache Society diagnostic groups.

NDPH may or may not be associated with medication overuse (4.7.1, 4.7.2). A diagnosis of NDPH takes precedence over one of TM or CTTH.

Chronic Tension-Type Headache

Daily headaches may also develop in patients with a history of ETTH (Table 12.5). These headaches are more often diffuse or bilateral, frequently involving the posterior aspect of the head and neck. In CTTH, in contrast to TM, prior or coexistent episodic migraine and most features of migraine are absent.

We propose several modifications to the current classification of CTTH. CTTH (2.2) requires head pain on at least 15 days a month for at least 6 months; patients often have daily headaches. Although the pain criteria are identical to ETTH, the IHS classification allows nausea but not vomiting. There is a need for operational rules regarding nausea, photophobia, and phonophobia, and for the decision about whether or not these features are prominent.[7] Mild nausea or mild photophobia and phonophobia may prove to be compatible with the diagnosis of CTTH if better measures of symptom severity are developed.[3,7,13] However, the need to include any of these migrainous features in the IHS definition of CTTH may be a result of including cases of TM under the rubric of CTTH. If TM is classified separately, it may not be necessary to include migrainous features in the diagnostic criteria for CTTH. For the present, the criteria we propose continue to permit only one of nausea, photophobia, and phonophobia (but these features need to be further tested).

CTTH evolving from ETTH requires a prior diagnosis of ETTH. Diagnostic confidence increases if ETTH increases in frequency until the criteria of CTTH are met. As with TM, the methods used for ascertaining and defining the evolutive process need to be better specified. The requirement of a history of TTH and a period of escalation needs to be tested. The IHS definition of CTTH includes no explicit time durations of headache. CTTH criteria should be modified to include an average headache duration of more than 4 hours (see Table 12.5). CTTH can exist in two varieties: headaches associated with (2.2.0.1) and not associated with (2.2.0.2) medication overuse. One could argue that CTTH could begin without preceding ETTH, in a scenario analogous to the development of chronic cluster headache (i.e., unrelenting from onset). However, cluster headache involves a series of episodic attacks, not a constant headache. Does CTTH, if unremitting from onset, differ from NDPH? We believe that there is a biological difference between them, but this has not been proven.

Pfaffenrath and Isler[7] proposed alternative modifications of the CTTH criteria to allow some migrainous features such as pulsatile pain, predominantly one-sided pain location, photophobia and phonophobia, and mild nausea and anorexia, but not severe nausea or vomiting. They recognized that there are patients with CDH who cannot be classified within the current IHS system. They advocate expanding the CTTH group instead of expanding the migraine group. We prefer to expand the migraine group, because of the arguments outlined previously that tie TM to migraine. In the absence of a definitive biological marker or gold standard for migraine diagnosis, it is difficult to argue absolutely for either position. Classification rules for patients with current migraine or current ETTH and the hierarchy that relates these disorders require further definition. As genetic markers emerge, biologically homogeneous subgroups of CDH may well be defined.

DRUG OVERUSE AND REBOUND HEADACHE

Patients with frequent headaches often overuse analgesics, narcotics, ergotamine, and sumatriptan. Medication overuse by headache-prone patients frequently produces CDH (drug-induced rebound headache) accompanied by dependence on symptomatic medication. In addition, medication overuse can make headaches refractory to prophylactic medication.[18,22–26] Stopping the symptomatic medication may result in the development of withdrawal symptoms and a period of increased headache. Subsequently, the rule is headache improvement.[26,27–30] For example, in two studies, hospitalized patients were withdrawn from ergotamine and analgesics without further therapy. Migraine prophylaxis was delayed for at least 3 months. More than 60% of these patients no longer had daily headaches, although approximately 40% still had some migraine attacks.[31,32]

Most patients with drug-induced headache seen in subspecialty centers have a history of episodic migraine that has been converted into TM as a result of medication overuse.[13,26,29,33–35] Patients with TTH, HC, and NDPH may also overuse symptomatic medications. Drug-induced CDH, or, as Isler[36] has termed it, "painkiller headache," has been reported since the seventeenth century, and occurrences reached epidemic proportions in Switzerland after World War II.

Epidemiology of Drug-Induced Headache

The epidemiology of chronic drug-induced headache is uncertain. In European headache centers, 5–10% of the patients have drug-induced headache. One series of 3,000 consecutive headache patients reported that 4.3% had drug-induced headaches.[37] In some American specialty headache clinics, as many as 80% of patients who presented with CDH used analgesics on a daily or near daily basis.[24] Other headache clinics report a smaller percentage but a majority nonetheless.[38]

Diener and Tfelt-Hansen[39] summarized 29 studies that included 2,612 patients with chronic drug-induced headache. Migraine was the primary headache in 65%, TTH in 27%, and mixed or other headaches in 8% (e.g., cluster headache). Women had more drug-induced headache than men (by a ratio of 3.5 to 1; 1,533 women, 442 men). The mean duration of primary headache was 20.4 years. The mean admitted time of frequent drug intake was 10.3 years in one study, and the mean duration of daily headache was 5.9 years. Results from headache diaries show that the number of tablets or suppositories taken per day averaged 4.9 (range, 0.25–25.00). Patients took, on average, 2.5–5.8 different pharmacologic components simultaneously (range, 1–14).[39]

Patients attending an outpatient neurology clinic in Austria reported taking, on average, 6.3 different headache pain drugs.[40] Of these patients, 26.5% reported using both prescription and over-the-counter (OTC) medications, 31.3% used OTC medications only, and 27.7% used prescription drugs only. Acetaminophen (average dose, 500 mg) was the most frequently used analgesic. Most patients attending a London migraine clinic used multiple medications.[41] Acetaminophen, again, was the most commonly used analgesic (34.9%), followed by aspirin (22.9%).

In a cross-sectional survey carried out in 1986–1987 in Tromsø, Norway, 19,137 men and women (aged 12–56 years) from the general population were asked about their drug use over the preceding 14 days. On average, 28% of the women and 13% of the men had used analgesics. The most significant predictor of analgesic use was headache; a lesser association was found with infections. Drug use in women was associated with symptoms of depression. Drug use in men was associated with sleeplessness. Higher drug use was associated with smoking and high coffee consumption, but not with frequent alcohol intake.[42]

In a representative sample of the Swiss population, 4.4% of men and 6.8% of women took analgesics at least once a week; 2.3% took them daily.[43] Analgesic dependency was more frequent than dependence on tranquilizers, hypnotics, or stimulating drugs in psychiatric inpatients in Switzerland.[44] In Germany, possibly 1% of the population take up to 10 pain tablets every day.[45]

In the United States, 20.2% of a national sample survey of 20,468 individuals reported "severe headache." OTC medications were used by 62.6% of the women and 74.6% of the men; prescription drugs were used by 34.5% of women and 21.3% of the men. OTC analgesic use was greater than prescription medication use among migraineurs as well as among those suffering from severe headache that was not further defined.[46]

A random telephone survey of 24,159 households in Canada produced a sample of 1,573 households with one or more eligible headache sufferers. Ninety percent of the IHS-diagnosed migraineurs reported using OTC drugs and 44% reported using prescription drugs. In the same sample, 1.5% of migraineurs had rebound headache resulting from ergotamine tartrate or analgesic overuse. Drug-induced rebound headache presents a major public health problem in both the clinic and the community.[47]

Clinical Features of Rebound Headache

Analgesic rebound headache has not been demonstrated in placebo-controlled trials. However, stopping daily low-dose caffeine frequently results in withdrawal headache.[48] In a controlled study of caffeine withdrawal, 64 normal adults (71% women) with low-to-moderate caffeine intake (the equivalent of about 2.5 cups of coffee a day) were given a two-day caffeine-free diet and either placebo or replacement caffeine. Under double-blind conditions, 50% of the patients who were given placebo had a headache by day two, compared with 6% of those given caffeine. Nausea, depression, and flu-like symptoms were very common in the placebo group. This study is relevant because caffeine is frequently used by headache sufferers for pain relief, often in combination with analgesics or ergotamine. The study is a model for short-term caffeine withdrawal but does not demonstrate the long-term consequences of detoxification.

The actual dose limits and time needed to develop rebound headaches have not been defined in rigorous studies. In addition, the relationship of drug half-life to the development of rebound is unknown. Our clinical knowledge is derived from observing patterns of medication use in patients who present with rebound headaches. Because there may be large individual differences in susceptibility to rebound headaches, anecdotal data must be generalized cautiously. It is believed that overuse occurs when patients take three or more simple analgesics a day more often than 5 days a week, combination analgesics containing barbiturates, sedatives, or caffeine more often than 3 days per week, or narcotics or ergotamine tartrate more often than 2 days per week.[13,18,26]

Specific limits are necessary to prevent overuse of analgesics, ergotamine, and sumatriptan. Wilkinson,[24] Saper,[27] Mathew et al.,[13] and Scholz et al.[49] compared ergotamine intake in patients with and without CDH. In the groups without CDH the maximum ergotamine intake was 24 mg per month. However, one patient with CDH consumed only 7 mg of ergotamine per month. The frequency of days of ergotamine use (treatment days or events) is as important as, if not more important than, the total monthly dose.[25,27] Rebound can develop in patients taking as little as 0.5–1.0 mg of ergotamine three times a week.[3,24,25,30]

Scholz et al.[49] studied the consumption of simple analgesics, comparing patients with and without rebound headache. Patients with rebound headache consumed between 1,200 and 1,500 mg of analgesics a day. Increased consumption of caffeine, but not of codeine, was correlated with the development of CDH. Barbiturate consumption was significantly higher in patients with CDH (60–500 mg per day; mean, 160 mg per day) than in those without CDH (mean < 60 mg per day). Recently, sumatriptan, a selective 5-HT$_1$ agonist that is effective in acute migraine treatment, has been reported to induce rebound headache.[50] We recommend limiting the use of sumatriptan to 3 days per week.

Most daily headache patients overuse symptomatic medication.[18] Psychological dependence, tolerance, and abstinence syndromes may develop. Medication overuse may be responsible in part for the transformation of episodic migraine or ETTH into daily headache and for the perpetuation of the syndrome. However, medication overuse is not a sine qua non of TM or CTTH. Some patients develop TM or CTTH without overusing medication, and others continue to have daily headaches long after the overused medication is discontinued. Medication overuse is usually motivated by a patient's desire to treat the headaches. However, some headache patients may overuse combination analgesics to treat their mood disturbance, and, in rare instances, medication overuse represents a form of primary substance abuse.

There are those who doubt the existence of drug-induced headache.[51] When Fisher[51] failed to find analgesic rebound headache in patients who were using analgesics for their arthritis, he attempted to refute the concept. His work has been reinterpreted to suggest that headache-prone patients are especially vulnerable to the rebound phenomenon. Headache-prone patients often develop daily headaches if put on analgesics for a nonheadache indication.[52,53]

In addition to exacerbating the headache disorder, drug overuse has other serious effects. The overuse of symptomatic drugs may interfere with the effectiveness of preventive headache medications. Long-duration use of large amounts of medication may cause renal or hepatic toxicity in addition to tolerance, habituation, or dependence. (Tolerance refers to the decreased effectiveness of the same dose of an analgesic, often leading to the use of higher doses to achieve the same degree of effectiveness. Habituation and dependence are, respectively, the psychological and physical need to repeatedly use drugs.)

PSYCHIATRIC COMORBIDITY WITH CHRONIC DAILY HEADACHE

Anxiety, depression, and bipolar disease are more frequent in migraine patients than in nonmigraine control subjects.[54,55] Because TM evolves from migraine, one would also expect psychiatric comorbidity in TM. In a clinic-based study of 630 patients with CDH, including patients with TM, CTTH, NDPH, and posttraumatic headache, the Minnesota Multiphasic Personality Inventory was abnormal in 61%, compared with 12.2% of patients with episodic migraine. Zung and Beck Depression Scale scores were significantly higher in the CDH patients than in migraine controls.[56] In several subspecialty center–based studies, depression occurred in about 80% of TM patients.[13,17,25] Clinical experience suggests that comorbid depression often improves when the cycle of daily head pain is broken.[57] The biological relationships between migraine, vulnerability to rebound headache, and psychiatric comorbidity remain to be clarified.

Psychiatric comorbidity is a predictor of headache intractability. The Minnesota Multiphasic Personality Inventory was abnormal in 100% of patients with CDH who failed to respond to aggressive management (31% of the CDH group), compared with 48% of the responders. Physical, emotional, or sexual abuse, parental alcohol abuse, and a positive dexamethasone suppression test were also highly correlated with poor response to aggressive management.

PATHOPHYSIOLOGY OF CHRONIC DAILY HEADACHE

Usually the pain from intensive stimulation or injury diminishes as healing progresses. Chronic continuous pain is often due to ongoing peripheral activation of nociceptors (e.g., chronic inflammation), although at times chronic pain may occur in the absence of painful stimuli. Although the pathophysiology of CDH is unknown, recent work suggests several mechanisms that could contribute to the process. CDH may be due to: (1) abnormal excitation of peripheral nociceptive afferent fibers, perhaps due to chronic neurogenic inflammation; (2) enhanced responsiveness of the nucleus caudalis (NC) neurons, i.e., central sensitization; (3) decreased pain modulation; (4) spontaneous central pain; or (5) a combination of these.

Peripheral Mechanisms

In migraine, trigeminal nerve activation is accompanied by the release of vasoactive neuropeptides, including calcitonin gene-related peptides (CGRP), substance P (SP), and neurokinin A from the nerve terminals. These mediators produce mast cell activation, sensitization of the nerve terminals, and extravasation of fluid into the perivascular space around the dural blood vessels. Intense neuronal stimulation causes induction of c-*fos* (an immediate early gene product) in the trigeminal NC of the brain stem. SP and CGRP further amplify the trigeminal terminal sensitivity by stimulating the release of bradykinin and other inflammatory mediators from nonneuronal cells.[58] Inflammatory mediators not only increase the responsiveness of, but also turn on, silent, or sleeping, nociceptors. Neurotropins such as NGF are synthesized locally and can also activate mast cells and sensitize nerve terminals.[59] Bradykinin and kallidin, both acting through the B_1 and B_2 receptors, can activate primary afferent nociceptors.[60] Prostaglandins and nitric oxide (a diffusible gas that acts as a neurotransmitter)[61] are both endogenous mediators that can be produced locally and can sensitize nociceptors. Repeated episodes of neurogenic inflammation may chronically sensitize nociceptors and thus contribute to the development of daily headache.

Central sensitization is a phenomenon well described in animal research. It is manifested by increased spontaneous impulse discharges, increased responsiveness to noxious and nonnoxious peripheral stimuli, and expanded receptive fields of nociceptive neurons. In animal models, conditioning stimuli that activate C (unmyelinated) fibers result in a marked and prolonged increase in the flexion withdrawal reflex in rats. Repetitive C-fiber stimulation at constant intensity induces the phenomenon of windup, which is the increase in dorsal horn nociceptive neuron responsiveness in both magnitude and duration with each subsequent stimulus above a certain frequency.[62]

Windup is sensitive to NMDA receptor antagonists. Neurons that exhibit windup are less sensitive to opioids than are neurons that do not.[63] Windup is a short-lasting phenomenon and cannot explain the phenomenon of sensitization, which is of longer duration and may involve changes in neuronal plasticity. Windup is mediated by NMDA and tachykinin receptors, blocked by morphine pretreatment, and accompanied by calcium entry via NMDA channels. It may be the trigger to long-lasting neuronal sensitization. The increased intracellular calcium induces translocation (from cytosolic to membrane-bound form) and activation of protein kinase C and phosphorylation of the NMDA channel, which relieves the Mg^{+2} block on the ion channel.[63] The increased calcium may also be responsible for the induction of the genes whose products are c-*fos* and c-*jun*.[63] This results in increased glutamate sensitivity. NGF and inflammatory cytokines may change the phenotype of sensory neurons, making them more sensitive to nociception.[64] NGF increases the synthesis, transport, and neuronal content of SP and CGRP. It also regulates two ion channels in sensory neurons: the capsaicin receptor ion channel and the tetrodotoxin-resistant Na^+ channel.[65]

Does central sensitization play a role in headache? In animal models of head pain, there is good evidence for c-*fos* activation in the trigeminal NC. In the NC superior dorsal horn, c-*fos* is a marker for nociceptive stimulation and may be one signal for the adaptive responses of the nervous system to insult.[66] C-*fos* and c-*jun*, two early gene products, can alter other peptides, proteins, and receptors, perhaps accounting for long-lasting neuronal sensitization. Sensitization of the NC neurons may result in increased activation of the trigeminal vascular system.

Pain Modulation

The mammalian nervous system contains networks that modulate nociceptive transmission. In the rostroventromedial medulla are so-called off-cells that inhibit and on-cells that facilitate nociception.[67] These cells are believed to modulate the activity of the trigeminal NC and dorsal horn neurons. Increased on-cell activity in the brain stem's pain modulation system could enhance the response to both painful and nonpainful stimuli. Opiate withdrawal results in increased firing of the on-cells, decreased firing of the off-cells, and enhanced nociception.[67] A similar mechanism may be at work during drug-induced headaches. CDH may result, in part, from enhanced neuronal activity in the NC as a result of enhanced on-cell or decreased off-cell activity. Other conditioned stimuli associated with pain and stress can also turn on the system and may account for some of the association between pain and stress.

Spontaneous Central Pain Activation

Post et al.[68] have suggested the kindling model for epilepsy as a model for nonepileptic progressive disorders such as mania. In kindling, low-level electrical stimulation induces a complex series of neurochemical and anatomic changes. C-*fos* activation provides evidence of transcription, and other early and late gene products may be expressed. Post and Silberstein[68] suggested that in the process of headache transformation, spontaneous recurrent migraine headaches may be analogous to the low levels of electrical stimulation in the kindling model. Preventive treatment of migraine could provide a dual benefit by preventing the occurrence of episodes and blocking the sensitization process that could lead to syndrome progression.

Drug-Induced Headache Mechanisms

Overuse of analgesics, barbiturates, or ergotamine-containing compounds may contribute to the transformation of episodic migraine into TM. Some believe drug-induced CDH is due to a rebound effect. Medication withdrawal triggers the next headache, which in turn leads to the consumption of more drug. This may produce a vicious cycle resulting in more frequent drug use and drug-induced CDH. Formulations of drugs that maintain sustained, nonfluctuating levels might avoid the development of drug-induced headache.[68]

CDH may be a result of enhanced nociception in the headache-prone individual. Continued high, fluctuating doses of ergots, analgesics, or narcotics could result in resetting of the pain control mechanisms in susceptible individuals, perhaps by enhancing on-cell activity, enhancing central sensitization through NMDA receptors, or blocking adaptive antinociceptive changes. The consequences of drug discontinuation depend on the type of therapeutic response the drug engenders. Different drugs are effective in different phases of migraine. Some drugs are effective only abortively, others only preventively, and some are effective only for infrequent episodic headache and not for frequent intractable migraine. Compensatory adaptive changes associated with frequent headaches, if they do occur, may not be enough to allow continued drug effectiveness. If tolerance has decreased drug effectiveness, a drug holiday could renew the response.[68] Drug overuse may, in part, prevent the occurrence of antinociceptive adaptive changes. The analgesic washout period could be a result of the time required for the system to reset. The failure of preventive drugs could result from the lack of endogenous antinociceptive agents. A similar phenomenon occurs in contingent tolerance in the seizure kindling model (described in the next section).

It has recently been demonstrated that cerebral blood flow increases in the brain stem and cortex of patients with migraine without aura. During the headache, the increased cerebral blood flow in the cortex, but not in the brain stem, is reversed by sumatriptan, as is the headache. This area of the brain stem is rich in opioids and includes the pain control centers. Dihydroergotamine and 311C90 (a selective 5-HT$_{1D}$ agonist effective in migraine treatment) selectively bind to this area of the brain stem, whereas sumatriptan may not. Perhaps this area of the brain stem integrates the phenomenon we call migraine. Ongoing activity in this area of the brain stem may produce recurrent or daily headache. Acute migraine medications may induce daily headache by preventing the development of adaptive changes and perhaps by maintaining brain stem activation.[69]

Contingent Tolerance Phenomena

The long-term effectiveness of anticonvulsants can be studied in amygdala-kindled animals. Repeated pretreatment with carbamazepine before kindling results in a loss of drug efficacy and constitutes a unique form of associative or contingent tolerance. Animals treated with carbamazepine after seizures occur do not show tolerance. Tolerance, once developed, can be reversed by giving the drug after seizures occur.[70] Some neurobiological alterations following seizures may thus be adaptive, or anticonvulsant, in contrast to more enduring changes related to the primary pathophysiology of the kindled process.[68]

Clinical strategies based on these concepts might be used to reverse tolerance in the long-term treatment of migraine or TM. Switching a patient to a drug that has a different mechanism of action and does not show cross-tolerance, or discontinuing the ineffective drug and reintroducing it later, may be effective in some migraine or TM patients.

TREATMENT

Patients suffering from CDH (especially drug-induced headache) can be difficult to treat, especially when they exhibit comorbid depression, low frustration tolerance, and physical and emotional dependency.[18,26] We recommend the following steps. First, exclude secondary headache disorders and reassure yourself and the patient; second, diagnose the specific primary headache disorder (e.g., TM, HC); and third, identify comorbid medical and psychiatric conditions and exacerbating factors, especially medication overuse. Limit all symptomatic medications (with the possible exception of the long-acting nonsteroidal anti-inflammatory drugs [NSAIDs]). For outpatients, we gradually taper the overused medications, often replacing them with NSAIDs. Patients should be started on a program of preventive medication (to decrease reliance on symptomatic medication), with the explicit understanding that the drugs may not become fully effective until medication overuse has been eliminated and the washout period completed.[41]

Inpatient and outpatient detoxification options are available. Withdrawal symptoms, including severely exacerbated headache accompanied by nausea, vomiting, agitation, restlessness, sleep disorder, and (rarely) seizures, may occur and may persist for as long as 2 weeks. Barbiturates and benzodiazepines must be tapered gradually to avoid a serious withdrawal syndrome. The washout period may last 3–8 weeks; once it is over, headaches are very often considerably improved.[11,13,30,71]

Detoxification can be difficult and sometimes requires hospitalization. Diener et al.[72] were able to detoxify only 1.5% of 200 patients on an outpatient basis. Hering and Steiner,[73] in contrast, successfully used outpatient detoxification in 37 of 46 patients who were taking simple analgesics or ergotamine. Based on the experience of many clinicians, it appears that the detoxification process may require hospitalization and can last up to 2 weeks. A recent consensus paper by the German Migraine Society recommends outpatient withdrawal for highly motivated patients who do not take barbiturates or tranquilizers with their analgesics. Inpatient treatment is recommended for patients who fail outpatient treatment, have high depression scores, or take tranquilizers, codeine, or barbiturates.[74]

Disturbances in mood and function are common and require management with behavioral methods of pain management and supportive psychotherapy (including biofeedback, stress management, and cognitive-behavioral therapy). Treatment of the comorbid psychiatric illness is often necessary before the CDH comes under control. Chronobiological interventions, such as encouraging regular habits of sleep, exercise, and meals, are often useful.[41]

Symptomatic Pharmacotherapy

Patients who do not overuse symptomatic medication can treat acute headache exacerbations with antimigraine drugs including sumatriptan, dihydroergotamine (DHE), and ergotamine, as well as narcotics. Use of these drugs must be strictly limited to prevent the development of superimposed rebound headache that will complicate treatment and require detoxification. The risk of rebound is much lower for DHE and sumatriptan than for analgesics, narcotics, and ergotamine.

Preventive Pharmacotherapy

Patients with daily headaches should be treated primarily with preventive medications, with the explicit understanding that the medications may not become fully effective until any overused medications have been eliminated. It may take 3–6 weeks for treatment effects to develop.

The following principles should guide the use of preventive treatment: (1) From among the first-line drugs, choose preventive agents based on their side-effect profiles, comorbid conditions, and specific indications (e.g., indomethacin for HC). (2) Start at a low dose. (3) Gradually increase the dose until you achieve efficacy, until the patient develops side effects, or until the ceiling dose for the drug in question is reached. (4) Treatment effects develop over weeks, and treatment may not become fully effective until rebound is eliminated. (5) If one agent fails and if all other things are equal, choose an agent from another therapeutic class. (6) Prefer monotherapy, but be willing to use combination therapy. (7) Communicate realistic expectations.[75]

Most preventive agents used for CDH have not been examined in well-designed double-blind studies. Table 12.6 summarizes an assessment of the efficacy, safety, and evidence for a number of agents.[76]

Antidepressants are attractive agents for use in CDH (TM, CTTH, NDPH), because many patients have comorbid depression and anxiety. The most widely used tricyclic antidepressants are nortriptyline (Aventyl, Pamelor), amitriptyline[77–86] (Elavil), and doxepin[87] (Sinequan), starting at 10–25 mg at bedtime and gradually increasing. Fluoxetine (Prozac), a selective serotonin reuptake inhibitor (SSRI), is coming into wider use for daily headaches; evidence from a double-blind study demonstrates its efficacy in CDH.[77,88] Fluvoxamine appears to be effective[89] and may have analgesic properties.[90] Other SSRIs and monoamine oxidase inhibitors may have a therapeutic role, but none has been proven to date.[91]

Beta-blockers (propranolol, nadolol) remain a mainstay of therapy for migraine[41] and are also used for CDH.[84,92] Though clinicians fear that beta-blockers may exacerbate depression, that relationship is controversial.[93] Beta-blockers are relatively contraindicated in patients with asthma and Raynaud's disease.

Calcium channel blockers are well tolerated;[41] anecdotal evidence supports their use for TM. Verapamil (Calan) is the most widely prescribed agent in this family. Diltiazem (Cardizem) and nifedipine (Procardia) may also be considered. Flunarazine[41,57] is widely used in Canada and Europe but is not available in the United States.

Table 12.6   Summary of prophylactic drugs for use in chronic daily headache[a]

Drug	Clinical efficacy	Side effects	Clinical evidence[b]
Antidepressants			
Amitriptyline	+++	++	+++
Doxepin	+++	++	++
Fluoxetine	++	+	+++
Anticonvulsants			
Divalproex	+++	++	++
Beta-blockers			
Propranolol, nadolol, etc.	++	+	+
Calcium channel blockers			
Verapamil	++	+	+
Miscellaneous			
Methysergide	+++	+++	+

[a]All categories are rated from + to ++++ based on a combination of published literature and clinical experience.
[b]Ratings of +++ for clinical evidence indicate at least one double-blind, placebo-controlled study. A rating of ++ indicates open well-designed studies and + indicates ratings based on clinical experience. A rating of ++++ requires at least two double-blind placebo-controlled trials.

The anticonvulsant divalproex sodium (Depakote)[94] is an important drug in migraine prophylaxis, even in patients in whom other agents have failed. Four double-blind placebo-controlled studies demonstrate its efficacy in migraine.[94–97] Smaller open studies support its utility in TM.[98] Doses lower than those used in epilepsy (250 mg twice a day) may be sufficient. Divalproex sodium is an especially useful agent in patients with comorbid epilepsy and manic-depressive illness and, possibly, anxiety disorders.

The ergot derivative methysergide[41] is the first Food and Drug Administration–approved migraine prophylactic drug, and one that is sometimes unreasonably feared. It is an effective migraine preventive agent and can be safely combined with tricyclic antidepressants, SSRIs, or calcium channel blockers. The usual initial dose of methysergide is 2 mg twice a day. It can be increased to a maximum of 8 mg a day (2 mg four times a day); higher doses, though not recommended by the *Physicians' Desk Reference*, are sometimes useful.

The NSAIDs can be used for both symptomatic and preventive headache treatment. Naproxen sodium is effective in prevention at a dose of one or two 275-mg tablets twice a day.[99] Other NSAIDs found to be effective include tolfenamic acid, ketoprofen, mefenamic acid, fenoprofen, and ibuprofen.[100,101] Aspirin was found to be effective in one study[102] and equal to placebo in another.[103] We believe that the short-acting NSAIDs such as ibuprofen and aspirin cause rebound and their use should be limited. It is not clear whether the other NSAIDs cause rebound. Indomethacin is the drug of choice for HC; the response to it in fact defines the disorder. We give indomethacin a therapeutic trial to rule out HC but otherwise limit the use of NSAIDs for preventive treatment.

Although monotherapy is preferred, it is sometimes necessary to combine preventive medications. Antidepressants are often used with beta-blockers or calcium channel blockers, and divalproex sodium may be used in combination with any of these medications.

Detoxification

Outpatient

There are two general outpatient detoxification strategies. One approach is to taper the overused medication, gradually substituting a long-acting NSAID for symptomatic treatment as effective preventive therapy is established. The alternative strategy is to abruptly discontinue the overused drug and either substitute an NSAID or use intramuscular DHE or corticosteroids. Serious withdrawal syndromes that can be produced by the overused drug must be prevented. For example, if high doses of a butalbital-containing analgesic combination are abruptly discontinued, phenobarbital should be used to prevent barbiturate withdrawal. Similarly, benzodiazepines must be tapered gradually. Outpatient treatment is preferred for motivated patients but is not always safe or effective.

Inpatient

If outpatient treatment fails or is not safe, or if significant medical or psychiatric comorbidity is present, inpatient treatment may be needed.[41] Patients with CDH often require inpatient treatment with repetitive intravenous DHE or alternative parenteral agents. The goals of inpatient headache treatment include (1) detoxification and rehydration, (2) pain control with parenteral therapy, (3) establishment of effective prophylaxis, (4) interruption of the cycle of pain, (5) patient education, and (6) establishment of outpatient methods of pain control.[17,41] Raskin[71] and Silberstein et al.[11] have shown that the detoxification process can be enhanced and shortened and the patient's symptoms made more tolerable by the use of repetitive intravenous DHE coadministered with metoclopramide (Figure 12.1),[71] which helps control nausea and is an effective antimigraine drug in its own right. Following 10 mg of intravenous metoclopramide, DHE, 0.5 mg, is administered intravenously. Subsequent doses are adjusted based on pain relief and side effects. Patients who are not candidates for DHE or are truly intolerant of the drug may require repetitive intravenous neuroleptics, corticosteroids, or both. These agents may also supplement repetitive intravenous DHE in patients with refractory headache.[41] Hospitalization is also used as a time for patient education, introducing behavioral methods of pain control, and adjusting an outpatient program of preventive and symptomatic therapy.

Our experience[11] with more than 300 patients has shown that repetitive intravenous DHE is a safe and effective means of rapidly controlling intractable headache. Of 214 patients suffering from daily headache with rebound, 92% became headache-free, usually within 2–3 days, with an average hospital stay of 7.3 days. Our initial overall response rate in hospitalized patients (91%) was similar to that reported by Raskin.[71] Like Raskin's patients, but unlike others described in the literature, our patients usually became comfortable and

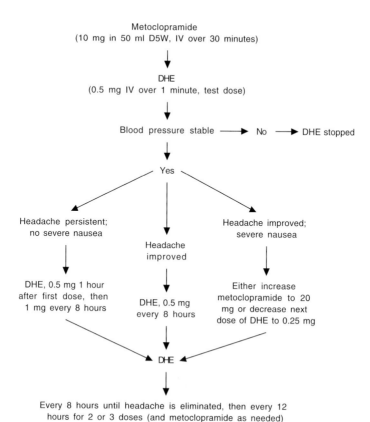

Figure 12.1 Dihydroergotamine (DHE) protocol.

headache-free within 2–3 days. Approximately 10% of our patients did not become headache-free for reasons that are unclear.

PROGNOSIS

The natural history of CDH, and of rebound headache in particular, has never been studied, and probably never will be, for ethical and technical reasons. Recognition of the rebound process is probably therapeutic in itself and can affect the patient's behavior or the physician's approach. Retrospective analysis suggests that there may be periods of stable drug consumption and phases of accelerated medication use. Patients who are treated aggressively generally improve. There are no literature reports of spontaneous improvement of rebound headache, although it may happen. We performed follow-up evaluations on 50 hospitalized CDH drug overuse patients who were treated with repetitive intravenous DHE and became headache-free.[12] Once detoxified, treated, and discharged, most patients did not

Table 12.7   Drug-induced headache: long-term follow-up

Year	Author	Drug	No. of patients	Follow-up (months)	Positive results (%)
1975	Andersson[108]	E	44	6	91
1981	Tfelt-Hansen and Krabbe[109]	E	40	12	47.6
1982	Ala-Hurula[105]	E	23	3–6	78
1984	Dichgans[104]	E/A	52	16	77
1985	Henry et al.[107]	E/A	22	3	78
1986	Rapoport et al.[29]	A	90	4	82
1988	Diener et al.[39]	E/A	85	35	69
1988	Andersson[28]	E	32	6	50
1989	Baumgartner et al.[30]	E/A	38	16	60.5
1990	Lake and Saper[106]	E/A	100	3–12	87
1991	Hering and Steiner[73]	E/A	46	6	80.4
1992	Silberstein and Silberstein[12]	E/A	50	24	87

E = ergotamine tartrate; A = analgesics.
Source: Modified from H-C Diener, WD Gerber, S Geiselhart, J Dichgans, et al. Short- and Long-term Effects of Withdrawal Therapy in Drug-Induced Headache. In H-C Diener, M Wilkinson (eds), Drug-Induced Headache. Berlin: Springer, 1988;133; and SD Silberstein, JR Silberstein. Chronic daily headache: Prognosis following inpatient treatment with repetitive IV DHE. Headache 1992;32:439.

resume daily analgesic or ergotamine use. Seventy-two percent continued to show significant improvement at 3 months, and 87% continued to show significant improvement after 2 years. This would suggest at least a 70% improvement at 2 years in the initial group (35 of 50), allowing for patients lost to follow-up.

Our[100] 2-year success rate of 87% is consistent with the long-term success rates reported in the literature. In a series of 11 papers[18,28,29,34,39,104–108] published between 1975 and 1991, the success rate of withdrawal therapy (often accompanied by pharmacologic and behavioral intervention) in patients overusing analgesics, ergotamine, or both was between 48% and 91%, and was reported as 77% or higher in eight papers (Table 12.7).

Henry et al.[107] hospitalized, detoxified, and followed 22 CDH drug overuse patients for 4–24 months after treatment. Nine of 15 patients showed marked improvement, one showed slight improvement, and five did not improve. Rapoport et al.[29] studied 90 patients with CDH who discontinued analgesics. After 1 month, 30% were significantly improved; 67% were significantly improved within 2 months, 80% after 3 months, and 82% after 4 months. The authors suggested that an "analgesic washout period" exists and may be as long as 3 months for some patients.

Diener et al.[34] hospitalized 85 patients overusing analgesics or various migraine drugs (including ergotamine) for 14 days. They detoxified the patients and followed them for 10–75 months (mean, 35 months) after discharge. Sixty-nine percent had at least 50% improvement; 29.4% were unchanged, and one patient had deteriorated. Baumgartner et al.[30] hospitalized 54 patients with drug-induced headache for 2 weeks, detoxified them, and started them on a prophylactic drug. At an average of 16.8 months (± 13.6 months) after treatment and discharge, 38 patients were evaluated: 76.3% had reduced their analgesic intake, and 60.5% had experienced a significant relief of headache intensity and frequency.

Lake et al.[106] reported on 100 patients who had been hospitalized with severe refractory CDH frequently complicated by symptomatic medication overuse. At follow-up between 3 and 12 months after discharge, the mean number of severe headaches was reduced by 64% and the mean number of dysfunctional days was reduced by 70%. Overall, 87% of patients reported at least a 50% headache reduction.

Hering and Steiner[73] followed 46 migraineurs who developed CDH as a result of analgesic overuse. Six months after analgesic and ergotamine withdrawal, 80.4% (37) were no longer overusing the agents and no longer had CDH.

Mathew et al.[14] studied 200 patients who were overusing daily symptomatic medication, 58% of whom were taking prophylactic medication without achieving a benefit. At the 3-month follow-up, among those in whom the analgesics had been discontinued and prophylactic medication started or modified, a reduction of approximately 86% in the weekly headache index was achieved, with a dropout rate of 10.3%. If symptomatic medication had been continued, only 21% improvement was achieved. It is interesting to note that merely discontinuing symptomatic medication resulted in 58% improvement.

PREVENTION

Headache sufferers often do not realize that excessive or frequent self-treatment may perpetuate or exacerbate their headaches. Because most headache sufferers do not seek medical advice until and unless the pain becomes frequent or intense, the opportunity for diagnosis and physician intervention to interrupt the cycle is often missed. Physicians should screen CDH patients for analgesic overuse. Headache patients must be informed about the risks of analgesic overuse and rebound headache. Yet, even when patients are aware of the risks, they may still overmedicate. For this reason, CDH is a condition that requires continued vigilance on the part of the treating physician.

Because patients who overuse medication may feel ashamed and out of control, an accurate history may be difficult to obtain. To facilitate this process, the clinician should explain the condition of medication rebound as a part of the natural history of migraine. Even if the patient is not rebounding at the time, doses of all symptomatic headache medications, with the possible exception of the long-acting NSAIDs, should be limited to prevent rebound.

Patients with drug-induced CDH, though difficult to treat, often return to a state of intermittent episodic headache after detoxification and treatment with preventive medication.

REFERENCES

1. Newman LC, Lipton RB, Solomon S, Stewart WF. Daily headache in a population sample: Results from the American Migraine Study. Headache 1994;34:295.

2. Rasmussen BK. Migraine and tension-type headache in a general population: Psychosocial factors. Int J Epidemiol 1992;21:1138.
3. Silberstein SD, Lipton R, Solomon S, Mathew N. Classification of daily and near daily headaches: Proposed revisions to the IHS classification. Headache 1994;34:1.
4. Solomon S, Lipton RB, Newman LC. Evaluation of chronic daily headache: Comparison to criteria for chronic tension-type headache. Cephalalgia 1992;12:365.
5. Sanin LC, Mathew NT, Bellmyer LR, Ali S. The International Headache Society (IHS) headache classification as applied to a headache clinic population. Cephalalgia 1994;14:443.
6. Messinger HB, Spierings ELH, Vincent AJP. Overlap of migraine and tension-type headache in the International Headache Society classification. Cephalalgia 1991;11:233.
7. Pfaffenrath V, Isler H. Evaluation of the nosology of chronic tension-type headache. Cephalalgia 1993;13:60.
8. Silberstein SD, Lipton RB, Sliwinski M. Assessment for revised criteria of chronic daily headache. Neurology 1995;45:A394.
9. Sandrini G, Manzoni GC, Zanferrari C, Nappi G. An epidemiological approach to the nosography of chronic daily headache. Cephalalgia 1993;13:72.
10. Olesen J, Tfelt-Hansen P, Welch KMA. The Headaches. New York: Raven, 1993.
11. Silberstein SD, Schulman EA, Hopkins MM. Repetitive intravenous DHE in the treatment of refractory headache. Headache 1990;30:334.
12. Silberstein SD, Silberstein JR. Chronic daily headache: Prognosis following inpatient treatment with repetitive IV DHE. Headache 1992;32:439.
13. Mathew NT. Transformed migraine. Cephalalgia 1993;13:78.
14. Mathew NT, Stubits E, Nigam MR. Transformation of episodic migraine into daily headache: Analysis of factors. Headache 1982;22:66.
15. Mathew NT, Reuveni U, Perez F. Transformed or evolutive migraine. Headache 1987;27:102.
16. Saper JR. Headache Disorders: Current Concepts in Treatment Strategies. Littleton, Massachusetts: Wright-PSG, 1983.
17. Silberstein SD. Chronic daily headache and tension-type headache. Neurology 1993;43:1644.
17a. Silberstein SD, Lipton RB, Sliwinski M. Classification of daily and near daily headaches: Field trial of revised IHS criteria. Neurology 1996;47:871.
18. Mathew NT, Kurman R, Perez F. Drug-induced refractory headache: Clinical features and management. Headache 1990;30:634.
19. Newman LC, Lipton RB, Solomon S. Hemicrania continua: 7 new cases and a literature review. Headache 1993;32:267.
20. Bordini C, Antonaci F, Stovner LJ, Schrader H, et al. "Hemicrania continua": A clinical review. Headache 1991;31:20.
21. Vanast WJ. New daily persistent headaches: Definition of a benign syndrome. Headache 1986;26:317.
22. Mathew NT. Drug-induced headache. Neurol Clin 1990;8:903.
23. Diamond S, Dalessio DJ. Drug Abuse in Headache. In The Practicing Physician's Approach to Headache (3rd ed). Baltimore: Williams & Wilkins, 1982;114.
24. Wilkinson M. Introduction. In H-C Diener, M Wilkinson (eds), Drug-Induced Headache. Berlin: Springer, 1988;1.
25. Saper JR. Ergotamine dependency: A review. Headache 1987;27:435.
26. Saper JR. Chronic headache syndromes. Neurol Clin 1989;7:387.
27. Saper JR, Jones JM. Ergotamine tartrate dependency: Features and possible mechanisms. Clin Neuropharmacol 1986;9:244.
28. Andersson PG. Ergotism: The Clinical Picture. In H-C Diener, M Wilkinson (eds), Drug-Induced Headache. Berlin: Springer, 1988;16.
29. Rapoport AM, Weeks RE, Sheftell FD, Baskin SM, et al. The "analgesic washout period": A critical variable in the evaluation of headache treatment efficacy. Neurology 1986;36(Suppl 1):100.
30. Baumgartner C, Wessely P, Bingol C, Maly J, et al. Long-term prognosis of analgesic withdrawal in patients with drug-induced headaches. Headache 1989;29:510.
31. Dichgans J, Diener HC, Gerber WD, Verspohl EJ, et al. Analgetika-induzierter Dauerkopfschmerz. Dtsch Med Wochenschr 1984;109:369.
32. Rapoport AM. Analgesic rebound headache. Headache 1988;28:662.
33. Kudrow L. Paradoxical effects of frequent analgesic use. Adv Neurol 1982;33:335.
34. Diener HC, Dichgans J, Scholz E, Geiselhart S, et al. Analgesic-induced chronic headache: Long-term results of withdrawal therapy. J Neurol 1989;236:9.
35. Rasmussen BK, Jensen R, Olesen J. Impact of headache on sickness absence and utilization of medical services: A Danish population study. J Epidemiol Community Health 1992;46:443.

36. Isler H. Headache Drugs Provoking Chronic Headache: Historical Aspects and Common Misunderstandings. In H-C Diener, M Wilkinson (eds), Drug-Induced Headache. Berlin: Springer, 1988;87.

37. Micieli G, Manzoni GC, Granella F, Martignoni E, et al. Clinical and Epidemiological Observations on Drug Abuse in Headache Patients. In H-C Diener, M Wilkinson (eds), Drug-Induced Headache. Berlin: Springer, 1988;20.

38. Solomon S, Lipton RB, Newman LC. Clinical features of chronic daily headache. Headache 1992;32:325.

39. Diener HC, Tfelt-Hansen P. Headache Associated with Chronic Use of Substances. In J Olesen, P Tfelt-Hansen, KMA Welch (eds), The Headaches. New York: Raven, 1993;721.

40. Schnider P, Aull S, Feucht M, et al. Use and abuse of analgesics in tension-type headache. Cephalalgia 1994;14:162.

41. Silberstein SD, Saper J. Migraine: Diagnosis and Treatment. In D Dalessio, SD Silberstein (eds), Wolff's Headache and Other Head Pain (6th ed). New York: Oxford University Press, 1993;96.

42. Eggen AE. The Tromsø study: Frequency and predicting factors of analgesic drug use in a free-living population (12–56 years). J Clin Epidemiol 1993;46:1297.

43. Gutzwiller F, Zemp E. Der analgetikakonsum in der Bevölkerung und socioökonomische aspekte des analgetikaabusus. In MJ Mihatsch (ed), Das Analgetikasyndrom. Stuttgart: Thieme, 1986;197.

44. Kielholz P, Ladewig D. Probleme des medikamentenmissbrauches. Schweiz Arztezeitung 1981;62:2866.

45. Schwarz A, Farber U, Glaeske G, et al. Daten zu analgetikakonsum and analgetikanephropathie in der bundesrepublik. Offentiches Gesundheitswesen 1985;47:298.

46. Celentano DD, Stewart WF, Lipton RB, Reed ML. Medication use and disability among migraineurs: A national probability sample. Headache 1992;32:223.

47. Robinson RG. Pain relief for headaches. Can Fam Physician 1993;39:867.

48. Silverman K, Evans SM, Strain EC, Griffiths RR. Withdrawal syndrome after the double-blind cessation of caffeine consumption. N Engl J Med 1992;327:1109.

49. Scholz E, Diener H-C, Geiselhart S. Drug-Induced Headache: Does a Critical Dosage Exist? In H-C Diener, M Wilkinson (eds), Drug-Induced Headache. Berlin: Springer, 1988;29.

50. Catarci T, Fiacco F, Argentino C, et al. Ergotamine-induced headache can be sustained by sumatriptan daily intake. Cephalalgia 1994;14:374.

51. Fisher CM. Analgesic rebound headache refuted. Headache 1988;28:666.

52. Bowdler I, Killian J, Gänsslen-Blumberg S. The association between analgesic abuse and headache: Coincidental or causal? Headache 1990;494.

53. Lance F, Parkes C, Wilkinson M. Does analgesic abuse cause headache de novo? Headache 1988;28:61.

54. Merikangas KR, Angst J, Isler H. Migraine and psychopathology: Results of the Zurich cohort study of young adults. Arch Gen Psychiatry 1990;47:849.

55. Breslau N, Davis GC. Migraine, physical health, and psychiatric disorders: A prospective epidemiologic study of young adults. J Psychiatr Res 1993;27:211.

56. Mathew NT. Chronic Daily Headache: Clinical Features and Natural History. In G Nappi, G Bono, G Sandrini, E Martignoni, et al (eds), Headache and Depression: Serotonin Pathways as a Common Clue. New York: Raven, 1991;49.

57. Lake AE, Saper JR, Madden SF, Kreeger C. Comprehensive inpatient treatment for intractable migraine: A prospective long-term outcome study. Headache 1993;33:55.

58. Moskowitz MA. Neurogenic vs vascular mechanisms of sumatriptan and ergot alkaloids in migraine. Trends Pharmacol Sci 1992;13:307.

59. Montalcini RL, Daltoso R, Dellavalle F, Skaper SD, et al. Update of the NGF saga. J Neurol Sci 1995;130:119.

60. Rang HP, Urban L. New molecules in analgesia. Br J Anaesth 1995;75:145.

61. Edelman GM, Gally JA. Nitric oxide: Linking space and time in the brain. Proc Natl Acad Sci U S A 1992;89:11651.

62. Mendell LM. Physiologic properties of unmyelinated fibre projection to the spinal cord. Exp Neurol 1966;16:316.

63. Price DD, Mao J, Mayer DJ. Central Neural Mechanisms of Normal and Abnormal Pain States. In HL Fields, JC Liebeskind (eds), Progress in Pain Research and Management, Vol 1. Washington, DC: IASP Press, 1994;61.

64. Woolf CJ. Somatic pain: Pathogenesis and prevention. Br J Anaesth 1995;75:169.

65. Dray A, Urban L, Dickenson A. Pharmacology of chronic pain. Trends Pharmacol Sci 1994;15:190.

66. Mungliani R, Hunt SP. Molecular biology of pain. Br J Anaesth 1995;75:186.

67. Fields HL, Heinricher MM, Mason P. Neurotransmitters as nociceptive modulatory circuits. Annu Rev Neurosci 1991;219:245.

68. Post RM, Silberstein SD. Shared mechanisms in affective illness, epilepsy, and migraine. Neurology 1994;44:S37.
69. Weiller C, May A, Limmroth V, Jumner M, et al. Brainstem activation in spontaneous human migraine attacks. Nature Med 1995;1:858.
70. Pazzaglia PJ, Post RM. Contingent tolerance and reresponse to carbamazepine: A case study in a patient with trigeminal neuralgia and bipolar disorder. J Neuropsychiatry Clin Neurosci 1992;4:76.
71. Raskin NH. Repetitive intravenous dihydroergotamine as therapy for intractable migraine. Neurology 1986;36:995.
72. Diener H-C, Gerber WD, Geiselhart S, Dichgans J, et al. Short- and Long-term Effects of Withdrawal Therapy in Drug-Induced Headache. In H-C Diener, M Wilkinson (eds), Drug-Induced Headache. Berlin: Springer, 1988;133.
73. Hering R, Steiner TJ. Abrupt outpatient withdrawal of medication in analgesic-abusing migraineurs. Lancet 1991;337:1442.
74. Diener HC, Pfaffenrath V, Soyka D, Gerber WD. Therapie des medikamenten-induzierten dauerkopf-schmerzes. Münch Med Wochenschr 1992;134:159.
75. Silberstein SD, Lipton RB. Overview of diagnosis and treatment of migraine. Neurology 1994;44:S6.
76. Couch JR, Micieli G. Prophylactic Pharmacotherapy. In J Olesen, P Tfelt-Hansen, HMA Welch (eds), The Headaches. New York: Raven, 1993;537.
77. Bussone G, Sandrini G, Patruno G, Ruiz L, et al. Effectiveness of Fluoxetine on Pain and Depression in Chronic Headache Disorders. In G Nappi, G Bono, G Sandrini, E Martignoni, et al (eds), Headache and Depression: Serotonin Pathways as a Common Clue. New York: Raven, 1991;265.
78. Couch JR, Ziegler DK, Hassainein R. Amitriptyline in the prophylaxis of migraine. Arch Neurol 1976;26:121.
79. Diamond S, Baltes B. Chronic tension headache treated with amitriptyline: A double-blind study. Headache 1971;11:110.
80. Holland J, Holland C, Kudrow L. Low-Dose Amitriptyline Prophylaxis in Chronic Scalp Muscle Contraction Headache. In Proceedings of the First International Headache Congress, Munich, 1983.
81. Lance JW, Curran DA. Treatment of chronic tension headache. Lancet 1964;1:1236.
82. Pluvinage R. Le traitement des migraines et des cephalees psychogenes par l'amitriptyline. Paris: Sem Hop 1978;54:713.
83. Pfaffenrath V, Diener HC, Isler H, Meyer C, et al. Efficacy and tolerability of amitriptylinoxide in the treatment of chronic tension-type headache: A multicentre controlled study. Cephalalgia 1994;14:149.
84. Pfaffenrath V, Kellhammer U, Pollmann W. Combination headache: Practical experience with a combination of a beta-blocker and an antidepressive. Cephalalgia 1986;6:25.
85. Holroyd KA, Nash JM, Pingel JD. A comparison of pharmacologic (amitriptyline Hcl) and non-pharmacologic (cognitive-behavioral) therapies for chronic tension headaches. J Consult Clin Psychol 1991;59:387.
86. Gobel H, Hamouz V, Hansen C, Heininger K, et al. Effect of Amitriptyline Prophylaxis on Headache Symptoms and Neurophysiologic Parameters. In J Olesen, T Schoenen (eds), Tension-Type Headache: Classification, Mechanisms, and Treatment. New York: Raven 1993;275.
87. Morland TJ, Storli OV, Mogstad TE. Doxepin in the prophylactic treatment of mixed "vascular" and tension headache. Headache 1979;19:382.
88. Saper JR, Silberstein SD, Lake AE, Winters ME. Double-blind trial of fluoxetine: Chronic daily headache and migraine. Headache 1994;34:497.
89. Manna V, Bolino F, DiCicco L. Chronic tension-type headache, mood depression, and serotonin: Therapeutic effects of fluvoxamine and mianserine. Headache 1994;34:44.
90. Palmer KJ, Benfield P. Fluvoxamine: An overview of its pharmacologic properties and a review of its use in nondepressive disorders. CNS Drugs 1994;1:57.
91. Langemark M, Olesen J. Sulpiride and paroxetine in the treatment of chronic tension-type headache: An explanatory double-blind trial. Headache 1994;34:20.
92. Mathew NT. Prophylaxis of migraine and mixed headache: A randomized controlled study. Headache 1981;21:105.
93. Bright RA, Everitt DE. Beta-blockers and depression: Evidence against an association. JAMA 1992;267:1783.
94. Jensen R, Brinck T, Olesen J. Sodium valproate has a prophylactic effect in migraine without aura. Neurology 1994;44:647.
95. Mathew NT, Saper JR, Silberstein SD, Rankin L, et al. Migraine prophylaxis with divalproex. Arch Neurol 1995;52:281.

96. Hering R, Kuritzky A. Sodium valproate in the prophylactic treatment of migraine: A double-blind study versus placebo. Cephalalgia 1992;12:81.

97. Klapper J. Divalproex sodium in the prophylactic treatment of migraine [Abstract]. Headache 1995;35:290.

98. Mathew NT, Ali S. Valproate in the treatment of persistent chronic daily headache: An open label study. Headache 1991;31:71.

99. Miller DS, Talbot CA, Simpson W, Korey A. A comparison of naproxen sodium, acetaminophen, and placebo in the treatment of muscle contraction headache. Headache 1987;27:392.

100. Johnson ES, Tfelt-Hansen P. Nonsteroidal Anti-inflammatory Drugs. In J Olesen, P Tfelt-Hansen, KMA Welch (eds), The Headaches. New York: Raven, 1993;391.

101. Mylecharane EJ, Tfelt-Hansen P. Miscellaneous Drugs. In J Olesen, P Tfelt-Hansen, KMA Welch (eds), The Headaches. New York: Raven, 1993;397.

102. Kangasniemi PJ, Nyrke T, Lang AH, Petersen E. Femoxetine—a new 5-HT uptake inhibitor—and propranolol in the prophylactic treatment of migraine. Acta Neurol Scand 1983;68:262.

103. Scholz E, Gerber WD, Diener HC, Langohr HD, et al. Dihydroergotamine vs Flunarizine vs Nifedipine vs Metoprolol vs Propranolol in Migraine Prophylaxis: A Comparative Study Based on Time Series Analysis. In CF Rose (ed), Advances in Headache Research. London: Libbey, 1987;139.

104. Dichgans J, Diener H-C. Clinical Manifestations of Excessive Use of Analgesic Medication. In H-C Diener, M Wilkinson (eds), Drug-Induced Headache. Berlin: Springer, 1988;8.

105. Ala-Hurula V, Myllyla V, Hokkanen E. Ergotamine abuse: Results of ergotamine discontinuation, with special reference to the plasma concentrations. Cephalalgia 1982;2:189.

106. Lake A, Saper J, Madden S, Kreeger C. Comprehensive inpatient treatment for intractable migraine: A prospective long-term outcome study. Headache 1993;33:55.

107. Henry P, Dartigues JF, Benetier MP, et al. Ergotamine- and Analgesic-Induced Headaches. In C Rose (ed), Migraine: Proceedings from the Fifth International Migraine Symposium, London, 1984;197.

108. Andersson PG. Ergotamine headache. Headache 1975;15:118.

109. Tfelt-Hansen P, Krabbe A. Ergotamine abuse: Do patients benefit from withdrawal? Cephalalgia 1981;1:29.

13
Cluster Headache

Lee Kudrow

HISTORY AND CLASSIFICATION

Cluster headache has been described intermittently since as early as the seventeenth century. Koehler[1] and Isler[2] ascribe the earliest observations to Nicolas Tulp in 1641 and Willis in 1671, respectively. Eighteenth-century contributors include Gerhard van Swieten in 1745, according to Isler,[3] and Whytt (1764) and Morgagni (1761), as reported by Eadie.[4] In all cases, clinical descriptions were too incomplete to satisfy today's criteria. Included, however, was the proverbial daily, cyclic pattern of excruciating unilateral headaches; a combination of features seen only in cluster headache or its variants.

Heyck[5] credits Eulenburg (1878) with the earliest complete description of cluster headache. It was rediscovered by Sluder[6] in 1910, Harris[7] in 1926, and Horton et al.[8] in 1939. The periodic character of cluster headache was first reported by Ekbom[9] in 1947, and the term *cluster headache* was introduced by Kunkle et al.,[10] who noted the typical clustering pattern of attacks. Various names for cluster headache were based on suspected autonomic nervous system dysfunction, such as *angioparalytic hemicrania, autonomic faciocephalalgia,* and *sympathetic hemicephalic vasodilatation.* Still other names reflect the suspected involvement of specific seventh cranial nerve pathways: *sphenopalatine ganglion, ciliary, vidian,* and *greater superficial petrosal neuralgias.*

In 1962 the Ad Hoc Committee on the Classification of Headache defined cluster headache under the heading "vascular headaches of the migraine type."[11] It was subsequently reclassified as a singular entity, apart from migraine.[12] The most recent change was undertaken by the Classification Committee of the International Headache Society, published in 1988[13] (Table 13.1).

The two major types of cluster headaches are known as episodic and chronic. The ratio of episodic to chronic cluster headache is approximately 4 to 1. The episodic type is defined by periods of attack susceptibility, lasting an average of 1 to 3 months, followed by headache-free intervals (remission periods) of a few months to several years. Chronic cluster headache lacks remission periods, either

Table 13.1   Classification of cluster headache

Cluster headache	3.1
Periodicity undetermined	3.1.1
Episodic	3.1.2
Chronic	3.1.3
Primary chronic	3.1.3.1
Secondary chronic	3.1.3.2
Chronic paroxysmal hemicrania	3.2
Cluster headache–like syndrome	3.3

from its inception (primary chronic) or after it has converted from the episodic type (secondary chronic).

Chronic paroxysmal hemicrania is a variant of cluster headache, first described in 1974.[14] An episodic variety, episodic paroxysmal hemicrania, was recently described[15] and corroborated.[16–18] The paroxysmal hemicranias resemble cluster headache in the intensity, quality, and location of pain and in the associated autonomic signs and symptoms. The frequency of attacks is greater, however, and their duration is shorter than in cluster headache. Unlike cluster headache, the paroxysmal hemicranias are completely and dramatically responsive to indomethacin. Paroxysmal hemicranias are discussed in Chapter 14.

Disorders that fall under the heading of cluster headache–like syndromes include cluster-tic syndrome and symptomatic cluster headache. Cluster-tic syndrome is a disorder that features symptoms of both cluster headache and trigeminal neuralgia.[19–21] Trigeminal nerve root compression by posterior cerebral vessels has been found to be causative in many cases, and surgical decompression can be beneficial.[22] Symptomatic (nonidiopathic or secondary) cluster headache is an increasingly widely reported condition. Associated lesions are located in or around the cavernous sinuses and include vascular malformations, meningiomas, and aneurysms.[23–26]

CLINICAL PICTURE

Prevalence and Demographics

The major sources of data on the prevalence of cluster headache include the study of 18-year-old Swedish army recruits by Ekbom et al.,[27] which found prevalence to be 0.09%. Extrapolation of these results to distribution of age at onset obtained from headache clinic data yielded a rate of approximately 0.4%.[28]

Cluster headache affects men more frequently than women by a ratio of 4.5–6.7 to 1. The mean age of onset is 27–31 years,[29–32] approximately 10 years later than that of migraine. In our clinic, cluster headache was found to be disproportionately more prevalent among blacks than among white patients, and particularly so among black women where the male-to-female ratio was 3 to 1,[32] corroborating an earlier finding of Lovshin.[33] Our survey found little difference between other ethnic groups, consistent with Italian[34] and Scandinavian[30] population data.

Familial History

In a recent study of 200 women with cluster headache, 24 (12%) were found to have at least one first-degree relative with the disorder. Indeed, three generations of cluster headache were found in seven of 24 kindreds (29.2%). Of 1,652 first-degree relatives of 300 male and female patients, 3.45% had cluster headache. This number represents 13 times the expected frequency of cluster headache in the general population.[35] These findings, which suggest a genetic role in the etiology of cluster headache, were recently corroborated by Russel et al.,[36] who reported a 14-fold increase in the risk of cluster headache among first-degree relatives of a cluster population.

Diagnostic Features

The following is a first-person account of an acute attack, modified from an earlier description[37]:

> Following a period of perhaps several hours of feeling quite elated and energetic, I experienced a fullness in my ears, somewhat more on the right side than the left, having a character similar to that which might occur during a rapidly descending airplane or elevator ride. I then became aware of a dull discomfort at the base of my skull, extending over the entire head, on both sides, although somewhat more on the right. Two or three minutes had elapsed— seemingly short, but long enough for me to know that a "cluster" had begun and, inexorably, would get worse. Such anticipation caused me considerable consternation about whether to continue my activities or cancel plans and find a place to be alone, giving way to a slowly increasing anxiety, fear, panic, and withdrawal. I became aware of myself "listening" for changes in my head. Is the cluster aborting itself early, progressing further, or unchanging? A sudden stab, only fleeting, struck my temple, then again—somewhat near the apex of my skull and upper molars in my face; always on the right side. It struck me again above my eyebrow. My nose was stuffed, yet ran simultaneously. Were I able to sneeze, I felt, the attack might have ended. But in spite of all tricks and gestures I was unable to induce a sneeze.
>
> While the sharp stabs continued, a slow crescendo of dull pain began, covering an area of a hand's length and breadth over my right eye and temple. As the painful area narrowed, it enlarged in intensity. I found myself bending my neck downward, although slightly, as if my head was being gently pushed from behind. My neck, up to the base of my skull, was tight as if I were wearing a neck collar. I felt compelled to remove my tie and loosen my shirt collar even though I knew it would not offer me even a modicum of relief.
>
> In an effort to alter this persistent discomfort I dropped my head between my legs while seated. My face and eyes seemed to fill with fluid while the pain continued unabated. I glanced at the mirror and barely recognized the gaunt,

tortured, and sickly face that peered back at me. My right eyelid drooped slightly and the white of my eye was charted with many red vessels lending it an overall pinkish hue. Having difficulty standing in one place too long, I left the mirror to continue alternating my pacing and sitting. I was suddenly terrorized by the possibility that the pain would never end, but dismissed it as impossible since if that were the case I would surely kill myself.

The pain, now located somewhere behind my eye and slightly above it, worsened. The pain is best described as an unseen "force," as with a hot boring iron, being pushed through my eye with incredible power. The "force" waxed and waned with, however, increased duration of successive exacerbations. The cluster attack had been at its peak for ten minutes and was celebrated by an outpouring of tears from solely my right eye, at which point my wife peeked into the room where I was holding forth. I looked up and in an instant saw her expression of pity, frustration, and helplessness. She saw my tortured face as I had seen it in the mirror at this stage before, with drooling mouth, agape; grey face wet on one side; an almost closed eyelid; and smelling of pain and anguish. She closed the door and left, hurt for me, angry at the impotence of medical science, and guilty—since within her mind is the suspicion that she is the cause of my suffering.

I cried for her, but more for myself. The pain was so intolerable. Suddenly, I was over whelmed by a fury. I lifted a chair high above my head and crashed it to the floor. With a doubled fist I struck the wall. But the pain persisted.

Waning periods became longer, and I allowed myself to suspect that the peak was behind me—but cautiously, since I had been tricked too often.

The pain was indeed ending. The descent from the mountain of pain was rapid. The "force" was gone, but considerable pain remained. My nose and eye continued to run. The road back, as with all travel, covers the same territory, but faster. A stabbing pain, yet easily tolerated, was felt. Then gone. Dull aching fullness, neck stiffness all disappeared, replaced in turn by a welcome sensation of pins and needles over my right scalp. Thus, my head awoke after a nightmare of torment.

Eye and nose dry, I let out a sigh. I collected my pile of wet tissues that had been strewn all over the floor and deposited them in a wastepaper basket. The innocent chair was uprighted and my bruised fist properly rubbed. Having ended the battle and cleaned up its field, I opened the door and entered a pain-free world—until tomorrow.

Frequency, Duration, Timing, and Provocation of Attacks

The mean frequency of cluster headache attacks ranges from one to three per day, but attacks may occur up to 15 times a day. Mean duration is 45 minutes, although they often last 1–2 hours.[31,32,38] The extreme range is from 5 minutes to 3 hours or more. Attacks occur most commonly on relaxing after a day's work. The second most common time is approximately 90 minutes after falling asleep, coincident to the first REM state of the night.[39,40] Attacks are least likely to occur during work or school hours.

During active cluster periods, vasodilators may induce cluster headache attacks. Alcohol, even in small amounts, and subcutaneous injections of histamine were noted to induce typical cluster attacks.[8] Ekbom[41] provoked cluster attacks in 10 of 10 patient-subjects by administration of 1 mg of sublingual nitroglycerin.

Location, Quality, and Intensity of Pain

The pain of cluster headache is exquisitely severe, constant, unrelenting, boring, hot, and tenaciously fixed to a small area in or about one eye, causing one to pace, rock forward and back in a chair, thrash about, or strike objects. In comparison, the pain of trigeminal neuralgia, while severely sharp and intense, is of only seconds' duration, and causes one to wince more than to wail. The cluster attack is accompanied by an agitated or colicky-like state in which neither position nor rest can offer relief, whereas the migraine attack is represented more as a vegetative state.

Associated Signs and Symptoms

Attacks are almost always associated with ipsilateral lacrimation, rhinorrhea or stuffiness, and conjunctival suffusion. Ipsilateral ptosis and miosis are associated features found in a lesser number of cases.

Periods of Susceptibility and Remission

In episodic cluster headache, spontaneous or provoked attacks occur solely during the cluster period, the attack-susceptible state. Cluster periods are frequently observed to occur cyclically, often during the same month each year. This pattern was confirmed in a prospective study in which almost 900 cluster period onsets, recorded by 400 patients, were plotted against month of the year.[42]

The frequency of cluster period onset was found to be related to photoperiod duration, increased in July and January, shortly after the longest and shortest days of the year, respectively. Cluster period onsets decreased following resetting of clocks 1 hour for daylight-saving and standard times in April and October, respectively (Figure 13.1).

Neither spontaneous nor provoked attacks occur during the remission period. Remission periods generally last several months to 1 or 2 years. Increased frequency of attacks, prolonged cluster periods, drug abuse, and treatment resistance were found among patients whose remissions lasted less than 6 months; the same features are found in many chronic patients. These observations prompted recognition of a third type of cluster headache, called subchronic, for which remission of less than 6 months is the major criterion.[43]

Differential Diagnosis

Few disorders resemble cluster headache. Its features are distinct and consistent from patient to patient and from cluster period to cluster period. A number of disorders, however, share features of cluster headache and may be confused with it.

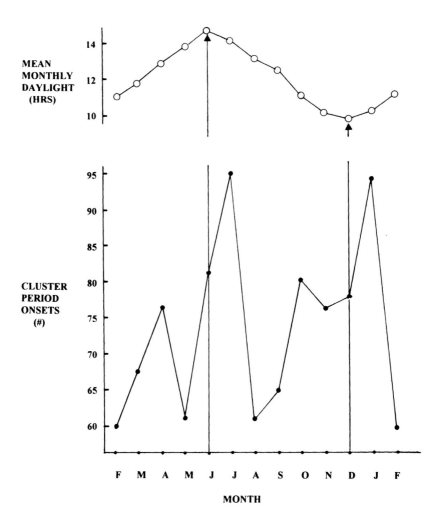

Figure 13.1 Cluster period onsets plotted against month of the year and mean monthly daylight duration. Data consisted of 892 cluster period onsets recorded by 404 male cluster headache patients over a span of 9 years. Peak frequencies of cluster period onset occurred in July and January, 2–3 weeks following the longest and shortest days of the year in June and December (arrows). Decreased frequencies in May and November followed the resetting of clocks by 1 hour at the end of April (to daylight-saving time) and October (to standard time).

Paroxysmal Hemicranias

In 1974, Sjaastad and Dale[14] described a condition they called chronic parox-ysmal hemicrania. It is characterized by cluster-like attacks, similarly associat-ed with autonomic signs and symptoms, but of greater frequency and shorter duration. Attack frequency has been reported to range from 4–38 per day, with a mean of 14 per day. Duration ranges from 3 minutes to 46 minutes, with a mean of 13 minutes.[44]

An episodic type of paroxysmal hemicrania has been described.[15–18] Episodic paroxysmal hemicrania is similar to chronic paroxysmal hemicrania except that the former is characterized by recurring remissions. Both types are totally responsive to prophylactic indomethacin. The initial dose is 25 mg four times a day; indomethacin maintenance may require as little as 25 mg daily.

Atypical Trigeminal Neuralgia

The syndrome known as atypical trigeminal neuralgia is characterized by the painful episodes, trigger zones, and hypesthesias, as in common trigeminal neuralgia, but untypically associated with autonomic symptoms and signs of cluster headache. Additionally, a dull, aching background pain is usually present.[45–47] Quality, intensity, and character of pain are similar in atypical and typical trigeminal neuralgia. The pain is often described as severe, having a lancinating, lightning-like or electric quality. It generally lasts only seconds or minutes and may recur several times a day. Attacks are generally provoked by even the lightest touch over facial trigger zones or by chewing, shaving, or brushing one's teeth.

Short-lasting unilateral neuralgiform headache attacks with conjunctival injection, tearing, sweating, and rhinorrhea (SUNCT)[48–49] may represent either a refinement or a variant of atypical trigeminal neuralgia.

Pheochromocytoma

Headache attacks in pheochromocytoma are similar to those of cluster headache in that they are severe, worsen in the supine position, last less than 1 hour, and may occur one to several times a day. In contrast to cluster headache, however, the headache is biooccipital, throbbing, and accompanied by sweating, pallor, tachycardia, and an increase in blood pressure.[50]

Raeder's Syndrome

The head pain of Raeder's paratrigeminal syndrome,[51] more recently called pericarotid syndrome,[52] is persistent and may last up to several months. It resembles cluster headache in that, early in the course of the disease, attacks may be severe and paroxysmal, often awakening the patient from sleep. Indeed, pain may be unilateral and supraorbital in location, burning in quality, and associated with a partial Horner's syndrome ipsilaterally. Later in the course of Raeder's syndrome, pain becomes constant and only dull to moderate in intensity.

Temporal Arteritis

As initially described by Horton,[53] the pain of temporal arteritis, located over one temple, is generally persistent, waxing and waning throughout the day.

The temporal artery may be enlarged, tortuous, nodular, and pulseless. Similarly, an enlarged and tortuous temporal artery may be noted during cluster attacks in some patients, but it is neither hard nor pulseless to palpation. Chewing claudication is a characteristic feature of temporal arteritis, and a highly elevated erythrocyte sedimentation rate is commonly found. Temporal arteritis should be regarded as a medical emergency, because it may rapidly lead to blindness.[54]

PATHOPHYSIOLOGY

The pathogenesis of cluster headache involves numerous systems, although it is basically a nervous system disorder. Through recent research advances, our understanding of cluster headache mechanisms has evolved to include the autonomic, chronobiological, neurohormonal, autoregulatory, and neuropeptide systems. To make sense of an ever-increasing spate of publications, we have separated the clinical aspects of cluster headache and their respective mechanisms into three major states, each dependent on the preceding one. These include (1) the cluster period and its attendant dysfunction in hypothalamic, sympathetic, and chronobiological systems; (2) cluster attack induction consequent to sustained hypoxemic episodes; and (3) cluster pain and autonomic signs and symptoms.

Cluster Period

Significantly lowered levels of plasma testosterone in male cluster headache patients during cluster periods compared with the same patients during remission periods or to control subjects provided the first evidence of hypothalamic involvement in cluster headache.[55–59] The role of the hypothalamus was confirmed in two studies of cluster populations that demonstrated a reduced response to stimulation by thyrotropin-releasing hormone.[60,61] Hypothalamic dysfunction leads to changes in chronobiological regulation and sympathetic neuronal activity.

Chronobiological Changes

During cluster periods, alteration or loss of circadian rhythmicity was found for plasma cortisol,[62–64] melatonin,[65,66] testosterone,[59] prolactin,[67,68] β-endorphins, and β-lipotropins[69] and for temperature and blood pressure.[70] In further support of cluster period–related dyschronia, cluster periods may be induced by photoperiod stress and may be prevented by manipulation of the sleep-wake cycle, that is, by resetting external clocks by 1 hour.[42]

Impaired Sympathetic Neuronal Activity

Impairment of vasomotor autonomic activity associated with cluster periods is suggested by changes in facial temperature as measured thermographically[71–74] and by changes in the internal carotid artery as demonstrated by Ekbom and Greitz.[75] Providing further evidence of impaired sympathetic activity associated with the cluster period, Fanciullacci et al.[76] and others[77,78] have demonstrated diminished ipsilateral pupillary responses following instillation of a tyramine solution. Findings during cluster periods of asymmetric sweating patterns,[79] and electrocardiographic evidence of asynchronous repolarization provoked by hyperventilation,[78] are further suggestive of sympathetic impairment.

Cluster Attack Induction

There are several theories regarding mechanisms responsible for the pain and autonomic symptoms of the cluster attack, but to date only one hypothesis attempts to explain possible mechanisms involved in the initiation of attacks.

Conditions commonly associated with induction of attacks include altitude exposure, the REM sleep state, postexertional relaxation, and vasodilators, all of which suggest a role for hypoxemia, particularly in the presence of impaired compensatory mechanisms. In addition, oxygen inhalation rapidly aborts cluster attacks.[80,81] This evidence led to the hypothesis that chemoreceptors may play a role in the induction of cluster attacks.[82] In this model, as a result of impaired autonomic activity, chemoreceptor responses during the cluster period are blunted, causing a buildup of activating substances. A sustained hypoxemic event may then exceed the altered threshold of chemoreceptor activation, resulting in a denervation-hyperactive response, conducted to the nucleus of the seventh cranial nerve via internuclear connections from the nucleus solitarius. This hypothesis has been supported indirectly by several studies that found attack-related oxygen desaturation during sleep[40] and sustained oxygen desaturation following nitroglycerin-provoked[83] and spontaneous attacks.[84] Other studies, however, have failed to demonstrate either carotid body dysfunction in cluster patients or provocation of attacks by an induced transient hypoxemia.[85,86]

In the hypothetical scheme just described,[82] the seventh cranial nerve serves as an intermediate pathway whereby impulses originating in the nucleus solitarius stimulate the superior salivary nucleus via nuclear interconnections. A role for seventh cranial nerve pathways in the pathogenesis of cluster attacks has been suggested by findings of partial to complete relief of cluster attacks following resection of the greater superficial petrosal nerve[87,88] or the nervus intermedius;[89] and by blockade of the sphenopalatine ganglion.[90] Kunkle[91] held that attack-associated autonomic features, including bradycardia, may be explained by parasympathetic storms involving the seventh and tenth cranial nerves.

Appenzeller et al.[92] suggested that the pain of cluster headache may result from histamine release associated with antidromal trigeminal nerve activity, because an increase in degranulated mast cells in proximity to cutaneous nerves was found on ipsilateral temporal skin biopsies. It was later shown that stimulation of the trigeminal ganglion increased vascular permeability in dura,[93] and increased mast cell degranulation.[94] More recently, it was suggested that cluster and migraine pain may be due to trigeminovascular neurogenic inflammatory changes mediated by neuropeptide release.[95] Indeed, Goadsby and Edvinsson[96] provided in vivo evidence for activation of trigeminovascular and parasympathetic systems associated with the acute cluster attack. Calcitonin gene-related peptide (CGRP), a marker for trigeminal activity, and vasoactive intestinal polypeptide (VIP), a marker for parasympathetic activity, were found to be increased in sampled ipsilateral jugular blood. CGRP levels returned to normal following treatment with sumatriptan or oxygen inhalation. Unexplained, however, was the failure to find an increase in substance P (SP), a major marker for pain and trigeminal activation.

Whether or not the attack is initiated by the trigeminovascular reflex, its final pathway remains within the seventh cranial nerve pathway, involving the sphenopalatine ganglion, from which efferent parasympathetic fibers pass with the ethmoid nerve via the ethmoid foramen to innervate cerebral blood vessels. These ganglia cells and nerves are rich in VIP and nitric oxide synthase, potent vasodilators,[97,98] as are internal carotid and cavernous sinus microganglia, described recently by Suzuki and Hardebo.[99,100] The latter findings are consistent with the likely site of pain in cluster headache, the cavernous sinus region.[23-26]

Many questions remain about the role of neuropeptides in cluster headache, such as the reason for the failure to demonstrate an increase in jugular blood SP (trigeminal activity) during cluster attacks.[96] Also, by what mechanism do both sumatriptan and oxygen inhalation reduce CGRP levels in external jugular blood and abort cluster attacks with a similar rapidity and distribution? Further, sensory neuropeptide measurements from saliva, during and between cluster attacks, though provocative, have proven more enigmatic than revealing. Nicolodi and Del Bianco[101] found that VIP, CGRP, and SP levels measured from the symptomatic side remained unchanged during attacks. VIP and CGRP, however, were significantly increased in saliva from the asymptomatic side. Finally, in saliva from both sides combined, CGRP levels during attacks were found to be significantly increased compared with interval periods.

TREATMENT OF CLUSTER HEADACHE

The cornerstones of successful treatment of cluster headache are patient education, effective prophylactic treatment, and symptomatic management. The following recommendations are based on many years of experience at the California Medical Clinic for Headache.

Patient Education

Patients should be instructed to avoid the following during cluster periods (in episodic and subchronic cluster headache) or at any time (in chronic cluster headache): alcohol, exposure to oil-based paints or solvents, afternoon napping, or work-shift changes. They should be cautioned that even moderately high-altitude exposure may increase the frequency of attacks. Attacks during weekend ski trips may be prevented by acetazolamide, 250 mg twice daily for 4 days beginning 2 days before reaching high altitude.

Prophylactic Treatment

Attacks occurring solely during sleep hours may be prevented by an oral dose of 1 mg of ergotamine tartrate 1 hour before bedtime. In general, however, the prophylactic treatment of choice is verapamil, 80 mg four times a day, equally spaced over waking hours. The efficacy of verapamil was first demonstrated by Meyer and Hardenberg in 1983.[102] Gabel and Spierings[103] reported an efficacy rate of 70% for verapamil as a sole agent in episodic and chronic cluster headache. The most troublesome side effect is constipation. Verapamil is contraindicated for patients in whom calcium channel blocking agents should be avoided.

Ekbom[104] reported the first successful treatment with lithium carbonate in five patients in 1978, and larger studies corroborated the finding.[105,106] In the latter studies, lithium carbonate alone, 300 mg two to three times daily, showed a 70–80% efficacy rate. Although rare, the most frequently seen side effect is gastrointestinal disturbance. Lithium should be avoided where diuretics are being used because the lithium ion competes with intracellular salt, which may lead to toxicity.

The addition of pre-bedtime ergotamine to daily prophylaxis with either verapamil or lithium increases the success rate by an additional 15%. In resistant cases, in which the frequency of attacks has not been satisfactorily reduced, triple therapy (a term coined at our clinic) is indicated. The regimen for treatment-resistant cluster headache includes verapamil, 80 mg four or five times daily; lithium, 300 mg twice or thrice daily; and ergotamine tartrate, 1–2 mg, 1 hour before bedtime. The larger doses represent the maximum at our clinic.

Treatment resistance is not uncommon in chronic or subchronic cluster headache.[43] It may be broken by a short course of corticosteroids alone: prednisone, 40 mg daily, tapered off over a 3-week period. Care should be taken not to exceed this period except in the most urgent circumstances, to avoid steroid-fastness and other complications. An alternative to steroids is sodium valproate, as demonstrated by Hering and Kuritzky.[107] In an open-label study, significant relief of attacks was achieved in 11 of 15 patients treated prophylactically with sodium valproate, 600–2,000 mg per day.

Surgical treatment may be indicated if all medical attempts have failed to significantly control cluster attacks. Patients selected for possible surgical treatment should undergo psychometric testing to rule out those with significant neuroses. The surgical procedure of choice, with the most favorable success rate, is radiofrequency trigeminal gangliolysis.[108] It should be noted, however, that facial sensory changes and eye dryness are common side effects, and anesthesia dolorosa is an uncommon complication.

Symptomatic Treatment

Oxygen Inhalation

The safest and most effective nonmedication treatment for the acute cluster attack is oxygen inhalation.[80,81] Given the following technique, 70% of attacks may be aborted within 10 minutes and 90% within 20 minutes. Equipment consists of a C (large) or E (portable) tank containing 100% oxygen, facial mask, tubing, and regulator. A facial mask is preferred over a nasal cannula because nasal stuffiness may impede proper ventilation. Oxygen inhalation should be initiated at the onset of the attack and may be continued for 20 minutes unless relief occurs sooner. If not successful, discontinue for 5 minutes, then resume for another 20 minutes. The patient should assume a sitting position, leaning forward with elbows on knees, facing the floor, a posture often assumed by patients during attacks even without instruction. In this position, gravity permits venous drainage from the congested cavernous sinus in the absence of valves. The patient should breathe normally. Hyperventilation during oxygen inhalation should be discouraged. It does not increase the rate of achieving peak oxygen saturation and indeed may have a paradoxical effect.[83]

Medication

As demonstrated by Ekbom et al.[109,110] in double-blind studies, the most effective medication for the acute cluster attack is sumatriptan, a 5-hydroxytryptamine (5-HT_1) receptor agonist. Subcutaneous treatment with 6 mg of sumatriptan was found to be no less effective than a 12-mg dose. Attacks were aborted in 49% of patients within 10 minutes and in 75% within 15 minutes, a distribution similar to that achieved with oxygen inhalation. No serious side effects or complications were reported. Subsequently, a long-term open-label study revealed no evidence of tachyphylaxis or rebound attacks.[111]

Prior to the introduction of sumatriptan, ergotamine preparations were the most widely used symptomatic medication for cluster headache. Sublingual and inhalant preparations offered effective rapid action but are no longer available in the United States. Intramuscular ergotamine tartrate is similarly fast-acting and effective but has the disadvantage of causing significant nausea. The ergotamine preparation of choice remains intramuscular or subcutaneous dihydroergotamine (DHE-45). Clinical experience suggests that it is as effective as sumatriptan. As a nonspecific 5-HT agonist, however, DHE-45 produces nausea (although less often than ergotamine tartrate), which can be prevented by adding an antiemetic agent.

Other effective sympathetic medications include intranasal administration of 5% cocaine hydrochloride[112] or 4% lidocaine solutions.[113] The action of these medications may be on the sphenopalatine ganglion, which may not be anatomically accessible in all patients. Cocaine has the additional disadvantage of addictiveness and tachyphylaxis.

REFERENCES

1. Koehler PJ. Prevalence of headache in Tulp's Observationes Medicae (1641) with a description of cluster headache. Cephalalgia 1993;13:318.
2. Isler H. Independent historical development of the concepts of cluster headache and trigeminal neuralgia. Funct Neurol 1987;2:141.
3. Isler H. Episodic cluster headache from a textbook of 1745: Van Swieten's classical description. Cephalalgia 1993;13:172.

4. Eadie MJ. Two mid-18th century descriptions of probable cluster headache. J Hist Neurosci 1992;1:125.
5. Heyck H. Der cluster-kopfschmerz. Dtsch Med Wochenschr 1975;100:1292.
6. Sluder G. The syndrome of sphenopalatine ganglion neuralgia. Am J Med Sci 1910;140:868.
7. Harris W. Neuritis and Neuralgia. London: Oxford University Press, 1926.
8. Horton BT, MacLean AR, Craig WM. A new syndrome of vascular headache: Results of treatment with histamine. Preliminary report. Mayo Clin Proc 1939;14:257.
9. Ekbom KA. Ergotamine tartrate orally in Horton's "histaminic cephalalgia" (also called Harris's "ciliary neuralgia"). Acta Psychiatr Scand 1947;46(Suppl):106.
10. Kunkle EC, Pfeiffer JB, Wilhoit WM, et al. Recurrent brief headache in "cluster" pattern. Trans Am Neurol Assoc 1952;77:240.
11. Friedman AP, Finley KM, Graham JR, et al. Classification of headache. The Ad Hoc Committee on the Classification of Headache. Arch Neurol 1962;6:173.
12. World Federation of Neurology's Research Group on Migraine and Headache. Classification of headaches. J Neurol Sci 1969;9:202.
13. Headache Classification Committee of the International Headache Society. Classification and diagnostic criteria for headache disorders, cranial neuralgias, and facial pain. Cephalalgia 1988;8(Suppl 7):35.
14. Sjaastad O, Dale I. Evidence for a new (?) treatable headache entity. Headache 1974;14:105.
15. Kudrow L, Esperanca P, Vijayan N. Episodic paroxysmal hemicrania? Cephalalgia 1987;7:197.
16. Spierings ELH. The chronic paroxysmal hemicrania concept expanded. Headache 1988;28:597.
17. Blau JN, Engel H. Episodic paroxysmal hemicrania: A further case and review of the literature. J Neurol Neurosurg Psychiatry 1990;53:343.
18. Newman LC, Gordon ML, Lipton RB, et al. Episodic paroxysmal hemicrania: Two new cases and a literature review. Neurology 1992;42:964.
19. Lance JW, Anthony M. Migrainous neuralgia or cluster headache? J Neurol Sci 971;13:401.
20. Diamond S, Freitag FG, Cohen JS. Cluster headache with trigeminal neuralgia. Postgrad Med 1984;2:165.
21. Watson P, Evans R. Cluster-tic syndrome. Headache 1985;25:123.
22. Solomon S, Apfelbaum RI, Guglielmo KM. The cluster-tic syndrome and its surgical therapy. Cephalalgia 1985;5:83.
23. Herzberg L, Lenman JAR, Victoratos G, et al. Cluster headache associated with vascular malformations. J Neurol Neurosurg Psychiatry 1975;38:648.
24. Thomas AL. Periodic migrainous neuralgia associated with an arteriovenous malformation. Postgrad Med J 1975;51:560.
25. Tfelt-Hansen P, Paulsen OB, Krabbe A. Invasive adenoma of the pituitary gland and chronic migrainous neuralgia: A rare coincidence or a causal relationship? Cephalalgia 1982;2:25.
26. Greve E, Mai J. Cluster headache-like headaches: A symptomatic feature? A report of three patients with intracranial pathologic findings. Cephalalgia 1988;8:79.
27. Ekbom K, Ahlborg B, Schele R. Prevalence of migraine and cluster headache in Swedish men of 18. Headache 1978;18:9.
28. Kudrow L. Cluster Headache. In JN Blau (ed), Headache: Clinical, Therapeutic, Conceptual, and Research Aspects. London: Chapman & Hall, 1987;113.
29. Friedman AP, Mikropoulos HE. Cluster headache. Neurology 1958;8:653.
30. Ekbom K. A clinical comparison of cluster headache and migraine. Acta Neurol Scand 1970;46(Suppl 41):1.
31. Lance JW. Mechanisms and Management of Headache (3rd ed). London: Butterworth, 1978.
32. Kudrow L. Cluster Headache: Mechanisms and Management. London: Oxford University Press, 1980;10.
33. Lovshin LL. Clinical caprices of histaminic cephalalgia. Headache 1961;1:3.
34. Manzoni GC, Terzano MG, Bono G, et al. Cluster headache: Clinical findings in 180 patients. Cephalalgia 1983;3:21.
35. Kudrow L, Kudrow DB. Inheritance of cluster headache and its possible link to migraine. Headache 1994;34:400.
36. Russel MB, Andersson PG, Thomsen LL, et al. The inheritance of cluster headache investigated by complex segregation analysis. Proceedings of the 7th International Headache Congress, Toronto, 1995.
37. Kudrow L. Cluster headache: Diagnosis and management. Headache 1979;19:142.
38. Ekbom K. Pattern of cluster headache with a note on the relation to angina pectoris and peptic ulcer. Acta Neurol Scand 1970;46:225.
39. Dexter JD, Riley TL. Studies in nocturnal migraine. Headache 1975;15:51.

40. Kudrow L, McGinty DS, Phillips ER, et al. Sleep apnea in cluster headache. Cephalalgia 1984;4:33.
41. Ekbom K. Nitroglycerin as a provocative agent in cluster headache. Arch Neurol 1968;19:487.
42. Kudrow L. The cyclic relationship of natural illumination to cluster period frequency [Abstract]. Cephalalgia 1987;7(Suppl 6):76.
43. Kudrow L. Subchronic cluster headache. Headache 1987;27:197.
44. Russell D. Chronic paroxysmal hemicrania: Severity, duration, and time of occurrences of attack. Cephalalgia 1984;4:53.
45. Sweet WH. Controlled thermocoagulation of trigeminal ganglion and rootlets for differential destruction of pain fibers: Facial pain other than trigeminal neuralgia. Clin Neurosurg 1976;23:96.
46. Yonas H, Jannetta PJ. Neurinoma of the trigeminal root and atypical trigeminal neuralgia: Their commonality. Neurosurgery 1980;6:273.
47. Cusick JF. Atypical trigeminal neuralgia. JAMA 1981;245:2328.
48. Sjaastad O, Russell D, Horven I, et al. Multiple, neuralgiform, unilateral headache attacks associated with conjunctival injection and appearing in clusters: A nosological problem. Proceedings of the Scandinavian Migraine Society, 1978;31.
49. Sjaastad O, Saunte C, Salvesen R, et al. Short-lasting, unilateral neuralgiform headache attacks with conjunctival injection, tearing, sweating, and rhinorrhea. Cephalalgia 1989;9:147.
50. Thomas JE, Rooke ED, Kvale WF. The neurologist's experience with pheochromocytoma: A review of 100 cases. JAMA 1966;197:754.
51. Raeder JG. "Paratrigeminal" paralysis of oculo-pupillary sympathetic. Brain 1924;47:149.
52. Vijayan N, Watson C. Pericarotid syndrome. Headache 1978;18:244.
53. Horton BT, Magath TB, Brown GE. An undescribed form of arteritis of the temporal vessels. Proc Staff Meet Mayo Clin 1932;7:700.
54. Huston KA, Hunder GG, Lie LT, et al. A 25-year epidemiologic, clinical, and pathologic study. Ann Intern Med 1978;88:162.
55. Kudrow L. Plasma testosterone levels in cluster headache: Preliminary results. Headache 1976;16:28.
56. Nelson RF. Testosterone levels in cluster and non-cluster migraine headache patients. Headache 1978;18:265.
57. Romiti A, Martelletti P, Gallo MF, et al. Low plasma testosterone levels in cluster headache. Cephalalgia 1982;3:41.
58. Klimek A. Plasma testosterone levels in patients with cluster headache. Headache 1982;22:162.
59. Facchinetti F, Nappi G, Cicoli C, et al. Reduced testosterone levels in cluster headache: A stress related phenomenon. Cephalalgia 1986;6:29.
60. Bussone G, Frediani F, Leone M, et al. TRH test in cluster headache. Headache 1988;7:43.
61. Leone M, Patrunko G, Vescovi A, et al. Neuroendocrine dysfunction in cluster headache. Cephalalgia 1990;10:235.
62. Nappi G, Ferrari E, Polleri A, et al. Chronobiological study of cluster headache. Chronobiologia 1981;2:140.
63. Ferrari E, Canepari C, Bossolo PA, et al. Changes of biological rhythms in primary headache syndromes. Cephalalgia 1983;3(Suppl 1):58.
64. Waldenlind E, Gustafsson SA, Ekbom K, et al. Circadian secretion of cortisol and melatonin in cluster headache during active cluster periods and remission. J Neurol Neurosurg Psychiatry 187;50:207.
65. Chazot G, Claustrat B, Brun J, et al. A chronobiological study of melatonin, cortisol, growth hormone, and prolactin secretion in cluster headache. Cephalalgia 1984;4:213.
66. Waldenlind E, Ekbom K, Friberg Y, et al. Decreased nocturnal serum melatonin levels during active cluster headache periods. Opusc Med 1984;29:109.
67. Polleri A, Nappi G, Murialdo G, et al. Changes in the 24-hour prolactin level in cluster headache. Cephalalgia 1982;2:1.
68. Waldenlind E, Gustafsson SA. Prolactin in cluster headache: Diurnal secretion, response to thyrotropin-releasing hormone, and relation to sex steroids and gonadotropins. Cephalalgia 1987;7:43.
69. Nappi G, Facchinetti F, Bono G, et al. Lack of β-Endorphin and β-Lipotropin Circadian Rhythmicity in Episodic Cluster Headache: A Model for Chronopathology. In V Pfaffenrath, P-O Lundberg, O Sjaastad (eds), Updating in Headache. Berlin: Springer, 1985.
70. Ferrari E, Martignoni E, Vailati A, et al. Chronobiological Aspects of Cluster Headache: Effects of Lithium Therapy. In F Savoldi, G Nappi (eds), Headache. Pavia: Palladio, 1979;152.
71. Fiedman AP, Wood EH. Thermography in Vascular Headache. In S Uema (ed), Medical Thermography. Los Angeles: Brentwood, 1976;80.
72. Kudrow L. Thermographic and Doppler flow asymmetry in cluster headache. Headache 1979;19:204.
73. Drummond PD, Anthony M. Extracranial vascular responses to sublingual nitroglycerin and oxygen inhalation in cluster headache patients. Headache 1985;25:70.

74. Drummond PD, Lance JW. Thermographic changes in cluster headache. Neurology 1984;34:1292.
75. Ekbom K, Greitz T. Carotid angiography in cluster headache. Acta Radiol Diagn 1970;10:177.
76. Fanciullacci M, Pietrini U, Gatto G, et al. Latent dysautonomic pupillary lateralization in cluster headache: A pupillometric study. Cephalalgia 1982;2:135.
77. Salvesen R, Bogucki A, Wysocka-Bakowska MM, et al. Cluster headache pathogenesis: A pupillometric study. Cephalalgia 1987;7:273.
78. Buccuni M, Murace G, Pietrini U, et al. Coexistence of pupillary and heart sympathergic asymmetries in cluster headache. Cephalalgia 1984;4:9.
79. Saunte C, Russell D, Sjaastad O. Cluster headache: On the mechanism behind attack-related sweating. Cephalalgia 1983;3:175.
80. Kudrow L. Response of cluster headache attacks to oxygen inhalation. Headache 1981;21:1.
81. Fogan L. Treatment of cluster headache: A double-blind comparison of oxygen v. air inhalation. Arch Neurol 1985;42:362.
82. Kudrow L. A possible role of the carotid body in the pathogenesis of cluster headache. Cephalalgia 1983;3:242.
83. Kudrow L, Kudrow DB. Association of sustained oxyhemoglobin desaturation and onset of cluster headache attacks. Headache 1990;30:474.
84. Kudrow L, Kudrow DB. The role of chemoreceptor activity and oxyhemoglobin desaturation in cluster headache. Headache 1993;33:483.
85. Zhao JM, Schaanning J, Sjaastad O. Cluster headache: The effect of low oxygen saturation. Headache 1990;30:656.
86. Shen JM, Schaanning J, White L, et al. Cluster headache: The ventilatory response to transient hypoxia with pure nitrogen. Headache 1993;33:476.
87. Gardiner WJ, Stowell A, Dutlinger R. Resection of the greater superficial petrosal nerve in the treatment of unilateral headache. J Neurosurg 1947;4:105.
88. Stowell A. Physiologic mechanisms and treatment of histaminic or petrosal neuralgia. Headache 1970;9:187.
89. Sachs E Jr. The role of the nervous intermedius in facial neuralgia: Report of four cases with observations on the pathways for taste, lacrimation, and pain in the face. J Neurosurg 1968;23:54.
90. Devoghel JC. Cluster headache and sphenopalatine block. Acta Anaesthesiol Belg 1981;1:101.
91. Kunkle EC. Acetylcholine in the mechanism of headaches of the migraine type. Arch Neurol Psychiatry 1959;84:135.
92. Appenzeller O, Becker WJ, Ragas A. Cluster headache: Ultrastructural aspects. Neurology 1978;28:371.
93. Moskowitz S, Saito S, Moskowitz MA. Neurogenically mediated leakage of plasma protein occurs from blood vessels in dura but not brain. J Neurosci 1987;7:4129.
94. Dimitriadou V, Buzzi MG, Lambracht-Hall M, et al. In vivo and in vitro ultrastructural evidence for stimulation of dural mast cells by neuropeptides. Proc Neurosci 1990;16:161.
95. Moskowitz MA. The neurobiology of vascular head pain. Ann Neurol 1984;16:157.
96. Goadsby PJ, Edvinsson L. Human in vivo evidence for trigeminovascular activation in cluster headache: Neuropeptide changes and effects of acute attack therapies. Brain 1994;117:427.
97. Noziaki K, Moskowitz MA, Maynard KI, et al. Possible origins and distribution of immunoreactive nitric oxide synthase-containing nerve fibers in cerebral arteries. J Cereb Blood Flow Metab 1993;13:70.
98. Goadsby PJ, Uddman R, Edvinsson L. Cerebral vasodilatation in the cat involves nitric oxide from parasympathetic nerves. Brain Res 1996;707:110.
99. Suzuki N, Hardebo JE. Anatomical basis for a parasympathetic and sensory innervation of the intracranial segment of the internal carotid artery in man: Possible implications for vascular headache. J Neurol Sci 1991;104:19.
100. Suzuki N, Hardebo JE. The cerebrovascular parasympathetic innervation. Cerebrovasc Brain Metab Rev 1993;5:33.
101. Nicolodi M, Del Bianco E. Sensory neuropeptides (substance P, calcitonin gene-related peptide) and vasoactive intestinal polypeptide in human saliva: Their pattern in migraine and cluster headache. Cephalalgia 1990;10:39.
102. Meyer JS, Hardenberg BA. Clinical effectiveness of calcium entry blockers in prophylactic treatment of migraine and cluster headache. Headache 1983;23:266.
103. Gabel IJ, Spierings ELH. Prophylactic treatment of cluster headache with verapamil. Headache 1989;29:167.
104. Ekbom K. Litium vid kroniska symptom av cluster headache. Opusc Med 1978;19:148.
105. Kudrow L. Lithium prophylaxis for chronic cluster headache. Headache 1977;17:15.

106. Mathew NT. Clinical subtypes of cluster headache and response to lithium therapy. Headache 1978;18:26.
107. Hering R, Kuritzky A. Sodium valproate in the treatment of cluster headache: An open clinical trial. Cephalalgia 1989;9:195.
108. Mathew NT, Hurt W. Radiofrequency trigeminal gangliolysis in the treatment of chronic intractable cluster headache. Headache 1985;25:166.
109. The Sumatriptan Cluster Headache Study Group. Treatment of acute cluster headache with sumatriptan. N Engl J Med 1991;31:322.
110. Ekbom K, et al. and the Sumatriptan Cluster Headache Study Group. Subcutaneous sumatriptan in the acute treatment of cluster headache: A dose comparison study. Acta Neurol Scand 1993;88:63.
111. Ekbom K, Krabbe A, Micelli G, et al., and the Sumatriptan Cluster Headache Long-term Study Group. Cluster headache attacks treated for up to three months with subcutaneous sumatriptan (6 mg). Cephalalgia 1995;15:230.
112. Barre F. Cocaine as an abortive agent in cluster headache. Headache 1982;22:69.
113. Kittrelle JP, Grouse DS, Seybold M. Cluster headache: Local anesthetic abortive agents. Arch Neurol 1985;42:496.

14
Paroxysmal Hemicranias

Lawrence C. Newman and Richard B. Lipton

The paroxysmal hemicranias are a group of rare, benign headache disorders that clinically resemble cluster headache but are resistant to typical cluster prophylaxis (see Chapter 13). They are, however, uniquely responsive to treatment with indomethacin.

Chronic paroxysmal hemicrania (CPH) was first described by Sjaastad and Dale in 1974.[1] The disorder was not named, however, until 1976.[2] The first cases were characterized by multiple, short-lived, unilateral attacks occurring on a daily basis for years without remission. Subsequently, it became apparent that not all patients experienced a chronic, unremitting course. In some patients, discrete headache phases were separated by prolonged pain-free remissions. This pattern was named episodic paroxysmal hemicrania (EPH) by Kudrow.[3] Still other patients experience an initially remitting course that over time evolves to become chronic.[4]

The nomenclature for the various forms of paroxysmal hemicrania has been controversial. Some authors prefer the terms *CPH, EPH,* and *CPH evolved from EPH* to describe the various syndromes.[3,5,6] These terms are analogous to the nomenclature for cluster headache.[7] Others prefer to label the paroxysmal hemicranias as types of CPH: chronic, either from onset or evolved from the remitting form; and nonchronic (remitting).[4] Currently, the International Headache Society recognizes only CPH.[7]

EPIDEMIOLOGY

A report by Antonaci and Sjaastad reviewed the clinical manifestations of 84 patients with the paroxysmal hemicranias.[4] Additional reports have subsequently been published.[5,6,8–12] To date there are more than 100 case reports of the paroxysmal hemicranias. For this chapter, we summarized data on 100 published cases, excluding reports that described atypical presentations, were incompletely documented, or appeared in languages other than English. The number of diagnosed

Table 14.1   Comparison of chronic and episodic paroxysmal hemicranias

	Chronic paroxysmal hemicrania	Episodic paroxysmal hemicrania
Age of onset (range)	6–81	12–51
Gender ratio (M:F)	1:2.8	1:1.45
Pain quality	Throbbing	Throbbing/stabbing
Pain severity	Excruciating	Excruciating
Location of maximal pain	Unilateral temple, orbit, jaw	Unilateral orbit, temple
Autonomic features	Present	Present
Attack frequency (daily)	1–40	6–30
Attack duration (minutes)	2–120	1–30
Nocturnal awakenings	Yes	Yes
Precipitated by alcohol	Yes	Yes
Response to indomethacin	Yes	Yes

cases is surely much higher; the disorder is no longer considered rare enough to warrant publication. We have pooled the data for cases of both EPH and CPH, whose clinical presentations are quite similar (Table 14.1). We have the impression that CPH is far more common than EPH, but systematic data are lacking.

Demographic Profile

In contrast to cluster headache, CPH shows a preponderance among women. To date, 68 women and 32 men with the disorder have been reported, thus the female-to-male ratio among reviewed cases is 2.13 to 1. The paroxysmal hemicranias typically begin in adulthood; Antonaci and Sjaastad reported a mean age of 34.1 ± 16.7 years.[4] In the more recent reports, the mean age when documented was 33 years.[5,6,8–12] The age of onset ranges from 6–81 years.

Family History of Headache

No family history of CPH or EPH was found in any of the reported cases. A family history of migraine occurred in 21% of the cases for which family history was reported. One patient reported a positive family history for cluster headache.[4]

CLINICAL FEATURES

Location of Pain

Pain is strictly unilateral and without side shift in the majority of patients. In one patient the pain was bilateral,[13] in three patients the headache may have demonstrated side shift.[4] A recent report—not included in the 100 cases we reviewed because of atypical features—described a patient with typical CPH, with recurring left hemicranial headaches associated with ipsilateral autonomic signs and absolute response to indomethacin treatment.[14] On withdrawal of indomethacin treatment, however, the patient noted occurrence of his usual left-sided autonomic symptoms but with little or no pain. Reinstituting treatment with indomethacin abolished this phenomenon, but when the drug was again discontinued, the patient noted two full-blown attacks on the contralateral side; these too resolved with reinstitution of therapy.

The maximum pain is most often experienced in the ocular, temporal, maxillary, and frontal regions; less often, the pain involves the nuchal, occipital, and retro-orbital areas. Pain may occasionally radiate into the ipsilateral shoulder and arm.

Pain Character

The pain is typically described as a throbbing, boring, pulsatile, sharp, or stabbing sensation ranging from moderate to excruciating in severity. Twenty-eight patients reported mild discomfort at the usual site of pain between attacks.[4] During episodes of pain, sufferers usually prefer to sit quietly or lie in bed in the fetal position; some patients, however, assume the pacing activity usually seen with cluster headaches.

Frequency and Duration of Attacks

In CPH, attacks recur from one to 40 times daily. Fluctuations in attack frequency have been well documented; the frequency of mild attacks ranges from two to 14 per day, and severe attacks recur six to 40 times daily. Most patients report 15 or more attacks per day. Attacks usually last between 2 and 25 minutes (range, 2–120 minutes).

In EPH, the daily attack frequency ranges from two to 30; attacks last from 3–30 minutes each. The duration of the headache phase lasts from 2 weeks to 4.5 months; remission periods range from 1–36 months. Attacks of both CPH and EPH may occur at night, awakening patients from sleep.

Associated Symptoms and Trigger Factors

During episodes of headache, ipsilateral lacrimation, conjunctival injection, nasal congestion, or rhinorrhea frequently accompany the headache. Ipsilateral eyelid edema, mild miosis, photophobia, and nausea have less frequently been reported. In one patient, there was a dissociation of the pain and autonomic features; i.e., lacrimation, conjunctival injection, and eyelid edema occurred in the absence of pain.[14] In another patient, bilateral tearing occurred during the headache episodes.[4]

Some patients report that attacks may be precipitated by bending or rotating the head, exerting pressure on the transverse processes of C4–5, the C2 root, or the ipsilateral greater occipital nerve. Alcohol ingestion triggered headaches in some patients.[4]

Table 14.2   Diagnostic criteria for chronic paroxysmal hemicrania

---

A. At least 50 attacks fulfilling B–E
B. Attacks of severe unilateral, orbital, supraorbital and/or temporal pain, always on the
    same side, lasting 2–45 minutes
C. Attack frequency > 5 per day for more than half of the time (periods with lower fre-
    quency may occur)
D. Pain is associated with at least one of the following signs or symptoms on the pain
    side:
    1. Conjunctival injection
    2. Lacrimation
    3. Nasal congestion
    4. Rhinorrhea
    5. Ptosis
    6. Eyelid edema
E. Absolute effectiveness of indomethacin (150 mg/day or less)
F. At least one of the following:
    1. History and physical and neurologic examinations do not suggest one of the disor-
        ders listed in groups 5–11, i.e., organic headaches, headaches associated with
        drug withdrawal, metabolic disorder, etc.
    2. History and/or physical and/or neurologic examinations do suggest such disorder,
        but it is ruled out by appropriate investigations
    3. Such disorder is present, but chronic paroxysmal hemicrania does not occur for
        the first time in close temporal relation to the disorder

---

Diagnostic Criteria and Differential Diagnosis

Of the various forms of the paroxysmal hemicranias, formal diagnostic criteria exist only for CPH.[7] The diagnostic criteria for CPH are shown in Table 14.2. The differential diagnosis of the paroxysmal hemicranias includes cluster headache,[15] hemicrania continua (HC),[16,17] trigeminal neuralgia (TN),[18] and the short-lasting, unilateral neuralgiform headache attacks with conjunctival injection and tearing (SUNCT) syndrome[19] (Table 14.3). Both EPH and CPH are characterized by throbbing or piercing headaches of excruciating intensity, localized predominantly in and around the orbit and temple and associated with the ipsilateral autonomic disturbances of cluster headache. Both disorders share the features of multiple, short-lived daily attacks, nocturnal attacks, precipitation by alcoholic beverages, and absolute response to treatment with indomethacin.

EPH is distinguished from CPH by its temporal profile; EPH is characterized by discrete attack and remission phases, whereas CPH occurs without remissions. EPH may be confused with the episodic form of cluster headache (ECH). Both EPH and ECH occur as active periods consisting of multiple attacks of brief, excruciating headaches with superimposed ipsilateral autonomic features, separated by periods of pain-free remission. Nocturnal attacks and alcohol precipitation are also seen in both conditions. EPH is distinguished from ECH by the higher frequency and shorter duration of the individual headaches as well as by its absolute response to treatment with indomethacin. Similarly, CPH must be differentiated from chronic cluster headache (CCH). Additionally, the female pre-

Table 14.3 Differential diagnosis of the paroxysmal hemicranias

	Paroxysmal hemicrania	Cluster	Hemicrania continua	Trigeminal neuralgia	SUNCT syndrome
Sex (F:M)	2.13:1	1:6	1.8:1	2:1	1:10
Age of onset (years)	6–81	20–40	11–58	50–60	30–68
Pain quality	Stabbing, pulsatile, throbbing	Stabbing, boring	Baseline dull ache, superimposed throbbing/stabbing	Lancinating	Lancinating
Site of maximal pain	Orbit/temple	Orbit/temple	Orbit/temple	V1–V2	Periorbital
Attacks per day	1–40	0–8	Varies	Varies	Varies
Duration of attacks	2–120 minutes (average, 2–25)	15–180 minutes (average, 20–45)	Minutes to days	Seconds	Seconds
Autonomic features	Yes	Yes	Yes (but less pronounced than cluster)	No	Yes
Alcohol trigger	Yes	Sometimes	Yes	No	No

SUNCT = short-lasting, unilateral neuralgiform headache attacks with conjunctival injection and tearing.

ponderance may help to separate the paroxysmal hemicranias from the over-whelmingly male-dominated cluster syndromes.

HC is another rare headache disorder that responds to indomethacin therapy. It too has clinical variants consisting of episodic (remitting), chronic (nonremit-ting), and evolved forms. HC is characterized by a constant, low-level, baseline hemicranial headache with superimposed exacerbations of more severe pain. These exacerbations last minutes to days and are associated at times with the ipsi-lateral autonomic features of cluster headache. Those autonomic features, when present, however, tend to be much less pronounced than those seen in either clus-ter headache or PH. HC is differentiated from cluster headache and PH by the presence of a constant, low-level, baseline headache. The painful exacerbations described in HC tend to be less severe than those of PH or cluster, and the ipsi-lateral autonomic features of HC are also less pronounced.

The PHs are occasionally confused with TN in the first division of the nerve. Both disorders are characterized by short-lived attacks of unilateral pain in and around the orbit. In contrast to the PHs, the attacks of TN are briefer in duration, with paroxysms of lancinating pain; and TN is not associated with autonomic fea-tures. In the cluster-tic syndrome, paroxysms of lancinating pain in the second and third divisions of the trigeminal nerve lasting seconds or minutes occur together with the excruciating, boring pain typical of cluster.[20] Autonomic fea-tures may accompany the cluster component of the disorder. Recently, Hannertz reported a patient with features of both CPH and TN, the CPH-tic syndrome.[21]

The SUNCT syndrome is a rare headache disorder characterized by strictly unilateral headaches accompanied by ipsilateral autonomic phenomena. Attacks consist of 30- to 120-second paroxysms of moderate- to high-intensity periorbital pains recurring up to 30 times per hour. SUNCT is differentiated from PH by the ultrashort duration and much higher frequency of daily attacks.

Rarely, intracranial lesions may mimic the clinical course of the paroxysmal hemicranias. The headaches of the paroxysmal hemicranias have been mimicked by aneurysms within the circle of Willis,[22] arteriovenous malformations,[23] cere-brovascular accidents,[23] collagen vascular disease,[22] and tumors of the frontal lobe,[22] sella turcica,[24] and cavernous sinus.[25] Because the paroxysmal hemicra-nias remain a relatively uncommon headache entity, neuroimaging procedures should be performed in all patients, especially those with atypical presentations or those requiring persistent high dosages of indomethacin to achieve response.

TREATMENT

Indomethacin is the treatment of choice for the paroxysmal hemicranias and, in fact, has been deemed the sine qua non for establishing the diagnosis. The ther-apy should be initiated at 25 mg three times per day. If no benefit is demonstrat-ed at that dose or if there is only a partial response after 1 week, the dose should be increased to 50 mg three times daily. Complete resolution of the headache is prompt, usually occurring within 1–2 days of initiating the effective dose. The typical maintenance dose ranges from 25–100 mg per day, but doses up to 300 mg per day are occasionally required; dosage adjustments may be necessary to address the clinical fluctuations seen occasionally in CPH. During active headache cycles, skipping or even delaying doses may result in the prompt reoccurrence of the headache. In patients with EPH, indomethacin should be given for slightly longer than the typical headache phase and then gradually tapered. In patients with CPH, long-term treatment is usually necessary; however, long-lasting remissions have been reported following cessation of indomethacin.[26]

In patients who do not respond to indomethacin, the diagnosis should be reconsidered. The need for constant, high doses of indomethacin may indicate underlying pathology.[25] The mechanism underlying the absolute indomethacin response is not known. It does not appear that indomethacin works in the PHs because of its effect on prostaglandin synthesis, because other nonsteroidal anti-inflammatory drugs with more potent antiprostaglandin actions have little or no effect. Quintana et al. suggest that indomethacin may affect the cerebral circulation without involving cyclo-oxygenase.[27] Short-term side effects of indomethacin therapy include gastrointestinal upset, and long-term use may induce ulcerations of the gastrointestinal tract. In cases where indomethacin may be required on a long-term basis, the concurrent use of antacids, misoprostol, or histamine H_2-receptor antagonists should be considered.

Other agents have demonstrated partial success in treating the paroxysmal hemicranias. Acetylsalicylic acid has been shown to be efficacious in the early phases of CPH[4] and possibly during the childhood phase of the disorder.[28] Partial success with calcium channel blockers (verapamil),[29] steroids, and other non-steroidal anti-inflammatory agents has also been reported.[4] Recently, a piroxicam derivative was found to be effective in some patients with CPH who had also responded to indomethacin.[30]

REFERENCES

1. Sjaastad O, Dale I. Evidence for a new (?) treatable headache entity. Headache 1974;14:105.
2. Sjaastad O, Dale I. A new (?) clinical headache entity "chronic paroxysmal hemicrania" 2. Acta Neurol Scand 1976;54:140.
3. Kudrow L, Esperanza P, Vijayan N. Episodic paroxysmal hemicrania? Cephalalgia 1987;7:197.
4. Antonaci F, Sjaastad O. Chronic paroxysmal hemicrania (CPH): A review of the clinical manifestations. Headache 1989;29:648.
5. Blau JN, Engel H. Episodic paroxysmal hemicrania: A further case and review of the literature. J Neurol Neurosurg Psychiatry 1990;53:343.
6. Newman LC, Gordon ML, Lipton RB, et al. Episodic paroxysmal hemicrania: Two new cases and a literature review. Neurology 1992;42:964.
7. Headache Classification Committee of the International Headache Society. Classification and diagnostic criteria for headache disorders, cranial neuralgias, and facial pain. Cephalalgia 1988;8(Suppl 7):1.
8. Spierings ELH. The chronic paroxysmal hemicrania concept expanded. Headache 1988;28:597.
9. Cummings WJK. Episodic paroxysmal hemicrania. J Neurol Neurosurg Psychiatry 1991;54:666.
10. Spierings ELH. Case report: Episodic paroxysmal hemicrania and chronic paroxysmal hemicrania. Clin J Pain 1992;8:44.
11. Newman LC, Lipton RB, Solomon S. Episodic paroxysmal hemicrania: Three new cases and a review of the literature. Headache 1993;3:195.
12. Sjaastad O, Antonaci F. A piroxicam derivative partially effective in chronic paroxysmal hemicrania and hemicrania continua. Headache 1995;35:549.
13. Pollmann W, Pfaffenrath V. Chronic paroxysmal hemicrania: The first possible bilateral case. Cephalalgia 1986;6:55.
14. Pareja JA. Chronic paroxysmal hemicrania: Dissociation of the pain and autonomic features. Headache 1995;35:111.

15. Sjaastad O. Cluster Headache Syndrome. London: Saunders, 1992.
16. Sjaastad O, Spierings ELH. "Hemicrania continua": Another headache absolutely responsive to indomethacin. Cephalalgia 1984;4:65.
17. Newman LC, Lipton RB, Solomon S. Hemicrania continua: Ten new cases and a review of the literature. Neurology 1994;44:2111.
18. Terrence CF, Fromm GH. Trigeminal Neuralgia and Other Facial Neuralgias. In J Olesen, P Tfelt-Hansen, KMA Welch (eds), The Headaches. New York: Raven, 1993;773.
19. Sjaastad O, Saunte C, Salvesen R, et al. Short-lasting, unilateral neuralgiform headache attacks with conjunctival injection, tearing, sweating, and rhinorrhea. Cephalalgia 1989;9:147.
20. Solomon S, Apfelbaum RI, Guglielmo KM. The cluster-tic syndrome and its surgical therapy. Cephalalgia 1985;5:83.
21. Hannerz J. Trigeminal neuralgia with chronic paroxysmal hemicrania: The CPH-tic syndrome. Cephalalgia 1993;13:361.
22. Medina JL. Organic headaches mimicking chronic paroxysmal hemicrania. Headache 1993;32:73.
23. Newman LC, Hershkovitz S, Lipton RB, Solomon S. Chronic paroxysmal headache: Two cases with cerebrovascular disease. Headache 1992;32:75.
24. Vijayan N. Symptomatic chronic paroxysmal hemicrania. Cephalalgia 1992;12:111.
25. Sjaastad O, Stovner LJ, Stolt-Nielsen A, et al. Case reports CPH and hemicrania continua: Requirements of high indomethacin dosages. An ominous sign? Headache 1995;35:363.
26. Sjaastad O, Antonaci F. Chronic paroxysmal hemicrania: A case report. Long-lasting remission in the chronic stage. Cephalalgia 1987;7:203.
27. Quintana A, Raczaka E, Giralt MT, et al. Effects of aspirin and indomethacin on cerebral circulation in the conscious rat: Evidence for a physiological role of endogenous prostaglandins. Prostaglandins 1983;25:549.
28. Kudrow DB, Kudrow L. Successful aspirin prophylaxis in a child with chronic paroxysmal hemicrania. Headache 1989;29:280.
29. Coria F, Claveria LE, Jimenez-Jimenez FJ, et al. Episodic paroxysmal hemicrania responsive to calcium channel blockers. J Neurol Neurosurg Psychiatry 1992;55:166.
30. Sjaastad O, Antonaci F. A piroxicam derivative partly effective in chronic paroxysmal hemicrania and hemicrania continua. Headache 1995;35:549.

THREE

ISSUES IN SECONDARY HEADACHE

15
Posttraumatic Headache and Posttraumatic Syndrome

William B. Young and Russell C. Packard

Posttraumatic syndrome (PTS) is a constellation of symptoms that may follow a mild-to-moderate closed head injury (HI). It is now clear that this syndrome can develop even without loss of consciousness; thus, the original term *postconcussion syndrome* is no longer appropriate. In addition to headache, symptoms include depression, irritability, memory impairment, loss of libido, dizziness or vertigo, alcohol intolerance, and attention and concentration difficulties. The association with compensation claims and litigation, the absence of diagnostically discriminatory testing, and the refractoriness of PTS have led to an unwarranted bias against the disorder in the health care community.

EPIDEMIOLOGY

Motor vehicle accidents account for 45% of HI, falls account for 30%, and occupational and recreational accidents for 20%.[1] Many HI patients suffer from PTS and have additional somatic and neuropsychological symptoms. Because many patients with mild head injuries (MHI) who subsequently develop posttraumatic headache (PTH) are never hospitalized, it is difficult to estimate the true burden of the disorder. Patients with MHI, defined as a Glasgow coma scale score of 13 to 15 (Table 15.1), are hospitalized at a rate of approximately 200 per 100,000 population per year.[2] PTH develops in 30–80% of such patients.[3–7] Seventy-nine percent to 90% of patients with postconcussion symptoms also have headache.[8,9]

The term *whiplash* refers to the sequence of extension, flexion, and lateral motions of the neck that follows impact, with or without direct trauma to the head. The symptomatology that follows whiplash is remarkably similar to that experienced by patients following HI. In addition to neck pain, headaches, dizziness, paresthesias, and cognitive and psychological sequelae are extremely common. In fact, we were unable to locate a published discussion of the *differences*

Table 15.1   Glasgow coma scale*

Eye opening (E)	
Spontaneous	4
To sound	3
To pain	2
None	1
Best motor response (M)	
Obeys	6
Localizes	5
Withdraws	4
Abnormal flexion	3
Extends	2
None	1
Verbal response (V)	
Oriented	5
Confused	4
Inappropriate	3
Incomprehensible	2
None	1

*Score equals sum of E + M + V and ranges between 3 and 15.

between HI and whiplash, although neck pain is more frequently seen after whiplash injury than HI. Ninety-seven percent of patients seeking help from a physician after whiplash have headache.[10] Because whiplash injury usually does not lead to hospitalization, its incidence is even more difficult to calculate than that of HI or PTH; however, it has been estimated at approximately 1 million cases per year in the United States.[11,12]

CLINICAL FEATURES

Symptoms of PTS (Table 15.2) may develop immediately or may be delayed (or not initially recognized) following trauma. Head, neck, and shoulder pain usually begins within 24–48 hours of the injury, whereas local occipital tenderness occurs immediately. Neuralgic symptoms can develop in the frontal or occipital region months after the injury. The International Headache Society (IHS) criteria for PTH (Table 15.3) require the onset of headache within 2 weeks of HI or of regaining consciousness. However, in clinical practice it is often difficult to determine when headache actually started, because head pain may be mild and other pains (particularly neck pain) more prominent. Furthermore, patients may develop chronic headaches as long as 24 months after the trauma. These late-onset headaches are clinically similar to chronic PTH (see Table 15.3). Brenner et al.[5] found that 6% of MHI patients had headaches that began within 16 months after discharge, and Cartlidge and Shaw found that 12% had late-acquired headache 6 and 24 months after discharge.[13] Such late-onset headaches (which do not meet IHS criteria for PTH) are more prevalent than would be expected by chance. Why the headaches begin late is uncertain. Their relationship to the pre-

Table 15.2   Sequelae of mild head injury

Headaches
    Tension-type
    Migraine
    Cluster
    Low cerebrospinal pressure
    Occipital neuralgia
    Idiopathic intracranial hypotension
    Supraorbital and infraorbital neuralgia
    Cervicogenic
    Temporomandibular joint syndrome or dysfunction
    Local neuroma
    Mixed
Cranial nerve symptoms and signs
    Dizziness
    Vertigo
    Tinnitus
    Hearing loss
    Blurred vision
    Diplopia
    Convergence insufficiency
    Light and noise sensitivity
    Diminished taste and smell
Psychological and somatic complaints
    Irritability
    Anxiety
    Depression
    Personality change
    Fatigue
    Sleep disturbance
    Decreased libido
    Decreased appetite
Rare sequelae
    Subdural and epidural hematomas
    Seizures
    Transient global amnesia
    Tremor
    Dystonia

ceding injury is highly controversial and difficult to establish with certainty. We believe these late-onset headaches may be due to a traumatically increased headache susceptibility that is not manifest until other factors ultimately push the patient over a headache threshold. The IHS criterion that PTH must begin within 2 weeks following injury or regaining consciousness may not have physiologic validity but instead may represent an arbitrary compromise useful in establishing causality for purposes of disability compensation, litigation, and insurance.

A variety of pain patterns may develop after HI; often they resemble the primary headache disorders (see Table 15.2). The most frequently seen pattern resembles tension-type headache (TTH) and occurs in 85% of patients. It is characterized by

Table 15.3   International Headache Society criteria for acute and chronic posttraumatic headache

---

5.1.1 With significant head trauma and/or confirmatory signs
Diagnostic criteria
  A. Significance of head trauma documented by at least one of the following:
    1. Loss of consciousness
    2. Posttraumatic amnesia lasting more than 10 minutes
    3. At least two of the following exhibit relevant abnormality: clinical neurologic examination, radiography of skull, neuroimaging, evoked potentials, spinal fluid examination, vestibular function test, neuropsychologic testing
  B. Headache occurs less than 14 days after regaining consciousness (or after trauma, if there has been no loss of consciousness)
  C. Headache disappears within 8 weeks after regaining consciousness (or after trauma, if there has been no loss of consciousness [acute]) or continues more than 8 weeks (chronic)
5.1.2 With minor head trauma and no confirmatory signs
Diagnostic criteria
  A. Head trauma that does not satisfy 5.1.1.A
  B. Headache occurs less than 14 days after injury
  C. Headache disappears within 8 weeks after injury (acute) or continues more than 8 weeks (chronic)

Source: Reprinted with permission from the Headache Classification Committee of the International Headache Society. Classification and diagnostic criteria for headache disorders, cranial neuralgia, and facial pain. Cephalalgia 1988;(Suppl 7):1.

generalized, persistent, bilateral, mild-to-moderate pain.[14] The headaches may be exacerbated by mild physical or mental activity.[15] In one study,[16] headaches were mild in 30%, moderate in 52%, and severe in 18% of patients, and the pain was occipital in 51%, frontal in 44%, and generalized in 11% of patients.

An otherwise typical migraine with or without aura may be triggered by impact.[17] Alternatively, a pattern of recurring migraine-like headaches may begin some time after a head injury.[3,14,18–20] In one study,[18] 35 patients had newly acquired migraine with or without aura beginning within a few days of MHI or whiplash injury. Twenty-seven were women and eight were men, and most patients experienced two or three attacks per week. Amitriptyline or propranolol was dramatically effective in 71%. Other patients have PTH with features of migraine or TTH that closely resembles transformed migraine.[21]

Neuralgic pain in the frontal or occipitocervical region may occur and may be associated with the other headache types. Mandel, Evans, and others have found cluster headache–like syndrome occurring in up to 10% of patients; these headaches may not undergo remissions.[3,14,21,22] Other authors find them to be quite rare.[23]

Haas used the IHS criteria for primary headache disorders to categorize 30 PTH patients. Eight patients were classified as migraine, 12 as chronic tension-type headache (CTTH), two as analgesic abuse headache, seven as "probable analgesic abuse headache," and one was unclassifiable.[24]

Orthostatic headache with features similar to those of a post–lumbar puncture headache can also occur after HI. In these cases, cerebrospinal fluid (CSF) hypotension could result from a CSF leak through a dural root sleeve tear or a cribriform plate fracture. Idiopathic intracranial hypertension (pseudotumor), with and without papilledema, has been reported as a consequence of HI.[25]

Dysautonomic cephalalgia, a rare type of PTH that occurs following injury to the anterior area of the carotid sheath, was described by Vijayan in 1977.[26] This severe, unilateral headache is localized to the frontotemporal area and is associated with ipsilateral increased facial sweating and pupillary dilation.

Temporomandibular joint (TMJ) injury may occur in conjunction with MHI. Symptoms include jaw pain with mastication or prolonged talking, incomplete jaw opening, clicking or lateral movements (which by themselves are not clinically relevant), and pain on palpation of the jaw joint or the muscles of mastication. TMJ dysfunction is thought to be a trigger for headache (see Chapter 23).

Trauma may also cause a fracture of the styloid process with symptoms resembling Eagle's syndrome: unilateral pain in the throat or neck or referred pain in the shoulder, chest, tongue, eye, cheek, TMJ, or ear. The pain is usually dull and continuous, but it may be neuralgic. The patient may complain of the sensation of a foreign body in the throat. Symptoms of carotid artery insufficiency may also occur. The fracture should be visualized radiographically. Treatment may involve local anesthetics or surgery.[27,28]

Most PTS patients have impaired memory and difficulty concentrating.[9] Some patients have neurocognitive deficits with a documented inability to process information.[29] Many have difficulty processing different stimuli simultaneously and appear absentminded because they must devote full concentration to the task at hand. If the information-processing capacity is overtaxed, the patient appears forgetful.[30] Patients with HI often appear distracted because of their inability to disregard irrelevant stimuli. Other frequently reported symptoms include anger, depression, irritability, and personality changes. A survey of high school and university students demonstrated that those with self-reported head injury had more cognitive and emotional symptoms than those without.[31] Constitutional abnormalities include changes in appetite, alterations in sexual drive, weight loss or gain, and menstrual irregularities. Patients may meet the criteria for posttraumatic stress disorder[32] (Table 15.4) with uncertain frequency.[33,34] Posttraumatic stress disorder, when present, often requires aggressive intervention.[33]

Nonspecific dizziness and episodic and positional vertigo are common among PTS patients.[35] Sleep disturbances, including insomnia and daytime drowsiness, are frequent. Nonrestorative sleep and hypersomnolence are common complaints; polysomnographic studies show increased fragmentation of nocturnal sleep.[36] Seizure-like events may occur, although few of these events appear to be epileptic, and the electroencephalograph (EEG) is usually normal. Spells such as nonspecific staring episodes, nonvestibular dizziness, and periodic loss of consciousness have been reported. Epilepsy and true syncope are rare. Narcolepsy- or cataplexy-like spells, episodic disorientation, and fugue-like states can occur.[37,38] The attacks are more common when there has been a loss of consciousness at the time of the initial injury.[39]

The symptoms of PTS are often present but unreported. Only 59% of patients hospitalized with HI who had headache complained of it spontaneously; the rest required prompting or direct questioning. At 6 months, only 33% of patients with headache after HI volunteered this information. Similar percentages of spontaneous complaints were noted for patients with dizziness, and the percentages of patients reporting symptoms of depression, anxiety, and irritability were much smaller.[13]

Table 15.4   Diagnostic and Statistical Manual classification for posttraumatic stress disorder

---

Person exposed to traumatic event
Traumatic event persistently re-experienced
Persistent avoidance of stimuli associated with trauma and numbing of general
    responsiveness
Persistent symptoms of increased arousal
Duration of the disturbance is more than 1 month
Disturbance causes clinically significant distress or impairment in social, occupational,
    or other important areas of functioning

Source: Modified from American Psychiatric Association. Diagnostic and Statistical Manual of Mental Disorders (4th ed). Washington, D.C.: American Psychiatric Association, 1994.

In the past, PTH was considered acute if it lasted less than 2 months and chronic if it lasted more than 2 months (see Table 15.3). Recently, Packard has suggested that PTH persisting more than 6 months should be considered chronic because continuous improvement is less likely to occur after that amount of time.[40] This criterion would also make the diagnosis of chronic PTH consistent with CTTH.

MYTH OF NONORGANICITY

Patients with PTS are often told by physicians, insurers, or employers that they are embellishing or malingering, that they have a primary psychiatric disorder, or that their condition is not related to their injury. However, most experts believe that few chronic PTS patients actually engage in such behavior. The presence of litigation does not appear to influence outcome, and patients are not cured by a verdict.[9,41,42] Symptoms of litigants are similar to those of nonlitigants.[43] Nonetheless, physicians are often placed in the position of having to justify an accurate diagnosis of PTS.

In 1961 Miller published a series of lectures in the *British Medical Journal* in which he ascribed chronic PTS to a desire for compensation or a desire not to work.[44,45] The same arguments continue to be used today, to the detriment of patients. Lidvall et al., however, prospectively studied patients and demonstrated that poor work adjustment did not predict PTS, but that patients with PTS subsequently demonstrated poor work adjustment.[35]

Arguing for nonorganicity, Mittenberg et al.[46] demonstrated that a control population, imagining they had symptoms after HI, identified the symptoms of PTS from a checklist in a similar manner to patients who complain of PTS. They concluded that the symptoms of PTS are due to the expectation of experiencing these symptoms. They suggested that education and reassurance of a favorable prognosis are adequate treatments and that some patients should be treated for anxiety. We find the evidence for organic pathology too strong to accept these conclusions. The findings of Mittenberg et al. suggest only that PTS is a common syndrome that most people are familiar with since the symptoms of chronic PTS and acute HI are similar and most people have sustained a mild acute HI at one time or another. The crux of PTS may be the organic magnification of symptoms commonly experienced by normal individuals, thus accounting for the easy recognizability of the symptoms by controls.

One of the arguments used against the organicity of PTS is that there are no abnormal studies or abnormal signs on examination. But "failure to understand the problem is no proof of psychogenecity."[47] Many neurologic diseases, such as migraine with aura, have no abnormal signs on examination. Another argument sometimes used to suggest that PTS is attributable to the perceived opportunity for gain is that sports injuries rarely cause PTS. However, the velocities and forces experienced during most sports injuries are much less than those that result from motor vehicle accidents and falls, which are the injuries that commonly cause PTS. In sports injuries, the head is often fixed, whereas in automobile accidents the head is freely mobile. The increased mobility results in more severe damage.

Similarly, the observation that seemingly trivial injuries can cause severe disability has led to the conclusion by some that such disability does not have a physiologic basis. But there are other disease states in which minor injuries cause severe pain. In particular, incomplete peripheral nerve injuries are often excruciatingly painful, whereas nerve transections are usually painless. In some injuries, skull fracture may dissipate the energy of impact and protect the brain from injury that might lead to PTS, producing fewer symptoms in a population that initially appears more severely injured.

Work factors have been hypothesized as a cause of prolonged disability. Miller[44,45] showed that unskilled workers and less intelligent persons suffer more prolonged disability due to PTS syndrome. The referral population, however, consisted of patients sent by an insurance company. Thus, it is likely that a marked referral bias was at work. Furthermore, jobs requiring certain cognitive skills are particularly difficult for patients suffering from PTS. Laborers whose jobs depend on sustained physical effort and mental vigilance have particular difficulty performing their jobs. Patients with jobs that allow more flexibility and do not require physical activity may be better able to cope with the disability. It has been noted that patients who blamed their employer for their injury and perceived the employer as a large impersonal body had more symptoms than those who did not. This observation has been interpreted as "clear evidence of nervous and emotional factors at work in the production of symptoms."[48] The other possibility—that patients who are anxious, depressed, irritable, and have more symptoms due to their PTS are more likely to blame others—was not addressed.

Some physicians argue that a patient who has psychiatric symptoms has an illness that does not have an organic cause. Many kinds of brain injuries, including stroke and neurodegenerative disease, produce psychiatric symptoms. Chronic pain by itself can induce depression and abnormal behavior; these symptoms do not mean organic pathology does not exist. Having a disabling illness that is not accepted by medical professionals, employers, or family members is a legitimate cause of anxiety, depression, and abnormal behaviors.

RISK FACTORS

Age, gender, and certain mechanical factors represent risks for a poor outcome after HI or whiplash injury. Women, compared with men, have a 1.9 times greater risk of PTH.[34] Increasing age is associated with less rapid and less complete recovery.[13,49,50] One study found that children under 15 years of age may develop acute, but not chronic, PTH.[51] Jensen and Nielsen, however, found no significant risk of PTH due to age.[34] Mechanical factors in the injury, apart from the force of impact, are important. If the head is rotated, increased stress is put on the cervical structures and more rotational forces are applied to the brain. Thus, PTH is more likely to occur if the head is inclined or rotated prior to impact. Other factors that correlate with PTS include a rear-end collision and an unprepared vehicle occupant.[41]

The relationship between the severity of injury and the severity of PTS has not been conclusively established. In general, the persistence of headache does not correlate with the duration of unconsciousness or with posttraumatic amnesia, skull fracture, EEG abnormalities, or bloody CSF.[16,35] Curiously, Yamaguchi[52] found an inverse relationship between the severity of the injury and the severity of the PTH. Since the study included patients with both moderate and severe HI, this finding may not apply within the MHI group.[52] In one study, the initially hospitalized MHI patients had similar symptoms to patients who were discharged from the emergency room. However, the hospitalized patients recovered more quickly. These findings could support the idea that the more severe MHI causes less PTH and PTS, although other explanations are possible.[53] Similarly, Wilkinson found that severe head injury may, in fact, reduce the incidence of PTH.[54]

On the other hand, a study found more depression and anger-control problems in patients with loss of consciousness than in those without.[39] The fact that diplopia, anosmia, and the presence of central nervous system abnormality at 24 hours correlate with the persistence of symptoms 6 weeks after injury suggests that a subset of patients with more severe injury have worse outcomes.[55] This difference suggests that more research using prospectively followed, stratified patient samples must be done before definitive conclusions can be reached.

Radanov et al.[56] studied patients 7 days after and again 2 years after whiplash injury. Patients who had high multiple-symptom scores shortly after their injury had a significantly greater chance of having symptoms 2 years after the injury. Patients who were still disabled 2 years after their injury had higher multiple-symptom scores at the initial examination compared with patients who were symptomatic but not disabled after 2 years. Radanov et al. believe that patients with more severe injuries have higher initial symptom scores and worse outcomes. Alternatively, individual vulnerability could lead to a greater number of initial symptoms and a poorer long-term outcome, regardless of the severity of the initial injury.

Some have speculated that a history of prior headache increases the risk for PTH. Jensen found that pretraumatic migraine was not a risk factor for developing PTH after hospitalization for cerebral concussion.[34] This study suffered from recall bias; the patients were interviewed 9–12 months after the injury. Weiss et al. reported that 31% of patients who developed migraine-like attacks following mild head or neck trauma had a family history of migraine in first-degree relatives. They suggested that head or neck trauma triggers the migraine process in a susceptible individual.[57] In another study in which patients were interviewed immediately following whiplash injury, pretraumatic headache was found to be a significant risk factor for developing PTH.[56] Early headache, occurring within 24 hours of injury, is a strong risk factor for PTS at 6 weeks.[55]

Lidvall et al. found that although lack of education was not a risk factor for acute PTS, unskilled laborers were more likely to develop symptoms.[35] Likewise, socioeconomic status predicts employment 3 months after minor HI. All the business managers and executives in Rimel's study were employed 3 months after injury, but only 57% of the unskilled laborers were still employed. Higher education also predicted continued employment. These studies do not differentiate between the effects of injury and those of premorbid factors such as lack of education, poor motivation to return to a menial job, poor resources to adjust to the effects of the injury, or—a factor we believe may play a role— employer intolerance.[9]

Preexisting psychopathology may influence the clinical evolution of PTS. Ross and McNaughton found that patients with localized PTH did not have pre-existing psychopathology, whereas those with "bizarre," generalized, or bilateral headaches had prior "unstable personalities."[58] In another study, the researchers assessed patients for premorbid psychopathology by interviewing them and their relatives within 1 month of HI. The patient's psychological state prior to the injury correlated with the subjective symptomatology. However, physical and social dysfunction correlated with the severity of injury, not with preexisting factors.[51] Another study found that patients with pretraumatic emotional problems had higher scores on scales of cognitive and emotional-vegetative dysfunction after MHI.[49] Disability was not measured. These three studies suggest that pre-existing psychopathology influences how symptoms are reported rather than affecting subsequent disability. Two additional studies do not support those conclusions. McClelland et al. found no difference in premorbid personality adjustment between chronic PTS sufferers and patients whose symptoms resolved.[50] Likewise, Lidvall et al.[35] found no differences in pretraumatic neuroticism or adjustment to work between similarly injured patients who developed PTS and those who did not. All of these studies have methodologic problems: the psychological assessments were retrospective, and the methods used to ascertain pre-existing psychopathology were often not well described.

Using the Freiburg Personality Inventory, Radanov assessed patients shortly after whiplash injury. Scores on the nervousness, depression, openness, neuroticism, and masculinity scales did not correlate with outcome 2 years after injury. In contrast, poor well-being scale scores correlated with the persistence of symptoms, but not with disability, among patients who were symptomatic 2 years after injury.[56]

PATHOPHYSIOLOGY

PTS is probably not a single pathologic entity, but a group of traumatically induced disorders with overlapping symptoms. The cognitive, sleep, and psychological deficits of PTS patients are manifestations of brain injury. We believe that the headache is mainly a manifestation of brain dysfunction, occasionally aggravated by persistent musculoskeletal injuries.

Injury to the neck, jaw, or tissues of the scalp may play a role in the development of acute PTH. Pain originating from these areas can be referred into the head. Injury to a peripheral nerve may result in neuralgic pain. Most such injuries heal completely and cannot, by themselves, account for chronic PTH or the associated neurocognitive symptoms of PTS. However, soft-tissue or skeletal injuries may initiate or trigger a transformation process in headache-prone patients similar to the process by which daily intermittent migraine or TTH evolves into chronic daily headache. Changes in the characteristics of wide-dynamic-range neurons (windup and sensitization) induced by peripheral painful injury could account for cervical pain syndromes, and perhaps for PTH itself. One model, based on the kindling phenomenon in experimental epilepsy,[59] could explain the evolution of peripheral injuries into chronic, centrally maintained pain. Nerve or musculoskeletal injuries could induce windup and sensitization, which could ultimately result in permanently altered neuronal function. Because these changes occur postsynaptically, neuronal function may be altered at distant brain sites involved in the production or experience of pain.[59]

As a result of HI or whiplash, shear forces are applied to the brain; such forces can result in diffuse axonal injury (DAI) that can be measured histologically. In experimental models, direct impact is not necessary to produce significant DAI.[60] DAI is most common in the corpus callosum, internal capsule, fornices, dorso-lateral midbrain, and pons.[61] Gennarelli et al. have suggested that there is a continuum of DAI, varying from functional abnormalities alone to structural lesions that become increasingly severe and result in widespread axonal disruption.[62] Although it is not clear what the minimal clinically relevant injury is and whether DAI can occur with subconcussive MHI, DAI has been demonstrated in concussive MHI.[63]

Because of unsynchronized rotations that may develop between the cerebral hemispheres and the cerebellum,[64] axons in the upper brain stem may be particularly vulnerable to DAI. Midbrain hemorrhage has been seen on magnetic resonance imaging (MRI) in a patient with MHI, again demonstrating that this area is vulnerable to injury.[65] The brain stem axons that are sheared in DAI are responsible for maintaining arousal, vigilance, and sleep.[66] Serotonergic projection fibers postulated to play a central role in pain control and "the migraine center," recently described by Diener's group,[67] are located in this area (see also Chapter 1). Both may be injured, resulting in head pain. Reactive synaptogenesis, a process of axonal sprouting that restores synaptic contact on denuded dendrites, has been demonstrated in at least one model of HI.[68] This process could account for both physiologic improvement through appropriate healing and new or worsening symptoms as aberrant connections are made.

HI usually involves a combination of translational and rotational forces. If rotation is restricted, it is more difficult to produce a concussion in animals.[64] Rotational forces occur even when movement is primarily translational. In studies using windows in cadaver skulls, the brain has been demonstrated to lag behind the skull when the head is accelerated due to inertia. As a result of the translational force, the brain is compressed near the point of impact, while negative pressures develop opposite to the site of impact.

There are several HI models. The angular acceleration model of Gennarelli, using subhuman primates, replicates many of the features of human HI. It reproduces the features of MHI, including axonal changes in the brain stem[69] similar to those found in the human autopsy cases of MHI.[70] In this model, DAI is a major neural response to severe HI and is probably the cause of coma.[71] In the cat fluid percussion model of experimental brain injury, a hydraulic pressure

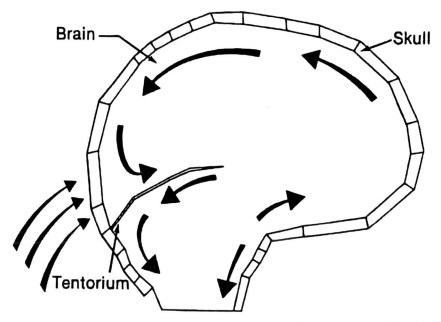

Figure 15.1   Brain motion. (Reprinted from C Ward. Status of Head Injury Modeling. Head and Neck Injury Criteria, Washington D.C.: U.S. Department of Transportation, 1981.)

pulse, lasting milliseconds, creates a physiologic response similar to that found in human moderate or mild HI. Based on microscopic changes observed after hydraulic injury, Povlishock and Coburn have speculated that stretching or compression, not shearing, is the cause of axonal injury in this model and possibly in human HI.[70] In rats, a fluid percussion pulse causes loss of cholinergic neurons in the forebrain, but not in the brain stem.[72]

The effects of various acceleration forces on the brain have been studied using a computerized structural analysis technique known as finite element modeling. By introducing an adjustment for brain tissue compressibility, Ward and coworkers have been able to create a model that fits with experimental data.[73] Finite element modeling has shown that rotational brain movements occur even when the motion of the head is primarily translational. It has also shown that various brain compartments are subject to different rotations (Figure 15.1). Shear stress in the brain stem is influenced by a number of factors, which include pressure release at the foramen magnum, the motion of the medulla due to the motion of the neck, the influence of individually rotating cerebral hemispheres and the cerebellum, the proximity of the brain stem to the skull, and restraint provided by the tentorium.[64,74]

Following severe HI, ischemic brain injury is common.[66] Abnormal cerebrovascular autoregulation and vasospasm may occur. The role of these phenomena in mild HI is unknown, but they may play a role in more severe brain injury or headache.

Table 15.5   Comparison of biochemical changes in mild head injury and migraine headache

Mild head injury	Migraine
Increased extracellular K^+ and intracellular Na^+, Ca^{2+}, and Cl^-	Increased extracellular K^+ and intracellular Na^+, Ca^{2+}, and Cl^-
Excessive release of excitatory amino acids (primarily glutamate)	Excessive release of excitatory amino acids (glutamate and aspartate)
Accumulation of platelet-derived 5-HT in CNS	Excessive firing of dorsal raphe leads to increased 5-HT release and depletion of available 5-HT pool
Increased levels of endogenous opioids (findings mixed)	Beta-endorphin content may be reduced in headache-free periods; high MET-endorphin levels during attacks
Decline in intracellular and total brain Mg	Deficiency of Mg levels between and during attacks
Influx of extracellular Ca^{2+} in compromised axolemmas	Increase in intracellular ratio Ca^{2+}/Mg^{2+} ratio
Nitric oxide may be converted to free oxygen radical, potentially leading to tissue injury	Nitric oxide may be involved in migraine pathogenesis; at the vascular endothelium, it is a potent vasodilator; in the spinal cord, it is pronociceptive

A series of neurochemical changes occur in HI (Table 15.5). In animal models these changes include increases in extracellular potassium, excitatory amino acids, and acetylcholine. The applicability of these findings to human HI and the role of such changes in the evolution of PTS are unknown. However, an altered chemical or electrical environment could account for immediate impact headache or aura. It could result in cellular injury and in PTS. The similarity between the biochemical changes of migraine headaches and those that are seen after HI suggests a shared physiology and possibly a role for similar treatment strategies.

The effectiveness of treatments such as repetitive intravenous dihydroergotamine in PTH suggests a similar or shared mechanism with the primary headache disorders. This could be due to a "final common pathway" of symptom expression, perhaps with central serotonergic dysfunction and trigeminovascular activation.[75,76]

Many authors uphold the "psychogenesis" of chronic PTH and PTS, but few point out specific mechanisms to account for it. Duckro et al.[77] used a "path analysis"—a directional multiple-regression analysis—to examine the relationship between posttraumatic pain, disability, depression, and anger. They concluded that depression might cause disability, and that expressed and unexpressed anger contribute to depression. However, this statistical technique cannot prove a causal relationship, and other explanations for the correlation between depression and disability could be equally valid.

Kelly posits that nonvalidation of real cognitive and physically painful symptoms by medical, legal, and employment authorities leads to an anxiety or depressive reaction that results in the persistence of originally organic symptoms. He relies on the now outdated concept that emotional tension is a principal cause of persistent headache.[15] Recent position emission tomography (PET) studies have shown a neurobiologic basis for many so-called psychological phenomena. Anxiety, pain, and even hallucinations can be imaged, which demonstrates that they all have a neural substrate. Perhaps the term *psychogenic* should refer to symptoms that are generated from ongoing neuronal activity in the associative cortex.

TESTING

Many studies have been performed in an attempt to establish the extent of the HI and the diagnosis of PTS. Unfortunately, no test has demonstrated enough sensitivity or specificity to reliably distinguish patients with PTS from normal controls or from patients with primary headache disorders.

Computed Tomography and Magnetic Resonance Imaging

Few studies have specifically evaluated brain imaging in PTS. Most series are published by radiologists and evaluate patients with HI who might require neurosurgical intervention. Kelly et al. specifically looked at a group of HI patients and found no MRI abnormalities among a subgroup of patients with PTS.[2,78] On the other hand, Levin et al. found MRI abnormalities within several weeks of injury[79] in 17 of 20 hospitalized patients with mild or moderate HI. MRI was clearly superior to computed tomography (CT) in identifying such abnormalities, which were located in the white matter or at the gray matter–white matter junction. Levin et al. went on to show a reduction, with time, in the mean parenchymal lesion size in patients admitted with mild-to-moderate HI. Most of the reductions occurred within the first month, and many had resolved by 1 month. Lesions that were present at 1 month remained at 3 months. Patients with HI who had abnormal MRIs had more cognitive deficits than did patients with HI and normal MRIs.[79,80] Although no radiologic or pathologic correlations were conducted, these lesions could represent DAI with resolving edema. It is possible that with less severe DAI the MRI changes resolve with the resolution of edema, whereas with more severe DAI the changes are permanent.

Mittl obtained MRIs on 20 consecutively hospitalized HI patients, which were then reviewed for DAI by two blinded readers. Both readers concurred that there was DAI in 30% of the patients. Only one radiologist diagnosed DAI in just 20% of the patients, indicating that even MRIs may not always provide an unequivocal diagnosis.[81] These MRI findings may not be characteristic of HI patients who were not hospitalized. Nevertheless, DAI of less severity (not producing MRI abnormalities) could still be present.

There are no prospective studies establishing the value of brain imaging in patients with PTH or PTS. In the acute setting it is prudent to image all patients with mild behavioral abnormalities or equivocal findings on examination or a Glasgow coma scale of less than 15 because of the risk of subsequent deterioration. In cases of subacute or chronic PTS, there is little information to guide the clinician. If neuroimaging was not done following the injury, it is prudent to obtain a brain CT or MRI to exclude chronic subdural hematoma, hydrocephalus, or a structural lesion unrelated to the trauma. If neck pain is prominent and persistent, a cervical MRI may be indicated, but in the absence of an abnormal neurologic examination or severe radicular symptoms, an abnormal result usually does not change therapy. In the acute setting, fracture or dislocation of the cervical spine is a concern that calls for cervical spine films.

Functional Imaging

Single-photon emission computed tomography (SPECT) observes the physiologic behavior of the brain. It can contribute information about the spatial distribution of radiolabeled ligands and the time course of ligand uptake and washout. It is analyzed by CT analysis to produce two-dimensional and three-dimensional images. SPECT has been used to study HI patients but has not been used specifically in PTH or PTS. In the acute phase of HI, SPECT, using technetium Tc 99m hexamethyl propyleneamine oxime (Tc-HMPAO), shows more lesions than CT and is helpful in predicting outcome.[82–84] Tc-HMPAO measures perfusion, so that abnormalities of hypoperfusion or hyperperfusion can be identified. In 20 patients with HI, Tc-HMPAO SPECT showed abnormalities in 60%, whereas only 25% had abnormalities on CT.[85] In 12 patients with mild-to-moderate HI tested 1–9 years after injury, Tc-HMPAO SPECT was abnormal in 10 and CT was abnormal in six patients.[86] The number of lesions correlates with the extent of disability.[87] Masdeu et al. suggest that two types of lesions may be seen on SPECT: circumscribed areas of hypoperfusion, representing contusion, and diffuse occipitotemporal hypoperfusion, representing multiple small contusions or DAI.[88] The Academy of Neurology's Therapeutics and Technology Assessment Subcommittee has determined the use of SPECT for the evaluation of head trauma to be "investigational" based on Class II evidence (one or more well-designed clinical studies).[89]

Using xenon-inhalation SPECT, one study showed a correlation between headache disability and cerebral blood flow using the mean asymmetry score. Both the emotional subscale score and the function subscale score of the headache disability inventory correlated with the mean asymmetry score.[90] This is the first test to show a physiologic abnormality in PTH.

Like SPECT, PET examines physiologic activity within the brain. It permits noninvasive measurement of the regional distribution of tracer and is analyzed by CT methods. In head trauma, PET has revealed widespread abnormalities in cerebral glucose metabolism.[91,92] In HI, it may demonstrate areas of diminished perfusion that tend to improve with clinical recovery.[91] In one study, these areas of perfusion abnormality corresponded to areas of abnormality identified by neuropsychological testing.[93] PET is limited by its expense and substantial technologic requirements (an on-site cyclotron is necessary).

Electroencephalography

The EEG is usually of little value in evaluating PTS with HI. Although it may be abnormal immediately after injury, it often normalizes within minutes to weeks. Persistent findings that were once considered abnormal are now considered normal variants that occur with the same frequency as in the general population.[94]

Quantitative EEG may be of use in HI, but its value is still uncertain. In one small study, quantitative EEG showed a statistically significant increase in both slow and fast activity over the temporal region of the skull. However, the author concluded that this test offers little benefit to the patient with PTH, because there is so much variability within the PTH group and because these findings are so common in both PTH and control patients.[95] Another study examined the ability of power spectra analysis to discriminate between 608 HI patients and 108 age-matched controls, and found that HI patients could be discriminated from age-matched controls with greater than 90% accuracy.[96] No correlation was made between the symptoms of PTH or PTS and abnormal test results. It is uncertain what the positive and negative predictive values of the study are. In general, these studies tell us that PTH patients, as a group, differ from nonheadache controls, but the studies cannot reliably differentiate an individual PTH patient from an idiopathic headache, nonheadache, or asymptomatic MHI control.

Evoked Potentials and Electronystagmography

Short-latency somatosensory evoked potentials have not been shown to be of value in HI or PTS.[97] On the other hand, brain stem auditory evoked potentials (BAEPs) have been found to be abnormal in 10–20% of patients with HI and postconcussion syndrome. The more prolonged the unconsciousness, the greater the incidence of abnormalities.[94] The BAEP can either improve or deteriorate from 2 days to 1 month after injury.[98] Symptomatic dizziness does not correlate with BAEP abnormalities. Although the BAEP separates groups of PTS patients from groups of controls, it is of no value in distinguishing an individual with PTS from one without PTS.

The P300 is an event-related potential manifested by a positive cortical potential that occurs after an infrequent stimulation to which the patient is attending, such as a loud sound in a train of soft sounds. It has been correlated with cognitive functions such as memory information delivery and decision making, and it decreases in amplitude with drowsiness or inattention. Studies of P300 in HI have yielded mixed results. One study demonstrated significant abnormalities of P300 amplitude and latency in 20 HI patients compared with 20 control subjects.[99] Another study[100] found that only one of 18 patients had an abnormal response. More recently, Kobylare and colleagues found a correlation between an abnormal P300 and an abnormal MRI.[101] The usefulness of the results of such testing is still uncertain in HI patients.

The electronystagmogram (ENG) is abnormal in 40–50% of patients with HI or "whiplash" in clinic-based studies. Toglia[102] examined 150 patients who complained of vestibular symptoms following either HI or whiplash injury. Spontaneous, latent, and positional nystagmus were searched for. Bithermal caloric tests and rotational tests were performed when possible. Abnormal caloric tests (including both canal paresis and directional preponderance) were found in 63% of whiplash patients and 68% of HI patients. Abnormal rotatory tests were found in 9 of 16 whiplash patients (56%) and 20 of 24 HI patients (83%). Rowe[103] studied 19 patients with postconcussive dizziness following HI and found that 11 patients (58%) had abnormalities of latent or positional nystagmus or of caloric-induced nystagmus. None of Rowe's patients with abnormal BAEP (three standard deviations) had normal ENG results. Conversely, most patients with abnormal ENG results had normal BAEPs. This suggests that the ENG may be more sensitive than the BAEP.

Brain Stem Inhibiting Reflex

Exteroceptive suppression (ES) is the inhibition of voluntary EMG activity of the temporalis muscle induced by trigeminal nerve stimulation. There are two successive suppressions, ES1 and ES2. The ES1 is thought to be an oligosynaptic brain stem response, whereas the ES2 is a polysynaptic response subject to limbic and other modulation. The duration of ES2 is reduced in dystonia, Parkinson's disease, and CTTH.[104,105] Keidel et al.[106] investigated the brain stem inhibiting reflex of temporal muscle contraction in patients with PTH and neck pain after whiplash injuries, and compared these results with age- and sex-matched controls. The ES2 was shortened in the PTH patients, whereas the ES1 and the interspersed EMG activity were slightly but significantly prolonged. These abnormalities resolved within 6 months. This test demonstrated reversible functional brain stem impairment in patients with whiplash, but it has not yet been shown to be of clinical value in PTH or PTS.

Neuropsychological Testing

Neuropsychological testing in HI often shows marked early abnormalities that improve or resolve with time. These involve information processing, auditory vigilance, reaction time, sustained divided and distributed attention, visual and verbal memory, design fluency imagination, and analytic capacity. Eisenberg reported that tests of design fluency and verbal memory showed improvement and normalization over 1–3 months, in parallel with MRI findings.[107] The paced auditory serial addition test is a widely used test of information processing that is often abnormal shortly after HI. Patients are presented with a random series of digits at intervals of either 1–2 or 2–4 seconds (same interval for entire test), and are asked to add the most recently presented number to the one before. The score is expressed as the percentage correct at each rate or as the mean correct response per second. It has been given serially over 8 weeks postinjury and demonstrates cognitive recovery to normal. Paced auditory serial addition test recovery, however, was delayed in HI patients with PTS compared with a non-PTS control group.[29]

Within 8 weeks of HI, one test of auditory vigilance (patients had to detect the rare instances in which the interval between elements in a string of numbers was longer than in the other instances) showed normalization.[108] However, "recovered" HI patients performed more poorly than normal controls at simulated high altitude,[109] demonstrating that deficits may reappear under physiologic stress. Several measures of reaction time, which are believed to be indicators of attention deficits, also reveal impairment in patients with HI at various times after injury, although recovery was demonstrated in one study of MHI patients 10 years after injury compared with twin controls.[110] In a test of selective attention devised by Gentilini et al.,[111] HI patients were significantly slower but not less accurate than controls 3 months after injury. Tests of sustained and divided attention, again devised by Gentilini et al.,[111] showed significant differences from controls at 1 month, but were inconclusive 3 months after injury. However, Bohnen demonstrated that patients with MHI and PTS performed less well than MHI (without PTS) controls on a test of sustained attention 12–34 months after injury.[112] The tests of distributed attention by Gentilini et al. showed deficits 1 and 3 months after HI.[111] They point out that the most sensitive tests for revealing cerebral dysfunction are those that test the function of the greatest number of cortical and subcortical areas simultaneously.[111] Only one study (Bohnen's), however, has been shown to distinguish PTH or PTS from MHI alone.[112]

Keidel performed repeated neuropsychological tests on 30 patients with PTS after whiplash injury. Patients with deficits in attention and concentration recovered within 6 weeks. Visual memory, imagination, and analytic capacity were recovered within the next 6 weeks. Verbal memory abstraction, cognitive selectivity, and information processing speed took more than 12 weeks to recover.[113] These findings demonstrate a hierarchy of functional recovery occurring over a period of greater than 12 weeks after apparently mild injury.

Ham et al. studied patients with PTH and compared them with patients with chronic "combination headache," low-back pain patients, and pain-free controls.[114] PTH patients had the highest scale elevations on the Symptom Checklist 90–Revised, a brief screen for somatic and psychological symptoms, which are broken down into nine primary "dimensions" or scales. Elevations were significant in all scales except on the hostility and phobic anxiety scales. PTH patients scored significantly higher than pain-free controls in the Beck depression inventory, but did not differ significantly from other pain groups. State anxiety, a measure of acute anxiety, was significantly higher in PTH than in controls and in other pain states, but trait anxiety, a measure of anxious personality structure, differed significantly only from controls. Mean headache severity was higher (but not significantly so) in the PTH group than in the control headache group. These findings suggest that PTH patients exhibit more psychopathology than normal controls or individuals with other headache types. On some tests, patients with PTH showed more psychopathology than patients with low-back pain, but not on others. In general, these tests do not demonstrate any specific pattern to the psychopathology.[114]

DIAGNOSIS

The diagnosis of PTH and PTS is established by the presence of symptoms consistent with the syndrome and onset related to trauma. The IHS criteria for PTH requires the headache to occur within 14 days after consciousness is regained (or after the trauma if there is no loss of consciousness). There are no IHS criteria for late-onset PTH. The IHS differentiates between acute PTH, lasting less than 8 weeks, and chronic PTH, which lasts longer (see Table 15.3). A worsening of a preexisting headache disorder does not qualify as PTH. A substantial difference between headache features before and after injury must be present for the designation of PTH.

Other physiologic or psychological disorders must be meticulously excluded. The differential diagnoses include subdural or epidural hematoma, CSF hypotension, cerebral vein thrombosis, cavernous sinus thrombosis, cervical or carotid artery dissection, cerebral hemorrhage, epilepsy, and hydrocephalus.

Many patients diagnosed with PTS are portrayed as malingerers or are thought to profoundly embellish their symptoms; however, most experts believe such behavior is rare. Binder suggests that the diagnosis of malingering should be made actively by surreptitious observation of the patient performing a task he or she has stated he or she cannot accomplish.[19] Alternatively, simulators have been shown to perform worse on sensorimotor tests[115] and memory tests[116] than would be expected. Performance that is significantly worse than chance on a forced-choice memory test can be interpreted as the deliberate production of wrong answers. Binder notes that such a result may not distinguish between malingering and conversion reactions.[117] If one is suspected of "faking bad," the clinician should actively search for other clues such as antisocial or borderline personality, poor work record, prior claims for injury, random test performance, and excessive endorsement of symptoms, indicating that the patient may be malingering.[118]

TREATMENT

Patients with PTS are often distressed and misunderstood and require support and an objective, comprehensive approach to treatment. Treating them inappropriately may create pathologic resentment and disability that is refractory. The comprehensive approach to treatment uses medications, physical modalities, and biofeedback or counseling. Medina[119] found that 85% of patients had returned to work after being treated aggressively in individualized programs including medication, biofeedback, stress management, exercise, and neuromuscular relaxation.

In the absence of any known remediable mechanism, treatment should be directed at the identifiable components of PTS. The headache should be treated based on its similarity to IHS headache disorders. Cervical and soft-tissue injury should be identified and treated. Anxiety and depression should be meticulously identified and addressed. Cognitive dysfunction should also be addressed.

Few studies have evaluated specific drug treatments for PTH, and few have looked at which headache type responds to which drugs. Most have involved the use of the antidepressant amitriptyline. In an uncontrolled study, Tyler et al.[120] found amitriptyline effective in 90% of PTH patients, but did not distinguish between the various headache patterns of PTH. The average daily dose of amitriptyline varied from 75 mg to 250 mg. Saran[121] tried amitriptyline in two groups of psychiatrically hospitalized patients with depression, one with PTH and the other with idiopathic headaches. Outcome was based on average daily headache intensity calculated from a headache calendar. Amitriptyline, at an average dose of 175 mg per day, was effective for the uninjured patients but not for the PTS patients. This study is likely to have selected a particularly intractable subgroup of PTS patients and may not apply to the group as a whole. Other tricyclic antidepressants that may be effective in PTH are imipramine, doxepin, and nortriptyline. Based on anecdotal evidence, selective serotonin-reuptake inhibitors may be just as effective in treating PTH as the tricyclic antidepressants (authors' observation), and they have fewer side effects, which can result in better compliance.

Abortive medications are widely used in PTS. One must be on the lookout for analgesic and ergotamine overuse. Sumatriptan is effective for the migrainous exacerbation of PTH, but not for the baseline headache.[122] Repetitive intravenous dihydroergotamine is effective for PTH that meets the criteria for chronic daily headache,[75,76] and according to one study it appears to improve cognitive function.[76] Intravenous chlorpromazine has been effective in acute PTH.[123] In patients with daily or near daily headache, preventive medications should be used preferentially and the use of abortive medications limited.

In the presence of true epilepsy, anticonvulsant therapy is indicated. Divalproex sodium is our drug of first choice if the patient has PTH and a seizure disorder. The many other spells seen in the PTS population, unfortunately, rarely respond to anticonvulsant treatment.

Biofeedback and psychotherapy or behavior modification may be helpful for many patients. Biofeedback, in combination with medication, enables the patient to recognize muscle tension and bring it under voluntary control. A recent study[124] found that 53% of patients were able to moderately increase their ability to relax and cope with pain by using biofeedback, and 68% believed it was at least moderately helpful.

Physical modalities such as physical therapy and exercise, chiropractic treatment, and massage have been beneficial for some patients, particularly when headache is related to or occurs in association with cervical trauma. Cervical orthoses, cold, electrotherapy, and heat have been used successfully, particularly in the acute stage, to improve functioning. In one open study, manual therapy was more successful than cold packs in relieving chronic PTS.[125] After the initial, acute phase, exercise programs are important to prevent deconditioning resulting from a decrease in the overall level of functioning.

Behavior modification or cognitive therapy is often helpful in providing support and education and improving the patient's ability to cope. For patients with more severe psychopathology, long-term psychotherapy may be needed. Medication may be valuable in the treatment of anxiety and depression.

Cognitive retraining exercises, counseling, adaptive strategy programs, and vocational rehabilitation are useful treatments for neurocognitive dysfunction. Alexander[126] suggests that programs that purport to treat attention and memory problems are of uncertain value in HI in general and are inappropriate for MHI. Levin has demonstrated greater improvement in neuropsychological function in MHI patients treated with cytidine-5'-diphosphate-choline for the month after injury than placebo-treated controls.[127] The role for this treatment in the long-term management of PCS is uncertain.

OUTCOME

Prognostic studies have used various definitions of HI, different study designs, and varying subject characteristics. Results have varied, so that it is difficult to accurately ascertain the prognosis of patients presenting at various stages of PTS. At 1 month after MHI, 31%[128] to 90%[129] of patients had headache. At 2–3 months postinjury, 32%[130] to 78%[9] of patients had headache. One year after injury, the range was 8%[131] to 35%.[110] Two to 4 years after injury, three studies show that between 20% and 24% of patients have persistent headache. Dizziness, memory problems, and irritability are less likely to be noted within the first few months of injury but are more likely to persist.[132]

Approximately one-third of patients are unable to return to work after HI.[131] In one study, 34% of previously employed patients admitted to a hospital had not returned to work 3 months after injury. Older patients with higher levels of education and employment, greater income, and higher socioeconomic status were more likely to return to work.[9]

SYNTHESIS AND CONCLUSION

It is likely that there are at least two simultaneous processes occurring in the patient who presents with PTH or PTS. The first process is likely due to DAI and correlates with the acceleration and deceleration forces involved in the injury. When more severe, DAI is associated with abnormalities on MRI, PET, SPECT, and certain neuropsychological tests. Clinical improvement may occur over several months, along with normalization or improvement on these tests. There may also be residual deficits that are not identified on routine neuropsychological testing (intelligence, etc.), but may be detected more easily with tests that evaluate attention.

There appears to be a second process, separate from DAI, that is responsible for the persistent headache, much of the psychopathology, and some of the neurocognitive deficits that occur after HI. This second process is often heralded by more severe early headache. A preexisting factor or vulnerability may be a necessary precondition for this process to manifest fully in a given individual. A mechanism similar to the kindling model of epilepsy, or, perhaps, aberrant connections made by injured axons, may underlie this second mechanism and explain most of the symptoms of chronic PTS and PTH. Additional factors, perhaps psychological, may be present (or be generated by the second process) and can potentiate the other mechanisms or magnify symptom expression. It is rare for headaches to occur solely due to psychological factors.

For most patients with PTS, the clinical history of new onset or changed headache after an injury with associated new cognitive, emotional, and sleep disturbances is so characteristic that, once intracranial pathology is excluded, confirmatory tests are not required in order to proceed with treatment. Unfortunately, tests are often conducted for medicolegal reasons; and such tests, when they are negative, can increase anxiety and self-doubt in the patient. Negative test results are often taken to indicate no abnormality. It is important to remember, however, that no test has the specificity and sensitivity to make or exclude a diagnosis in a particular individual. Similarly, if PTS is, as we have suggested, not a single entity but a syndrome derived from several pathologic processes initiated by head trauma, no single test would be expected to diagnose all cases.

PTH and PTS are common and, if chronic, frequently disabling conditions. There is no specific symptom cluster or reliable diagnostic test to unequivocally establish a diagnosis. The diagnosis is thus most reliably made by establishing the onset of symptoms soon after injury. The absence of a generally accepted mechanism for the genesis of chronic symptoms has led to an unfortunate skepticism about the validity of those symptoms and in turn hindered the development of more effective treatments. The search for better treatment should continue; if new treatments can be based on interference with a putative mechanism of symptom genesis (e.g., windup, kindling, aberrant reinnervation, neurochemical cascade), they may provide insight into the causes of PTS. Relying on a so-called psychogenesis as an explanation of the syndrome reinforces a cultural pattern that is singularly harmful to individuals who have already been injured.

REFERENCES

1. Jennett B, Frankowski RF. The Epidemiology of Head Injury. In R Braakman (ed), Handbook of Clinical Neurology (Vol. 13). New York: Elsevier, 1990;1.
2. Kraus JF, McArthur DL, Silberman TA. Epidemiology of mild brain injury. Semin Neurol 1994;14:1.
3. Evans RW. The postconcussion syndrome and the sequelae of mild head injury. Neurol Clin 1992;10:815.
4. Raskin NH. Posttraumatic Headache: The Postconcussion Syndrome. In NH Rashkin (ed), Headache. New York: Churchill Livingstone, 1988.
5. Brenner C, Friedman AP, Merritt HH, et al. Posttraumatic headache. J Neurosurg 1944;1:379.
6. Elkind AH. Posttraumatic Headache. In S Diamond, DJ Dalessio (eds), The Practicing Physician's Approach to Headache (5th ed). Baltimore: Williams & Wilkins 1992;146.
7. Speed WG. Psychiatric Aspects of Posttraumatic Headaches. In C Adler, S Adler, R Packard (eds), Psychiatric Aspects of Headache. Baltimore: Williams & Wilkins, 1987;210.
8. Gfeller JD, Chibnall JT, Duckro PN. Postconcussion symptoms and cognitive functioning in posttraumatic headache patients. Headache 1994;34:503.
9. Rimel RW, Giordani B, Barth JT, Boll TJ, et al. Disability caused by minor head injury. Neurosurgery 1981;9:221.
10. Balla J, Iansek R. Headaches Arising from Disorders of the Cervical Spine. In A Hopkins (ed), Headache: Problems in Diagnosis and Management. London: Saunders, 1988;241.
11. O'Neill B, Haddon W, Kelley AB, et al. Automobile head restraints: Frequency of neck claims in relation to the presence of head restraints. Am J Public Health 1972;62:403.
12. Foreman S, Croft A. Whiplash injuries: The Cervical Acceleration/Deceleration Syndrome (2nd ed). Baltimore: Williams & Wilkins, 1995.
13. Cartlidge NEF, Shaw DA. Epidemiology of Whiplash. In Head Injury. London: Saunders, 1981.
14. Mandel S. Minor head injury may not be "minor." Postgrad Med 1989;85:213.
15. Kelly R. Headache after Cranial Trauma. In A Hopkins (ed), Headache: Problems in Diagnosis and Management. London: Saunders, 1988;219.
16. DeBenedittis G, DeSantis A. Chronic posttraumatic headache: Clinical, psychopathologic features and outcome determinants. J Neurosurg Sci 1983;27:177.
17. Haas DC, Lourie T. Trauma-triggered migraine: An explanation for common neurologic attacks after mild head injury. J Neurosurg 1988;68:181.
18. Weiss HD, Stern BJ, Goldbert J. Posttraumatic migraine: Chronic migraine precipitated by minor head or neck trauma. Headache 1991;31:451.
19. Binder LM. Persisting symptoms after mild head injury: A review of the postconcussive syndrome. J Clin Exp Neuropsychol 1986;8:323.
20. Winston KR. Whiplash and its relationship to migraine. Headache 1987;27:452.
21. Saper JR. Headache Disorders: Current Concepts and Treatment Strategies. Boston: John Wright, 1983.
22. Duckro PN, Greenberg M, Schultz KT, et al. Clinical features of chronic posttraumatic headache. Headache Quarterly 1992;3:295.
23. Packard RC, Ham LP. Incidence of cluster-like posttraumatic headache: An inconsistency. Headache Quarterly 1996;7:139.
24. Haas DC. Classification of chronic posttraumatic headache. Cephalalgia 1995;15:162.
25. Silberstein S, Marcelis J. Pseudotumor cerebri without papilledema. Headache 1990;30:304.
26. Vijayan N. A new posttraumatic headache syndrome. Headache 1977;17:19.
27. Montalbetti L, Ferrandi D, Pergami P, Savoldi F. Elongated styloid process and Eagle's syndrome. Cephalalgia 1995;15:80.

28. Wong E, Lee G, Mason DT. Temporal headaches and associated symptoms relating to the styloid process and its attachments. Ann Acad Med Singapore 1995;24:124.
29. Gronwall D, Wrightson P. Delayed recovery of intellectual function after minor head injury. Lancet 1974;2:605.
30. Andrasik F, Wincze JP. Emotional and psychologic aspects of mild head injury. Semin Neurol 1994;14:60.
31. Segalowitz SJ, Lawson S. Subtle symptoms associated with self-reported mild head injury. J Learn Disabil 1995;28:309.
32. Hickling EJ, Blanchard EB, Silverman DJ, Schwarz SP. Motor vehicle accidents, headaches, and posttraumatic stress disorder: Assessment findings in a consecutive series. Headache 1992;32:147.
33. Sbordone RJ, Liter JC. Mild traumatic brain injury does not produce posttraumatic stress disorder. Brain Injury 1995;9:405.
34. Jensen OK, Nielsen FF. The influence of sex and pretraumatic headache on the incidence and severity of headache after head injury. Cephalalgia 1990;10:285.
35. Lidvall HF, Linderoth B, Norlin B. Causes of the postconcussional syndrome. Acta Neurol Scand 1974;50:1.
36. Prigatano GP, Stahl ML, Orr WC, et al. Sleep and dreaming disturbances in closed head injury patients. J Neurol Neurosurg Psychiatry 1982;45:78.
37. Silberstein SD, Lipton RB, Saper JR, Solomon S, et al. Headache and facial pain: Part A. Continuum 1995;1:8.
38. Lankford DA, Wellman JJ, O'Hara C. Posttraumatic narcolepsy in mild to moderate closed head injury. Sleep 1994;17:25.
39. Lake AE, Branca B, Lutz T, Hamel R, et al. Comorbid symptoms in chronic posttraumatic headache. I: Comparison to intractable migraine. II: Relationship to severity of injury and litigation [Abstract]. Headache 1995;35:302.
40. Packard RC, Ham LP. Posttraumatic headache: Determining chronicity. Headache 1993;33:133.
41. Mendelson G. Not "cured by a verdict." Med J Aust 1982;2:132.
42. Packard RC. Posttraumatic headache. Permanency and relationship to legal settlement. Headache 1992;32:496.
43. Davies RA, Luxon LM. Dizziness following head injury: A neurootologic study. J Neurol 1995;242:222.
44. Miller H. Accident neurosis: Lecture I. BMJ 1961;1:918.
45. Miller H. Accident neurosis: Lecture II. BMJ 1961;1:992.
46. Mittenberg W, DiGiulio D, Perrin S, Bass A. Symptoms following mild head injury: Expectation as etiology. J Neurol Neurosurg Psych 1992;55:200.
47. Strauss I, Savitsky N. Head injury. Arch Neurol Psychiatry 1934;31:893.
48. Rutherford WH, Merrett JD, McDonald JR. Sequelae of concussion caused by minor head injuries. Lancet 1977;1:1.
49. Bohnen N, Twijnstra A, Jolles J. Posttraumatic and emotional symptoms in different subgroups of patients with mild head injury. Brain Injury 1992;6:481.
50. McClelland RJ, Fenton GW, Rutherford W. The postconcussional syndrome revisited. J R Soc Med 1994;87:508.
51. Keshavan MS, Channabasavanna SM, Reddy GNN. Posttraumatic psychiatric disturbances: Patterns and predictors of outcome. Br J Psychiatry 1981;131:157.
52. Yamaguchi M. Incidence of headache and severity of head injury. Headache 1992;32:422.
53. Barrett K, Ward AB, Boughey A, Jones M, et al. Sequelae of minor head injury: The natural consciousness and follow-up. J Accid Emerg Med 1994;11:79.
54. Wilkinson M, Gilchrist E. Posttraumatic headache. Ups J Med Sci 1980;31:48.
55. Rutherford WH. Postconcussion Symptoms. In HS Levin, HM Eisenberg, AZ Beriton (eds), Mild Head Injury. New York: Oxford University Press, 1989;217.
56. Radanov BP, Sturzenegger M, DiStefano G. Long-term outcome after whiplash injury: A 2-year follow-up considering features of injury mechanism and somatic, radiologic, and psychosocial findings. Medicine 1995;74:281.
57. Weiss HD, Stern BJ, Goldberg J. Post-traumatic migraine: Chronic migraine precipitated by minor head or neck trauma. Headache 1991;31:451.
58. Ross WD, McNaughton FL. Head injury: A study of patients with chronic posttraumatic complaints. Arch Neurol Psychiatry 1944;52:255.
59. Post RM, Silberstein SD. Shared mechanisms in affective illness, epilepsy, and migraine. Neurology 1994;44:37.
60. Gennarelli TA. Mechanisms of brain injury. J. Emerg Med 1993;1:5.

61. Blumbergs PC, Jones NR, North JB. Diffuse axonal injury in head trauma. J Neurol Neurosurg Psychiatry 1989;52:838.
62. Gennarelli TA, Thibault LE, Adams JH, Graham DI, et al. Diffuse Axonal Injury and Traumatic Coma in the Primate. In RG Dacey, et al. (eds), Trauma of the Central Nervous System. New York: Raven, 1985;169.
63. Blumbergs PC, Scott G, Manavis J, Wainwright H, et al. Staining of amyloid precursor protein to study axonal damage in mild head injury. Lancet 1994;344:1055.
64. Elson LM, Ward CC. Mechanisms and pathophysiology of mild head injury. Semin Neurol 1994;14:8.
65. Servadei P, Vergoni G, Pasini A, Fagioli L, et al. Diffuse axonal injury with brainstem localization: Report of a case in a mild head injured patient. J Neurosurg Sci 1994;38:129.
66. Goodman JC. Pathologic changes in mild head injury. Semin Neurol 1994;14:19.
67. Weiller C, May A, Limmroth V, et al. Brainstem activation in spontaneous human migraine attacks. Nature Med 1995;1:658.
68. Erb DE, Povlishock JT. Neuroplasticity following traumatic brain injury: A study of GABAergic terminal loss and recovery in the cat dorsal lateral vestibular nucleus. Exp Brain Res 1991;83:253.
69. Jane JA, Steward O, Gennarelli TA. Axonal degeneration induced by experimental noninvasive minor head injury. J. Neurosurg 1985;62;96.
70. Povlishock JT, Coburn TH. Morphopathologic Change Associated with Mild Head Injury. In HS Levin, HM Eisenberg, AL Benton (eds), Mild Head Injury. New York: Oxford University Press, 1989.
71. Gennarelli TA, Thibault LE, Adams JH, Graham DI, et al. Diffuse axonal injury and traumatic coma in the primate. Ann Neurol 1975;12:564.
72. Schmidt RH, Grady MS. Loss of forebrain cholinergic neurons following fluid-percussion injury: Implications for cognitive impairment in closed head injury. J Neurosurg 1995;83:496.
73. Ward CC, Nahum AM. Correlation Between Brain Injury and Intracranial Pressures in Experimental Head Impacts. Proceedings of the 4th International Conference on the Biomechanics of Trauma, Gotebog, Sweden, 1979;133.
74. Ward CC. Finite Element Modeling of the Head and Neck. In R Ewing, et al. (eds), Impact Injury of the Head and Spine. Springfield, IL: Thomas, 1982;421.
75. McBeath JG, Nanda A. Use of dihydroergotamine in patients with postconcussion syndrome. Headache 1994;34:148.
76. Young WB, Hopkins MM, Janyszek B, Primavera JP. Repetitive intravenous DHE in the treatment of refractory posttraumatic headache [abstract]. Headache 1994;34:297.
77. Duckro PN, Chibnall JT, Tomazic TJ. Anger, depression, and disability: A path analysis of relationships in a sample of chronic posttraumatic headache patients. Headache 1995;35:7.
78. Kelly AB, Zimmerman RD, Gandy SE, Deck MD. Comparison of magnetic resonance imaging and computed tomography in the evaluation of head injury. Neurosurgery 1986;18:45.
79. Levin HS, Amparo E, Eisenberg HM, et al. Magnetic resonance imaging and computerized tomography in relation to the neurobehavioral sequelae of mild and moderate head injuries. J Neurosurg 1987;66:706.
80. Levin HS, Williams DH, Eisenberg HM, et al. Serial MRI and neurobehavioral findings after mild to moderate head injuries. J Neurol Neurosurg Psychiatry 1992;55:255.
81. Mittl RL, Grossman RI, Hiehl JF, Hurst RW, et al. Prevalence of MR evidence of diffuse axonal injury in patients with mild head injury and normal head CT findings. Am J Neuroradiol 1994;15:1583.
82. Abdel-Dayem HM, Sadek SA, Kouris K, et al. Changes in cerebral perfusion after acute head injury: Comparison of CT with Tc-99m-PAO SPECT. Radiology 1987;165:221.
83. Reid RH, Gulenchyn K, Ballinger JR, et al. Cerebral perfusion imaging with Tc-HM-PAO following cerebral trauma. Clin Nucl Med 1990;15:383.
84. Abdel-Dayem H, Masdeu J, O'Connell R, et al. Brain perfusion abnormalities following minor/moderate closed head injury: Comparison between early and late imaging in two groups of patients. Eur J Nucl Med 1994;21:750.
85. Gray BG, Ichise M, Chung D, et al. Technetium-99m-HMPAO SPECT in the evaluation of patients with a remote history of traumatic brain injury: A comparison with X-ray computed tomography. J Nucl Med 1992;33:52.
86. Krelina M, Reid R, Ballinger J. Regional cerebral blood flow in patients with remote close-head injuries [abstract]. Can J Neurol Sci 1989;2:279.
87. Newton MR, Greenwood RJ, Britton KF, et al. A study comparing SPECT with CT and MRI after closed head injury. J Neurol Neurosurg Psychiatry 1992;55:92.

88. Masdeu JC, Abdel-Dayhem H, VanHeertum RL. Head trauma: Use of SPECT. J Neuroimaging 1995;5:53.
89. Report of the Therapeutics and Technology Assessment Subcommittee of the American Academy of Neurology. Assessment of brain SPECT. Neurology 1996;46:278.
90. Ramadan NM, Norris LL, Shultz LR. Abnormal cerebral flood flow correlates with disability due to chronic posttraumatic headache [abstract]. J Neuroimaging 1995;5:68.
91. Alavi A, Fazekas T, Alves W, et al. Positron emission tomography in the evaluation of head injury. J Cereb Blood Flow Metab 1987;7:646.
92. George JK, Alavi A, Zimmerman RA, et al. Metabolic (PET) correlates of anatomic lesions (CT/MRI) produced by head trauma [abstract]. J Nucl Med 1989;30:802.
93. Rao N, Turski PA, Polcyn RE, et al. [18]F Positron emission computed tomography in closed head injury. Arch Phys Med Rehab 1984;65:780.
94. Schoenhuber R, Gentilini M. Neurophysiologic Assessment of Mild Head Injury. In HS Levin, HM Eisenberg, AL Benton (eds), Mild Head Injury. New York: Oxford University Press, 1989;142.
95. Hughes JR, Robbins LD. Brain mapping in migraine. Clin Electroencephalog 1990;21:14.
96. Thatcher RW, Walker RA, Gerson I, et al. EEG discriminant analyses of mild head trauma. Electroencephalogr Clin Neurophysiol 1989;73:94.
97. Bricolo AP, Turella GS. Electrophysiology of Head Injury. In R Braakman (ed), Handbook of Clinical Neurology (Vol. 13): Head Injury. New York: Elsevier 1990;181.
98. Geets W, Louette N. EEG et potentials évoqués du tronc cérébral dans 125 commotions récentes. Rev Electroencephalogr Neurophysiol Clin 1983;13:253.
99. Pratap-Chand R, Sinniah M, Salem FA. Cognitive evoked potential (P300): A metric for cerebral concussion. Acta Neurol Scand 1988;78:185.
100. Werner RA, Vanderzant CW. Multimodality evoked potential testing in acute mild closed head injury. Arch Phys Med Rehabil 1991;72:31.
101. Kobylare EJ, Dunford J, Jabbari B, Salazar A, et al. Auditory event-related potentials in head injury patients. Neurology 1995;45:358P.
102. Toglia JU. Dizziness After Whiplash Injury of the Neck and Closed Head Injury: Electronystagmographic Correlations. In AE Walker, WF Caveness, M Critchley (eds), The Late Effects of Head Injury. Springfield, IL: Thomas, 1969;72.
103. Rowe MJ, Carlson C. Brainstem auditory evoked potentials in postconcussion dizziness. Arch Neurol 1980;37:679.
104. Schoenen J, Jamart B, Geard P, Lenarduzzi P, et al. Exteroceptive suppression of temporalis muscle activity in chronic headache. Neurology 1987;37:1834.
105. Nakashima K, Takahashi K. Exteroceptive suppression of the masseter, temporalis, and trapezius muscles produced by mental nerve stimulation in patients with chronic headaches. Cephalalgia 1991;11:23.
106. Keidel M, Rieschke P, Juptner M, Diener HC. Pathologic jaw opening reflex after whiplash injury. Neurologische Universitatsklinik Essen, Nervenarzt 1994;65:241.
107. Eisenberg HM. CT and MRI Finding in Mild to Moderate Head Injury. In HS Levin, HM Eisenberg, AL Benton (eds), Mild Head Injury. New York: Oxford University Press, 1989;133.
108. McCarthy D. Memory and vigilance after concussion. Master's thesis, University of Auckland, 1977.
109. Ewing R, McCarthy D, Gronwall D, Wrightson P. Persisting effects of minor head injury observable during hypoxic stress. J Clin Neuropsychol 1980;2:147.
110. Dencker SJ, Lofving BA. A psychometric study of identical twins discordant for closed head injury. Acta Psychiatr Neurol Scand 1958;(Suppl):33.
111. Gentilini TM, Michelli P, Schoenhuber R. Assessment of Attention in Mild Head Injury. In HS Levin, HM Eisenberg, AL Benton (eds), Mild Head Injury. New York: Oxford University Press, 1989;163.
112. Bohnen NI, Jolles J, Twijnstra A, Mellink R, et al. Late neurobehavioural symptoms after mild head injury. Brain Injury 1995;9:27.
113. Keidel M, Yaguez L, Wilhelm H, Diener HC. Prospective follow-up of neuropsychologic deficits after cervicocephalic acceleration trauma. Neurologische Klinik and Poliklinik, Universitat Essen. Nervenarzt 1992;63:731.
114. Ham LP, Andrasik F, Packard RC, Bundrick CM. Psychopathology in individuals with posttraumatic headaches and other pain types. Cephalalgia 1994;14:118.
115. Heaton RK, Smith HH, Lehman RA, Vogt AJ. Prospects for faking believable deficits on neuropsychologic testing. J Consult Clin Psychol 1978;46:892.
116. Benton AL, Spreen O. Visual memory test: The simulation of mental incompetence. Arch Gen Psychiatry 1961;4:79.

117. Binder LM. Malingering following minor head trauma. Clin Neuropsychol 1990;4:25.
118. Ruff, MR, Willie T, Tennant W. Malingering and malingering-like aspects of mild closed head injury. J Head Trauma Rehab 1993;8:60.
119. Medina JL. Efficacy of an individualized outpatient program in the treatment of chronic posttraumatic headache. Headache 1992;32:180.
120. Tyler GS, McNeely HE, Dick ML. Treatment of posttraumatic headache with amitriptyline. Headache 1980;20:213.
121. Saran A. Antidepressants not effective in headache associated with minor closed head injury. Int J Psychiatry Med 1988;18:75.
122. Gawel MJ, Rothbart P, Jacobs H. Subcutaneous sumatriptan in the treatment of acute episodes of posttraumatic headache. Headache 1993;33:96.
123. Herd A, Ludwig L. Relief of posttraumatic headache by intravenous chlorpromazine. J Emerg Med 1994;12:849.
124. Ham LP, Packard RC. A retrospective, follow-up study of biofeedback-assisted relaxation therapy in patients with post-traumatic headache. Biofeedback and Self Regulation, in press.
125. Jensen OK, Nielsen FF, Vosmar L. An open study comparing manual therapy with the use of cold packs in the treatment of posttraumatic headache. Cephalalgia 1990;10:241.
126. Alexander MP. Mild traumatic brain injury: Pathophysiology, natural history, and clinical management. Neurology 1995;45:1253.
127. Levin HS, Williams D, Eisenberg HM. Treatment of postconcussional symptoms with CDP-Choline. Neurology 1990;40:326.
128. Munderhoud JM, Boclens ME, Huizenga J, et al. Treatment of minor head injuries. Clin Neurol Neurosurg 1980;82:127.
129. Denker PG. The postconcussion syndrome: Prognosis and evaluation of the organic factors. NY State J Med 1944;44:379.
130. Denny-Brown D. Disability arising from closed head injury. JAMA 1945;127:429.
131. Rutherford WH, Merrett JD, McDonald JR. Symptoms of one year following concussion from minor head injuries. Injury 1978;10:225.
132. Evans RW. The postconcussion syndrome: 130 years of controversy. Semin Neurol 1994;14:32.

16
Headache Due to Idiopathic Intracranial Hypertension

James J. Corbett

The association of headache with intracranial pressure due to intracranial mass lesions, hydrocephalus, and pseudotumor cerebri (idiopathic intracranial hypertension [IIH]) has always been a source of great concern to those who are faced with patients complaining of headache. The problem is whether it is possible to distinguish the head pain of an intracranial process such as tumor, pseudotumor, or hydrocephalus from the pain due to migraine or tension-type headache. Clearly, this is not an important problem in those patients who have focal neurologic signs, papilledema, or other evidence of intracranial disease. This chapter characterizes the headache due to IIH and discusses its management.

It is known from direct-stimulation studies, conducted in the course of intracranial surgical procedures done on awake patients, that the arteries at the base of the brain are painful when stimulated or stretched (see Chapter 1).[1] Moskowitz has demonstrated substance P in these arterial vessels out to the second bifurcation as well as in the walls of the major venous sinuses.[2] Studies done in the early 1940s, using intrathecal administration of artificial cerebrospinal fluid (CSF) or removal of spinal fluid, demonstrated the key features of increased and decreased CSF pressure on head pain in normal volunteers.[3] Using this intrathecal infusion method, it was possible to rapidly vary pressure and volume. Researchers found that pain was experienced when the CSF pressure was lowered after having been artificially elevated. Furthermore, a headache produced by low CSF pressure could be alleviated by raising the pressure to normal levels. Of particular importance, CSF pressure could be raised to ten times normal levels (680–850 mm H_2O) without producing any head pain. From these studies and others[4] it can be inferred that the absolute height of the pressure alone is not the cause of head pain but that the pain occurs when painful structures are deformed because of pressure and volume changes between intracranial compartments.

The posterior fossa is innervated by vagus and glossopharyngeal nerves as well as branches of C2 and C3, which project to neurons of the caudal trigeminal nucleus (see Chapter 1). Stretch on dural structures in this location can be associated with pain in the occiput, neck, and shoulders. The roof of the posterior fossa, the tentorium cerebelli, when electrically stimulated, however, refers pain to the forehead ipsilateral to the stimulation or to the midline.[1] Thus, although an occipitonuchal headache strongly suggests a posterior fossa site, it is not unusual to see patients with posterior fossa lesions whose headaches are bifrontal or are unilateral over, behind, or around one eye.

Thus, the major mechanisms involved in the production of headache due to intracranial mass lesions and to high CSF pressure caused by IIH and hydrocephalus include (1) traction on pain-sensitive structures, especially venous sinuses and arteries at the base; (2) distension and traction on pain-sensitive areas associated with ventricular distension; and (3) direct pressure on pain-carrying cranial and cervical nerves.

Increased intracranial pressure due to IIH can cause headache unilaterally, bilaterally, frontally, or occipitally; however, bifrontotemporal headache is the most common.[5] Unilateral headache with increased CSF pressure due to IIH may be explained by exacerbation of a migraine diathesis, or such a headache may reflect a new local phenomenon caused by irritation of painful structures through stretch and deformation. Many patients with IIH complain of occipitonuchal and shoulder pain, which may be due to posterior fossa or cervical root irritation.[5–7]

HEADACHE IN IDIOPATHIC INTRACRANIAL HYPERTENSION

Headache due to IIH occurs in about 75% of idiopathic cases. It is more common in patients who present to neurologists (in Weisberg's series, 100% had headache) than in those who present to ophthalmologists with visual loss or to otolaryngologists with noise in the ears.[8] Patients with IIH are, on the whole, not particularly ill, although headache may be severe; somnolence, fever, systemic symptoms, or obvious malaise should suggest venous sinus occlusion or some other primary cause of increased pressure. If the patient has been prone to headaches in the past, the headaches of IIH may be qualitatively similar but more constant and more severe. In patients with IIH the headaches are usually daily and continuous and qualify for the designation of chronic daily headache.

ASSOCIATED SIGNS AND SYMPTOMS

IIH is associated with papilledema in most recognized cases, although IIH without papilledema has been well described.[9] Papilledema is associated with transient visual obscurations (seconds-long loss of vision in one or both eyes), "blurry" vision (loss of clarity without loss of acuity), and, in severe or long-standing cases, loss of visual field or degradation of central visual acuity. Sixth-nerve paresis as a nonspecific and false localizing sign of increased intracranial pressure occurs in about one-third of cases.[7,10] Much less common are facial nerve paralysis, facial pain, hearing loss,[11,12] and even Lhermitte's phenomenon as a manifestation of IIH.[13] Nausea and vomiting are variably reported in the major case series, but both are fairly common. Pain on eye movement is not a common feature of migraine headache, but with IIH it is reported in up to 20%

of patients.[5,7] The typical ocular pain with IIH is retrobulbar and bilateral, as contrasted with the unilateral pain on eye movement that occurs with optic neuritis and is associated with visual loss.

Another feature of the headache with IIH is cranial bruit, which may be objective at times. The noise is pulsatile and pulse synchronous, and stops with carotid compression. It is a common reason for a patient with IIH to seek otolaryngologic consultation. The bruit may be soft or high pitched, is best auscultated with the bell over the mastoid or the temporalis with the mouth held open, and is caused by turbulence in the major venous sinuses.

EFFECT OF SPINAL TAP ON HEADACHES OF IDIOPATHIC INTRACRANIAL HYPERTENSION

Spinal taps have been used therapeutically with good effect in patients with IIH. Headache almost always improves, at least temporarily, following spinal tap, but there are problems related to frequent spinal taps. Occasionally, a single spinal tap will "cure" the headache, and patients who are successfully treated this way will occasionally return asking for another spinal tap if headache reappears. The bifrontal, holocranial headache due to high CSF pressure may, with repeated spinal tap, become an occipitonuchal headache associated with hindbrain herniation, or a posture-dependent post–spinal tap headache. Frequent spinal taps cause back pain that may become chronic. Repeated lumbar puncture as a treatment for IIH-related headache seems a reasonable approach, but it is an unusual patient who will want this as a long-term form of treatment. Furthermore, the long-term effect of repeated spinal taps may include a spinal epidermoid tumor, which can take 10–15 years to develop.[14]

TREATMENT OF HEADACHE DUE TO IDIOPATHIC INTRACRANIAL HYPERTENSION

It is clear that the increased CSF pressure is causally related in some way to the headache of IIH, but it is not clear just how it is related. Treatment of headache due to IIH with drugs that are solely aimed at reducing production of CSF seems reasonable theoretically, but neither of these medications (acetazolamide or furosemide) has been shown to effectively reduce CSF pressure for any length of time in the doses ordinarily used.

Acetazolamide is a potent carbonic anhydrase inhibitor that reduces CSF production at least for a time and, as a sole therapy, occasionally improves headache. The dose should start at 500 mg twice daily and can go to 2 g or even more daily. Side effects include nausea, depression, acral and perioral numbness and tingling, renal stones, and, *rarely,* hepatic failure. All patients will develop a compensated metabolic acidosis, which serves as a marker of compliance. Furosemide at 40–160 mg per day with potassium supplementation may also reduce headache by itself. Neither drug alone nor both together is the best way to treat the headache of IIH. The headache of IIH can be treated simply as head pain, without trying to keep the CSF pressure low. In a spinal fluid examination study of 85 patients with refractory transformed migraine, 12 patients were found to have CSF pressures ranging from 230–450 mm H_2O.[15] Ten of the 12 were women, and obesity was a feature in more than half. Thus, a subset of patients with chronic daily headache, who fit the stereotype of the obese woman of childbearing age seen in IIH, may be found without papilledema. These patients respond fairly well to migraine prophylaxis, but they respond better if acetazolamide or furosemide is added to the treatment regimen.[15] These patients would not have been discovered without a lumbar puncture.[16]

SURGICAL TREATMENT OF PAPILLEDEMA AND ITS EFFECT ON HEADACHE

The surgical treatment of papilledema includes optic nerve sheath fenestration and lumbar peritoneal shunt.[17,18] Both procedures are effective in reducing headache, although the reasons for improvement with optic nerve sheath fenestration are not entirely clear. Optic nerve sheath fenestration has a 50–65% rate of success in improving headache.[17] This result was observed in 1872 by DeWecker when he first reported treatment of papilledema by opening of the optic nerve sheath. Unilateral sheath fenestration is *not* associated with a decrease in CSF pressure as measured by 24-hour subdural bolt, but it *is* associated with defervescence of papilledema in both eyes in most cases.[17] This suggests that mean intracranial pressure must decrease even if the decrease is not reflected immediately in the 24-hour postoperative CSF-pressure profile.

Lumbar peritoneal shunt relieves headache, but the head pain is commonly replaced by a low-pressure postural headache. There is also the frequent, if not invariable, development of an acquired Chiari I malformation with lumbar peritoneal shunt. This may cause a number of different headache patterns including occipital, unilateral, and bifrontal migraine-like headache, which may be posture- or Valsalva-sensitive. Before considering lumbar peritoneal shunt as treatment for headache in IIH, the clinician should make sure that the patient has had a thorough trial of headache prophylaxis, that the picture is not complicated by analgesic rebound, and that the patient understands that the surgical treatment may trade one set of problems for another.

SUMMARY

Headache does not occur invariably with IIH, but when present, tends to be a new headache or worse than preexisting headaches. Large and frequent doses of analgesic self-medication can complicate the headache picture, as can post–lumbar puncture headache and, if lumbar peritoneal shunt is used, cerebellar tonsillar herniation.[19] Lumbar peritoneal shunt–induced headaches may exacerbate earlier headache syndromes or create whole new headache scenarios. The headache of IIH should not be treated as simply a manifestation of increased pressure. The combination of acetazolamide and furosemide, or a combination of one of the two diuretics with some form of migraine prophylaxis may provide the most satisfactory treatment regimen.[15]

REFERENCES

1. Ray BS, Wolff HG. Experimental studies on headache: Pain-sensitive structures of the head and their significance in headache. Arch Surg 1940;41:813.
2. Moskowitz MA. The neurobiology of vascular head pain. Ann Neurol 1984;16:157.
3. Kunkle EC, Ray BS, Wolff HG. Studies on headache: An analysis of the headache associated with changes in intracranial pressure. Arch Neurol Psychiatry 1943;49:323.
4. Johnston I, Paterson A. Benign intracranial hypertension. II: CSF pressure and circulation. Brain 1974;97:301.
5. Wall M. Headache profile of idiopathic intracranial hypertension. Cephalalgia 1990;10:331.
6. Bortoluzzi M, DiLauro L, Marini G. Benign intracranial hypertension with spinal and radicular pain. J Neurosurg 1982;57:833.
7. Giuseffi V, Wall M, Siegal PZ, Rojos PB. Symptoms and disease associations in idiopathic intracranial hypertension (pseudotumor cerebri): A case control study. Neurology 1991;41:239.
8. Weisberg LA. Benign intracranial hypertension. Medicine 1975;54:197.
9. Marcelis J, Silberstein SD. Idiopathic intracranial hypertension without papilledema. Arch Neurol 1991;48:397.
10. Corbett JJ, Savino PJ, Thompson HS, Kansu T, et al. Visual loss in pseudotumor cerebri: Follow-up of 57 patients from 5 to 41 years and a profile of 14 patients with permanent severe visual loss. Arch Neurol 1982;39:461.
11. Round R, Keane JR. The minor symptoms of increased intracranial pressure: 101 patients with benign intracranial hypertension. Neurology 1988;38:1461.
12. Dorman PJ, Campbell MJ, Maw AR. Hearing loss as a false localizing sign in raised intracranial pressure. J Neurol Neurosurg Psychiatry 1995;58:516.
13. Comabella M, Montalban J, Lozano M, Codina A. Lhermitte's sign in pseudotumor cerebri. J Neurol 1995;242:610.
14. Batnitzky S, Kencher TR, Mealey J Jr., Campbell RL. Iatrogenic intraspinal epidermoid tumors. JAMA 1977;237:148.
15. Mathew NT, Ravishankar K, Sanin LC. Co-existence of migraine and idiopathic intracranial hypertension without papilledema. Neurology 1996;46:1226.
16. Silberstein SD, Corbett JJ. The forgotten lumbar puncture. Cephalalgia 1993;13:212.
17. Corbett JJ, Nerad JA, Tse DT, Anderson RL. Results of optic nerve sheath fenestration for pseudotumor cerebri: The lateral orbitotomy approach. Arch Ophthalmol 1988;106:1391.
18. Sergott RC, Savino PJ, Bosley TM. Modified optic nerve sheath decompression provides long-term visual improvement for pseudotumor cerebri. Arch Ophthalmol 1988;106:1384.
19. Nightingale S, Williams B. Hindbrain herniation headache. Lancet 1987;1:731.

17
Painful Ophthalmoplegias, Tolosa-Hunt Syndrome, and Ophthalmoplegic Migraine

Lea Averbuch-Heller and Robert B. Daroff

CAUSES OF PAINFUL OPHTHALMOPLEGIA

Almost all types of ophthalmoplegia can be painful; the only exceptions are myasthenia gravis and chronic progressive external ophthalmoplegia, both characteristically painless. Thus, the association of ophthalmoplegia with pain only minimally narrows etiologic possibilities and does not greatly assist in localizing the pathologic process, except for its laterality.

Localization

Pathologic processes responsible for painful ophthalmoplegias may be located anywhere from the midbrain to the orbit.

Orbital

Any inflammatory, vascular, or neoplastic process that involves the orbit can cause painful ophthalmoplegia. One example is Brown's syndrome (superior oblique tendon sheath inflammation) in isolation or in the context of a generalized connective tissue disorder such as rheumatoid arthritis.[1,2] Orbital pseudotumor is an idiopathic inflammation involving different orbital structures; it can be either diffuse or localized to extraocular muscles, sclera, or the lacrimal gland, and may manifest with uveitis or optic neuropathy.[3] This syndrome overlaps clinically, pathologically, and radiologically with Tolosa-Hunt syndrome (THS). Lid swelling, proptosis, scleral injection, or ocular tenderness may suggest an orbital localization of the pathologic process.

Peripheral

The ocular motor nerves (third, fourth, and sixth) are the most common sites of lesions producing painful ophthalmoplegia. Involvement of several ocular motor nerves (combined ophthalmoplegia), in conjunction with ipsilaterally impaired facial sensation, usually implicates the cavernous sinus, where these nerves are together in a compact space and can be simultaneously affected. Such combined palsies can also occur in processes outside the cavernous sinus, such as tip of the petrous bone (Gradenigo's syndrome), tumors of the base of the skull such as chordomas and chondrosarcomas,[4] or inflammation involving proximal portions of the cranial nerves such as idiopathic cranial polyneuritis, which is often painful.[5]

Central

Hopf and Gutmann[6] suggested that an isolated diabetic third-nerve palsy, with or without pupillary sparing, is more likely to arise from a discrete mesencephalic infarct, as demonstrated by magnetic resonance imaging (MRI) in some of their patients. Given that eight out of 10 of their patients had an abnormal masseter reflex, the orbital pain may have been secondary to involvement of the trigeminal mesencephalic tract and the main sensory nucleus. Alternatively, the recurrent dural branches of the trigeminal nerve might be irritated, as in occipital infarctions.[7] Our experience, however, is that most painful ischemic third- or sixth-nerve palsies occurring in diabetic or hypertensive patients are peripheral, as originally postulated.[8] Nevertheless, unilateral orbitofrontal pain is not infrequent with midbrain infarctions and does not necessarily imply an extra-axial lesion. Similarly, oculomotor palsy with frontal headache can occur in nonischemic conditions affecting midbrain, such as tumors, arteriovenous malformations (in the authors' experience), and multiple sclerosis.[9]

Etiology

The numerous etiologies of painful ophthalmoplegia include inflammatory, vascular, and neoplastic processes affecting ocular motor nerves, extraocular muscles, or brain stem structures involved in ocular motor control (Table 17.1). Vascular lesions are the most common when a single ocular motor nerve is usually involved, such as in diabetic (hypertensive) third-nerve palsy.[3] When several ocular motor nerves are affected, structural lesions or inflammation within or near the cavernous sinus are the most likely causes.

Combined painful ophthalmoplegia can be produced by diverse processes (see Table 17.1): inflammatory (infectious and noninfectious), neoplastic (primary and metastatic), or vascular (arterial and venous; both ischemic and structural, i.e., carotid aneurysm, arteriovenous malformations). Within the cavernous sinus, the etiologies include infection (mucormycosis, aspergillosis), granulomatous inflammation (THS, sarcoidosis), cavernous sinus thrombosis,[3] carotid-cavernous fistula and low-flow dural-cavernous shunt,[10–12] giant aneurysms,[13] cavernous angiomas,[14] and tumors such as epidermoid, meningioma, chordoma, lymphoma, monoclonal gammopathy, and hemangiopericytoma.[3,15–17] Outside the cavernous sinus, combined painful ophthalmoplegia occurs with basal and pituitary tumors; pituitary apoplexy; and lymphoma, lymphoid hyperplasia, and solid tumors of the nasopharynx.[3,4,18]

Table 17.1 Conditions causing painful ophthalmoplegia[a]

Vascular
    Arterial: hypertension, diabetes, carotid dissection, internal carotid aneurysm, posterior
        communicating aneurysm,[b] pituitary apoplexy, midbrain infarction[b]
    Venous: cavernous sinus thrombosis, carotid-cavernous fistula, dural-cavernous shunt
Inflammatory
    Granulomatous: sarcoid, Wegener's granulomatosis, Tolosa-Hunt syndrome
    Dysimmune: systemic lupus erythematosus, rheumatoid arthritis,[b] mixed connective
        tissue disorder, necrotizing vasculitis, temporal arteritis, multiple sclerosis,[b] segmental
        Guillain-Barré syndrome, chronic inflammatory demyelinating polyneuropathy[b]
    Parainfectious/postinfectious: Epstein-Barr virus,[b] mycoplasma,[b] herpes simplex,[b] herpes
        zoster, idiopathic cranial polyneuropathy
    Infectious: mucormycosis, aspergillosis, syphilis, tuberculosis, Lyme disease
Neoplastic
    Solid: epidermoid, meningioma, craniopharyngioma, chordoma,[b] chondrosarcoma,
        hemangioma, hemangiopericytoma, pituitary adenoma, metastases
    Hematologic: lymphoma, macroglobulinemia, lymphoid hyperplasia
    Meningeal carcinomatosis
Other
    Ophthalmoplegic migraine

[a]All may result in combined painful ophthalmoplegia.
[b]This condition usually involves a single ocular motor nerve.

Idiopathic cranial polyneuropathy, an entity that overlaps with segmental Guillain-Barré syndrome and THS, most frequently involves the third and sixth nerves associated with facial or orbital pain.[5] Similar clinical manifestations are encountered in postinfectious painful ophthalmoplegia following mycoplasma, infectious mononucleosis, and herpes zoster[19–21]; or during the course of infectious or malignant diseases producing basal meningitis, e.g., syphilis, Lyme disease, tuberculosis, or meningeal carcinomatosis.[3,5,22]

Ischemia can be a cause of combined painful ophthalmoplegia. Although simultaneous involvement of several adjacent cranial nerves suggests a structural lesion, the same combination of nerves can be affected by ischemia. The explanation lies in the anatomy of the blood supply of the cranial nerves. The three nerves to the extraocular muscles and the ophthalmic division of the trigeminal nerve are all supplied by a single vessel: the inferolateral trunk (ILT), which arises from the intracavernous internal carotid siphon.[23] Lapresle and Lasjaunias[23] argue that concurrent trigeminal ischemia accounts for the pain accompanying ophthalmoplegia in ILT occlusion. This view is supported by reports of painful ophthalmoplegia when carotid dissection extends into the ILT.[24] Combined ischemic syndromes also occur in diabetic patients.[25,26] Painful ophthalmoplegia in these patients, occasionally associated with ischemic optic neuropathy,[25,27] is clinically indistinguishable from THS, but the response to treatment is different. Although pain improves following institution of corticosteroids in both syndromes, the course of ophthalmoplegia in the ischemic syndromes is unchanged.[25]

Pathophysiology of Pain

Why involvement of a single ocular motor nerve can be painful is unclear. Although Wolff[28] implied that the ocular motor nerves are not pain-sensitive, one of us (RBD), based on indirect evidence and clinical experience, believes they can be, at least within their cavernous sinus portions.

Some cases in diabetic or hypertensive patients may represent variants of partial intracavernous ILT occlusion; two of the three published pathologic studies of diabetic third-nerve palsies demonstrated infarctions within the intracavernous portion of the nerve.[29,30] None of the three reports of "diabetic thirds"[8,29,30] demonstrated major vessel occlusion; instead, there was hyalinization and proliferation of intimal endothelial cells in intraneural arterioles.

There is no direct evidence, however, that the vasa nervorum of ocular motor nerves are innervated by trigeminal fibers, although intracranial vessels of larger size are innervated by small, unmyelinated trigeminal sensory fibers.[31,32] Cranial blood vessels and the trigeminal nerve form a functional network, the trigeminovascular system.[31,32] The same applies to the dural venous sinuses, which are innervated by the trigeminal nerve.[33] Thus, any process affecting intracranial blood vessels and venous sinuses, either directly or indirectly, may cause pain in the distribution of the trigeminal nerve. This is the explanation for the painful nature of a variety of neurologic conditions, with or without ophthalmoplegia—from migraine and midbrain infarctions to THS.

TOLOSA-HUNT SYNDROME

THS usually refers to a granulomatous inflammation of the anterior cavernous sinus and orbital apex that may affect cranial nerves, from the second to the sixth, in any combination. The process is self-limited but recurrent; each relapse is characteristically steroid-responsive. The misleading use of the term "painful ophthalmoplegia syndrome" as synonymous with THS ignores the other myriad causes of pain and ophthalmoplegia.

History

In 1954, Eduardo Tolosa, a neurosurgeon in Barcelona (and the late father of the contemporary neurologist of the same name), reported a patient with complete unilateral ophthalmoplegia, progressive ipsilateral visual loss, and hypesthesia over the forehead, associated with severe retro-orbital pain.[34] Autopsy showed nonspecific granulomatous inflammation in the ipsilateral cavernous sinus, surrounding the carotid and intracavernous cranial nerves. In 1961, neurosurgeon William Hunt of Ohio State University described six patients (one his own wife), with recurrent unilateral painful ophthalmoplegia, variable hypesthesia of the upper face, and visual loss.[35] Treatment with corticosteroids resulted in prompt resolution of symptoms in all the patients. The neuro-ophthalmologist J. Lawton Smith first coined the eponym THS in 1966.[36]

Clinical Manifestations

Tolosa's and Hunt's original cases had visual impairment, implicating involvement of the optic nerve, which extends the pathologic process beyond the anterior cavernous sinus to the orbital apex. Thus, the THS might best be called an orbitocavernous syndrome. Indeed, there is no clear distinction between orbital pseudotumor[37] and THS, as both share the same pathologic process. THS is often heralded by steady, gnawing (but occasionally pulsating) retro-orbital pain that may precede the ophthalmoplegia by several days. Subsequently, ipsilateral optic, oculomotor, trochlear, abducens, and first two divisions of trigeminal nerve may become affected, singly or in different combinations. The pupil may be dilated with sluggish reactivity due to involvement of parasympathetic fibers in the third nerve; may be spared; or may be small, consequent to a Horner's syndrome caused by involvement of intracavernous sympathetic fibers. Parasympathetic and sympathetic pupillary dysfunction frequently coexist.

Clinical Course

If THS is untreated, partial or complete spontaneous recovery may occur after approximately 8 weeks,[38] but recurrences are common months or years after the initial recovery. In up to one-third of patients, the relapses manifest solely as unilateral periorbital pain, without ophthalmoplegia, and some develop chronic unilateral periorbital pain.[38]

Pathology

Pathologic findings in THS cases are only sparsely documented, because surgical exploration is not typically indicated. Since Tolosa's original description,[34] the few additional reports of pathology have disclosed granulomatous inflammation in the cavernous sinus and superior orbital fissure.[35,39–41] Goadsby and Lance[41] described a patient with recurrent painful ophthalmoplegia involving left sixth and third nerves, initially steroid-responsive, who, over a period of 6 years, underwent multiple surgeries, including retro-orbital and posterior fossa explorations and section of the ophthalmic division of the trigeminal nerve, until the removal of noncaseating granuloma from the cavernous sinus led to amelioration of the symptoms.

Pathophysiology

Painful ophthalmoplegia is a syndrome and not a single etiologic entity; it can be produced by any inflammatory process involving the cavernous sinus–orbital apex region, including sarcoidosis, vasculitides, systemic lupus erythematosus, rheumatoid arthritis, and Wegener's granulomatosis.[3,42–45] Yet, there is a subgroup of patients with orbitocavernous granulomatous inflammation that may share similar pathophysiology, and we restrict the term *THS* to this subgroup. The nature of the process responsible for THS is not fully elucidated, but the response to corticosteroids and the relapsing-remitting course of THS indicate a dysimmune disorder: This is further supported by an association between THS and systemic immunologic disorders such as lupus,[43,44] Wegener's granulomatosis,[45] and generalized vasculitis.[46] Laboratory tests in THS are often positive for immunologic markers including rheumatoid factor and antinuclear antibodies.[47,48] Montecucco et al.[49] reported two THS patients with positive antineutrophil cytoplasmic antibody. These antibodies correlate with active Wegener's granulomatosis and with microscopic polyarteritis, and their presence led the authors to propose that THS may be a forme fruste of Wegener's granulomatosis. The frequency of antineutrophil cytoplasmic antibody in THS patients is unknown, because the antibody is only recently discovered.

Diagnosis

THS is in part a diagnosis of exclusion. There is nothing specific in the clinical presentation that distinguishes THS from other pathologic processes in the orbitocavernous region. The response to corticosteroids in THS prompted Smith and Taxdal,[36] in the era before computed tomography (CT), to recommend a 2-day corticosteroid trial as a diagnostic test; failure to improve would rule out THS, and rapid improvement would make THS likely and preclude angiography, at that time the radiographic procedure of first choice. This recommendation proved dangerous because of other steroid-responsive conditions such as sarcoidosis, lymphoma, plasma-cell dyscrasia, and solid tumors masquerading as THS. Prior to CT, the role of imaging was to rule out structural and vascular causes of painful ophthalmoplegia. The angiographic features of THS are nonspecific and consist of narrowing of the carotid siphon, occlusion of the superior ophthalmic vein, and nonvisualization of the cavernous sinus—all of which reverse following treatment with corticosteroids.[50,51] Orbital phlebograms are abnormal in up to 50% of the patients.[52]

With the advent of high-resolution CT and MRI, the inflammatory lesions responsible for THS in the cavernous sinus, superior orbital fissure, and orbital apex can be directly visualized.[15,53,54] The typical finding on CT is enhancing soft-tissue infiltration in either orbital apex or the cavernous sinus, unaccompanied by bony changes. The lateral wall of the involved cavernous sinus in THS has a concave contour, as opposed to the convex lateral margin seen with carotid aneurysm or neuroma.[15] The enhancement in THS is less prominent than with meningioma or giant aneurysm, and, in contrast to carotid-cavernous fistula and cavernous sinus thrombosis, the superior ophthalmic vein is not enlarged. MRI usually demonstrates abnormal signal in the cavernous sinus, which is either hypointense on T1-weighted images and isointense on T2-weighted images[53] (Figure 17.1) or hyperintense on T1-weighted and intermediate-weighted images.[54] In the majority of cases, the signal extends into the orbital apex. Postgadolinium MRI shows enhancement that can include the cisternal portion of the oculomotor nerve.[55]

Treatment

Once the diagnosis is made, oral corticosteroids should be started at a dose of 80–100 mg prednisone (or equivalent) per day. Corticosteroid responsiveness is

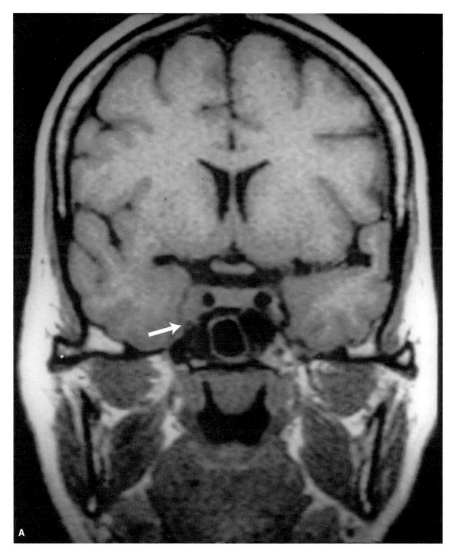

Figure 17.1 Magnetic resonance imaging of a patient with Tolosa-Hunt syndrome involving right ocular motor nerves. Coronal and axial T1-weighted images show a slightly hypointense signal (arrow) in the right cavernous sinus (A and B) that enhances with gadolinium (C). (Courtesy of Dr. John O. Susac.)

dramatic; symptoms resolve completely within days. However, the response is nonspecific: In patients with painful ophthalmoplegia due to idiopathic cranial polyneuropathy or malignant infiltration of the cavernous sinus, corticosteroids may also induce quick and complete resolution of symptoms.[3,5] Conversely, if the symptoms remain unchanged after a week on prednisone therapy, the diagnosis

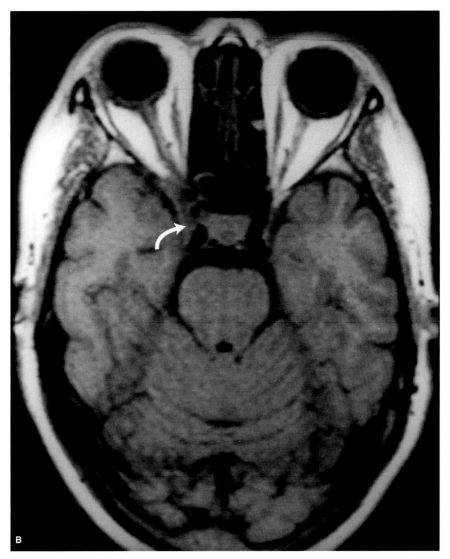

Figure 17.1   continued

of THS should be reconsidered and the imaging repeated, including angiography. Usually, corticosteroid therapy need not be prolonged; Hunt recommended discontinuation of the medication after 2 weeks,[56] but we start a slow taper after the patient has been symptom-free for 1 week; most patients are weaned in 4–6 weeks. Occasionally, patients with frequent relapses or those who later in the course develop chronic periorbital pain may require long-term corticosteroid therapy.[38,57] In such patients, steroid-sparing agents (azathioprine, methotrexate) may be used.

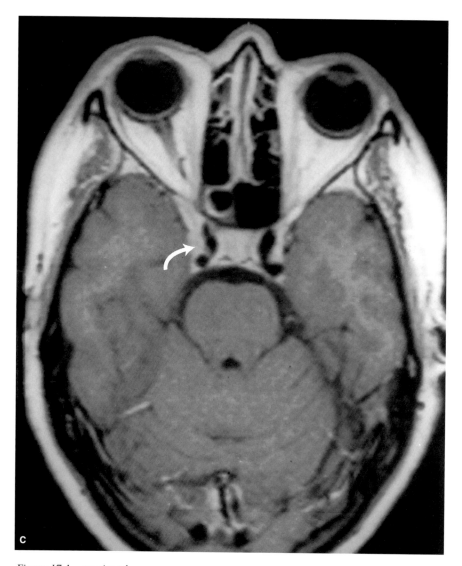

Figure 17.1   continued

Illustrative Case Reports of Tolosa-Hunt Syndrome and Other Causes of Painful Ophthalmoplegia

Case 1

A 23-year-old woman developed left retro-orbital pain, followed after 2 days by horizontal double vision. On examination there was a left sixth nerve palsy with only 60% of abduction, left Horner's pupil, and forehead hypesthesia. MRI showed abnormal signal in the left cavernous sinus, extending into the orbital apex. On presumptive diagnosis of THS, the patient was given 80 mg of prednisone a day. Two days later, the pain was gone; after a week on corticosteroids, diplopia occurred only on extreme left gaze; 3 weeks later, the examination was essentially normal, and the patient was tapered off the medication. Seven months later similar symptoms recurred, with prompt resolution on reinstitution of oral corticosteroids.

Case 2

A 75-year-old man presented with right supraorbital pain, diagonal double vision, and ptosis of 1 week's duration. He was diagnosed elsewhere with THS involving his right third, fourth, and sixth nerves. Brain CT demonstrated a soft-tissue swelling in the right orbital apex. Laboratory tests showed an erythrocyte sedimentation rate of 75 mm per hour and IgM kappa paraprotein of 4 g per dl. Bone marrow biopsy was consistent with Waldenström's macroglobulinemia. The patient was given chlorambucil, 2 mg per day, and experienced complete resolution of clinical and radiographic manifestations within 1 month. (This case was previously reported.[16])

Case 3

A 40-year-old woman developed left temporal and supraorbital pain, and horizontal diplopia that was initially intermittent. A tensilon test performed elsewhere resulted in transient amelioration of double vision; antibodies to acetylcholine receptor were negative. On examination, there was left sixth nerve palsy with slow limited abduction of about 80% of normal range, and left Horner's pupil. MRI demonstrated an enhancing lesion in the lateral aspect of the left cavernous sinus, surrounding the internal carotid artery. Biopsy from the lesion confirmed the diagnosis of meningioma.

Case 4

A 28-year-old woman presented with left supraorbital pain, followed 1 day later by diagonal double vision and droopy eyelid. Her examination showed complete left ptosis, poor adduction, supraduction, and infraduction, and dilated nonreactive pupil on the left, consistent with left third nerve palsy; sensation in the distribution of the first division of the left trigeminal nerve was mildly decreased. MRI and magnetic resonance angiography (MRA) performed in another hospital were reportedly normal; spinal tap was unrevealing. On the presumptive diagnosis of THS, the patient was started on 60 mg of prednisone per day; after 2 weeks without any response the dose was increased to 100 mg per day. Three weeks later, there was no change in pain or ocular motor signs. Because of severe steroid-induced acne, the dose of prednisone was gradually decreased to 30 mg per day, and methotrexate added. After 4 weeks on this regimen, there still was no improvement. The medications were discontinued. Repeat MRI/MRA showed a left internal carotid artery aneurysm at the level of the cavernous sinus; angiography demonstrated that the 5-mm aneurysm arose from the left posterior communicating artery. The patient underwent clipping of the aneurysm, which resulted in partial improvement of the third-nerve palsy.

OPHTHALMOPLEGIC MIGRAINE

The 1988 International Headache Society (IHS) classification of headaches stated: "Whether OM in fact has anything to do with migraine is uncertain."[58] The diagnosis of ophthalmoplegic migraine (OM), by IHS criteria, requires at least two attacks of headache coinciding with paralysis of third, fourth, or sixth cranial nerves, and exclusion of parasellar pathology by imaging studies. Migrainologists regard the condition as extremely rare,[59] and some believe that most instances of OM actually represent THS.[60,61]

OM can be mimicked by other conditions. Cano et al. reported a patient with pituitary adenoma, first presenting as painful intermittent third-nerve palsy that later became permanent.[62] Pituitary apoplexy in a migraineur may cause a complete oculomotor palsy reminiscent of OM.[63]

Hansen et al.[60] investigated the epidemiology of OM in Copenhagen over a period of 10 years. They identified four patients who satisfied the IHS criteria, providing an incidence of 0.7 per million inhabitants. After adding another four patients diagnosed outside the studied period, they found that only two out of the eight patients fulfilled the diagnostic criteria required for migraine. The authors argue that THS in a migraineur may induce headache with migrainous characteristics and may be misdiagnosed as OM, but unfortunately they provide no information about the steroid-responsiveness of the ophthalmoplegia in these migraineurs.[60] Straube et al.[61] described a patient diagnosed with OM (who, however, did not satisfy IHS criteria for the diagnosis) whose MRI showed enhancement of the precavernous portion of the third nerve. Spontaneous improvement started after 5 days, and became near complete 5 weeks after the administration of corticosteroids; the authors believed that the patient had THS.

Clinically, it has been difficult to differentiate between OM and THS because they have similar manifestations, both are recurrent, and both were traditionally diagnosed by exclusion. However, with further refinement of CT and MRI techniques, THS is becoming a diagnosis of inclusion and should be readily distinguished from OM.

CONCLUSION

There are multiple causes of painful ophthalmoplegia, with both peripheral and central localization. THS is responsible for only a minority of cases, but is readily diagnosed and treated. OM is an extremely rare cause.

REFERENCES

1. Fuller GN, Matthews TD, Maini RN, Kennard C. An unusual cause for diplopia: Acquired Brown's syndrome. J Neurol Neurosurg Psychiatry 1995;58:506.
2. Knopf HLS. An unusual case of painful ophthalmoplegia in a patient with rheumatoid arthritis. Ann Ophthalmol 1989;21:521.
3. Glaser JS, Bachynsky B. Infranuclear Disorders of Eye Movement. In JS Glaser (ed), Neuro-ophthalmology (2nd ed). Philadelphia: Lippincott, 1990;361.

4. Volpe NJ, Liebach NJ, Munzenrider JE, Lessell S. Neuro-ophthalmologic findings in chordoma and chondrosarcoma of the skull base. Am J Ophthalmol 1993;115:97.
5. Junkos JL, Beal MF. Idiopathic cranial polyneuropathy: A fifteen-year experience. Brain 1987;110:197.
6. Hopf HC, Gutmann L. Diabetic 3rd nerve palsy: Evidence for a mesencephalic lesion. Neurology 1990;40:1041.
7. Knox DL, Cogan DG. Eye pain and homonymous hemianopsia. Am J Ophthalmol 1962;54:1091.
8. Weber RB, Daroff RB, Mackey EA. Pathology of oculomotor nerve palsy in diabetes. Neurology 1970;20:835.
9. Galer BS, Lipton RB, Weinstein S, et al. Apoplectic headache and oculomotor nerve palsy: An unusual presentation of multiple sclerosis. Neurology 1990;40:1465.
10. Kosmorski GS, Hanson MR, Tomsak RL. Carotid-cavernous fistulae presenting as painful ophthalmoplegia without external ocular signs. J Clin Neuro-Ophthalmol 1988;8:131.
11. Hawke HB, Mullie MA, Hoyt WF, et al. Painful oculomotor nerve palsy due to dural-cavernous sinus shunt. Arch Neurol 1989;46:1252.
12. Brazis PW, Capobianco DJ, Chang F-LF, et al. Low-flow dural arteriovenous shunt: Another cause of "sinister" Tolosa-Hunt syndrome. Headache 1994;34:523.
13. FitzSimon JS, Toland J, Phillips J, et al. Giant aneurysms in the cavernous sinus. Neuro-Ophthalmology 1995;15:59.
14. Sepehrnia A, Tatagiba M, Brandis A, et al. Cavernous angioma of the cavernous sinus: Case report. Neurosurgery 1990;27:151.
15. Kwan ESK, Wolpert SM, Hedges TR III, Laucella M. Tolosa-Hunt syndrome revisited: Not necessarily a diagnosis of exclusion. AJR 1988;150:413.
16. Lossos A, Averbuch-Heller L, Reches A, Abramsky O. Complete unilateral ophthalmoplegia as the presenting manifestation of Waldenström's macroglobulinemia. Neurology 1990;40:1801.
17. McCall S, Wagenhorst BB. Painful ophthalmoplegia caused by hemangiopericytoma of the cavernous sinus. J Neuroophthalmol 1995;15:98.
18. Herishanu YO, Tovi F, Hertzanu Y, Goldstein J. Painful ophthalmoplegia with lymphoid hyperplasia of the nasopharynx. Neuro-Ophthalmology 1995;15:9.
19. Murray HW, Masur H, Senterfit LB, Roberts RB. The protean manifestations of mycoplasma pneumoniae infection in adults. Am J Med 1975;58:229.
20. Schnell RG, Dyck PJ, Bowie EJW, et al. Infectious mononucleosis: Neurologic and EEG findings. Medicine 1966;45:51.
21. Archambault P, Wise JS, Rosen J, et al. Herpes zoster ophthalmoplegia: Report of six cases. J Clin Neuro-Ophthalmol 1988;8:185.
22. Wintercorn JMS. Neuro-Ophthalmic Lyme Disease in Perspective. In RJ Tusa, SA Newman (eds), Neuro-Ophthalmological Disorders. Diagnostic Work-up and Management. New York: Dekker, 1995;561.
23. Lapresle J, Lasjaunias P. Cranial nerve ischaemic arterial syndromes: A review. Brain 1986;109:207.
24. Mokri B, Silbert PL, Schievink WI, Piepgras DG. Cranial nerve palsy in spontaneous dissection of the extracranial internal carotid artery. Neurology 1996;46:356.
25. Jabs DA, Miller NR, Green WR. Ischaemic optic neuropathy with painful ophthalmoplegia in diabetes mellitus. Br J Ophthalmol 1981;65:673.
26. Kosmorsky GS, Tomsak RL. Ischemic ("diabetic") cavernous sinus syndrome. J Clin Neuro-Ophthalmol 1986;6:96.
27. Annabi A, Lasjaunias P, Lapresle J. Paralysies de la IIIe paire au cours du diabete et vascularisation du moteur oculaire commun. J Neurol Sci 1979;41:359.
28. Dalessio DJ (ed). Wolff's Headache and Other Head Pain (4th ed). New York: Oxford University Press, 1980;24.
29. Dreyfus PM, Hakim S, Adams RD. Diabetic ophthalmoplegia: Report of case, with postmortem study and comments on vascular supply of human oculomotor nerve. Arch Neurol Psychiatry 1957;77:337.
30. Asbury AK, Aldredge H, Herschberg R, Fisher CM. Oculomotor palsy in diabetes mellitus: A clinico-pathological study. Brain 1970;93:555.
31. Moskowitz MA. Neurogenic inflammation in the pathophysiology and treatment of migraine. Neurology 1993;43(Suppl 3):S16.
32. Goadsby PJ, Edvinsson L. The trigeminovascular system and migraine: Studies characterizing cerebrovascular and neuropeptide changes seen in humans and cats. Ann Neurol 1993;33:48.
33. Kaube H, Hoskin KL, Goadsby PJ. Activation of the trigeminovascular system by mechanical distension of the superior sagittal sinus in the cat. Cephalalgia 1992;12:133.

34. Tolosa E. Periarteritic lesions of the carotid siphon with the clinical features of a carotid infraclinoid aneurysm. J Neurol Neurosurg Psychiatry 1954;17:300.

35. Hunt WE, Meagher JN, LeFever HE, Zeman W. Painful ophthalmoplegia: Its relation to indolent inflammation of the cavernous sinus. Neurology 1961;11:56.

36. Smith JL, Taxdal DSR. Painful ophthalmoplegia: The Tolosa-Hunt syndrome. Am J Ophthalmol 1966;61:1466.

37. Blodi FC, Gass JDM. Inflammatory pseudotumor of the orbit. Trans Am Acad Ophthalmol Oto-Laryngol 1967;71:303.

38. Hannerz J. Recurrent Tolosa-Hunt syndrome. Cephalalgia 1991;12:45.

39. Lakke JPWF. Superior orbital fissure syndrome. Report of a case caused by local pachymeningitis. Arch Neurol 1962;7:289.

40. Schatz NJ, Farmer P. Tolosa-Hunt Syndrome: The Pathology of Painful Ophthalmoplegia. In Smith JL (ed), Neuro-Ophthalmology: Symposium of the University of Miami and the Bascom Palmer Eye Institute, Vol. 6. St. Louis: Mosby, 1972;102.

41. Goadsby PJ, Lance JW. Clinicopathological correlation in a case of painful ophthalmoplegia: Tolosa-Hunt syndrome. J Neurol Neurosurg Psychiatry 1989;52:1290.

42. Campbell RJ, Okazaki H. Painful ophthalmoplegia (Tolosa-Hunt variant): Autopsy findings in a patient with necrotizing intracavernous vasculitis and inflammatory disease of the orbit. Mayo Clin Proc 1987;62:520.

43. Evans OB, Lexow SS. Painful ophthalmoplegia in systemic lupus erythematosus. Ann Neurol 1978;4:584.

44. Davalos A, Matias-Guiu J, Codina A. Painful ophthalmoplegia in systemic lupus erythematosus. J Neurol Neurosurg Psychiatry 1984;47:323.

45. Nishino H, Rubino FA, DeRemee RA, et al. Neurological involvement in Wegener's granulomatosis: An analysis of 324 consecutive patients at the Mayo Clinic. Ann Neurol 1993;33:4.

46. Hannerz J. Pathoanatomic studies in a case of Tolosa-Hunt syndrome. Cephalalgia 1987;8:25.

47. Mathew N, Chandy J. Painful ophthalmoplegia. J Neurol Sci 1970;11:243.

48. Hannerz J, Ericson K, Bergstrand G. A new etiology for visual impairment and chronic headache. Cephalalgia 1986;6:59.

49. Montecucco C, Caporali R, Pacchetti C, Turla M. Is Tolosa-Hunt syndrome a limited form of Wegener's granulomatosis? Report of two cases with anti-neutrophil cytoplasmic antibodies. Br J Rheumatol 1993;32:640.

50. Muhletahler CA, Gerlock AJ Jr. Orbital venography in painful ophthalmoplegia (Tolosa-Hunt syndrome). AJR Am J Roentgenol 1979;133:31.

51. Sondheimer FK, Knapp J. Angiographic findings in the Tolosa-Hunt syndrome: Painful ophthalmoplegia. Radiology 1973;106:105.

52. Hannerz J, Ericson K, Bergstrand G. Orbital venography in patients with Tolosa-Hunt syndrome in comparison with normal subjects. Acta Radiol Diagn 1984;25:457.

53. Yousem DM, Atlas SW, Grossman RI, et al. MR imaging of Tolosa-Hunt syndrome. AJNR 1989;10:1181.

54. Goto Y, Hosokawa S, Goto I, et al. Abnormality in the cavernous sinus in three patients with Tolosa-Hunt syndrome: MRI and CT findings. J Neurol Neurosurg Psychiatry 1990;53:231.

55. Mark AS, Blake P, Atlas SW, et al. Gd-DTPA enhancement of the cisternal portion of the oculomotor nerve on MR imaging. AJNR 1992;13:1463.

56. Hunt WE. Tolosa-Hunt syndrome: One cause of painful ophthalmoplegia. J Neurosurg 1976;44:544.

57. Kline LB. The Tolosa-Hunt syndrome. Surv Ophthalmol 1982;27:79.

58. International Headache Society Headache Classification Committee. Classification and diagnostic criteria for headache disorders, cranial neuralgias, and facial pain. Cephalalgia 1988;8(Suppl 7):1.

59. Daroff RB. The eye and headache. Headache Quarterly 1995;6:89.

60. Hansen SL, Borelli-Moller L, Strange P, et al. Ophthalmoplegic migraine: Diagnostic criteria, incidence of hospitalization, and possible etiology. Acta Neurol Scand 1990;81:54.

61. Straube A, Bandmann O, Büttner U, Schmidt H. A contrast enhanced lesion of the III nerve on MR of a patient with ophthalmoplegic migraine as evidence for a Tolosa-Hunt syndrome. Headache 1993;33:446.

62. Cano M, Lainez JM, Escudero J, Barcia C. Pituitary adenoma presenting as painful intermittent third nerve palsy. Headache 1989;29:451.

63. Silvestrini M, Matteis M, Cupini LM, Troisis E, et al. Ophthalmoplegic migraine-like syndrome due to pituitary apoplexy. Headache 1994;34:484.

18
Giant-Cell (Temporal) Arteritis as a Cause of Headache in the Elderly

Richard J. Caselli and Gene G. Hunder

The new onset of headache in an elderly patient is a common presenting symptom of giant-cell (temporal) arteritis (GCA). The headache is usually generalized, throbbing, and continuous, with focally worse pain in the temporal or, less often, occipital regions. Most patients show clinical evidence of superficial temporal artery inflammation on examination. An elevated erythrocyte sedimentation rate (ESR) further supports the diagnosis, and temporal artery biopsy is confirmatory. Corticosteroid therapy generally produces symptomatic relief and normalization of the ESR within days, though active vasculitis probably continues for at least several weeks. Superficial temporal artery involvement in GCA is frequent, but GCA is more properly viewed as a vasculitis of the aortic arch and its branches. GCA, therefore, can cause a wide variety of vascular complications, including anterior ischemic optic neuropathy, cerebral infarction, myocardial infarction, and aortic rupture, making prompt diagnosis and treatment imperative. Duration of corticosteroid therapy is generally 1–2 years. Complications related to corticosteroid treatment are frequent, so it is important to confirm the diagnosis by temporal artery biopsy before committing the patient to long-term corticosteroid therapy.

GCA occurs primarily in the elderly, and headache is the most frequent reason such patients are referred to a neurologist.[1] Headache is a prominent symptom in approximately 70% of patients and is the initial symptom in one-third.[2] Headache is a nonspecific symptom, but it must be carefully evaluated, because GCA can lead to a variety of disabling and sometimes life-threatening complications.

PATHOPHYSIOLOGY

The vasculitic damage of GCA results from activated CD4+ T-helper cells responding to an antigen presented by macrophages, and it therefore repre-

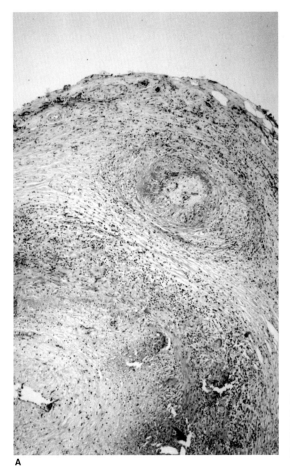

A

Figure 18.1   A. Temporal arteritis. Low magnification, lumen at bottom left. Small branch of temporal artery also involved, top right. Original × 40.

sents a disease of cellular immune mechanisms.[3–6] The inflammatory response is centered around the internal elastic lamina[7] and results in the formation of multinucleated giant cells, which are a histologic hallmark of GCA (Figure 18.1). The multinucleated giant cells contain elastic fiber fragments,[3] and although the specific antigen inciting the inflammatory response is unknown, elastin is suspected.[8,9]

The superficial temporal artery is involved in most patients. However, GCA also affects the aortic arch[10–14] and its branches (Figure 18.2), including the coronary arteries,[10,13] subclavian, axillary, and proximal brachial arteries,[11–13,15–18] and cervicocephalic arteries, including the carotid and vertebral arteries.[7,10–25] Vertebral arteries are involved as frequently as are the superficial temporal arteries in fatal cases[7,11,21] (Figure 18.3). Vertebral arteritis is extracranial, but it may extend intracranially for roughly 5 mm beyond dural penetration.[7] Basilar artery involvement is rare.[11,26] Intraorbital branches, especially posterior ciliary and ophthalmic arteries, are commonly affected.[7,21,27,28] Perhaps because

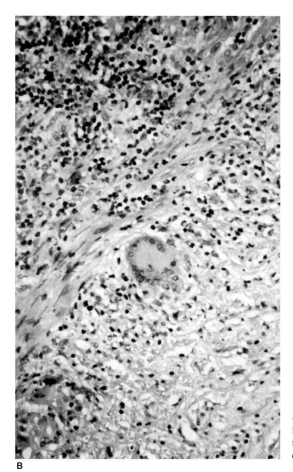

Figure 18.1 B. High-power magnification of same specimen shows lymphocytes and giant cells in media of artery.

B

intracranial arteries lack an internal elastic lamina, GCA does not cause a widespread intracranial cerebral vasculitis. Less often, the descending aorta,[12,13,14,29] mesenteric,[12] renal,[12] iliac, or femoral arteries[10–13,30] are affected. Pulmonary arterial involvement also has been described.[11,12]

HEADACHE AND OTHER CRANIOFACIAL PAIN SYNDROMES DUE TO GIANT-CELL ARTERITIS

The headache of GCA often has no pathognomonic features, but some qualities may be diagnostically suggestive. Perhaps most important is that the headache is either new in a patient without a history of headaches or of a new type in a patient with a history of chronic headaches. The headache is most commonly throbbing, generalized, and continuous. The temples are often cited by the patient as focal-

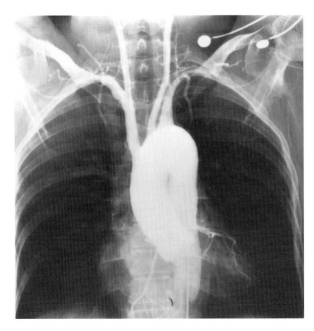

Figure 18.2   Aortic arch syndrome in patient with giant-cell arteritis. Left subclavian and axillary arteries are diffusely narrowed over a lengthy segment.

ly painful, and generally hurt to touch. Patients occasionally describe tender red cords in their temples (Figure 18.4), or scalp tenderness when combing their hair. Rarely, the headache is predominantly occipital. One-third of patients have no clinical signs of temporal or occipital artery inflammation. Approximately 5% of patients experience visual scintillations,[2,31] though not specifically in a fixed temporal relationship with the headache. The significance of these scintillations is not known, but they should be viewed as a possible sign of retinal or optic nerve ischemia due to the vasculitis rather than as benign migrainous auras.

Occipitonuchal pain may result from vasculitic involvement of the occipital arteries; or it may be part of the more generalized proximal limb, spine, and torso pain that typifies polymyalgia rheumatica (PMR). PMR occurs in approximately 50% and is the initial symptom in one-fourth of GCA patients.[2]

Ischemia of jaw and tongue muscles results in jaw and tongue claudication. Jaw claudication occurs in approximately 40% of patients and is the initial symptom in roughly 4%.[2] Tongue claudication occurs in approximately 4% of patients and is rarely the initial symptom.[2]

Rare cranial neuropathic syndromes that may be a source of discomfort to patients include transient hemianesthesia of the tongue,[2] lingual paralysis,[32] and facial pain due to facial artery vasculitis[33] (which might be mistaken for trigeminal neuralgia).

Approximately 15% of patients with GCA have carotodynia.[2] Presumably this reflects carotid vasculitis, but there are no angiographic studies of such patients. Finally, intracerebral hemorrhage has rarely occurred in patients with GCA,[4] but its infrequency suggests that it is probably unrelated to vasculitis.

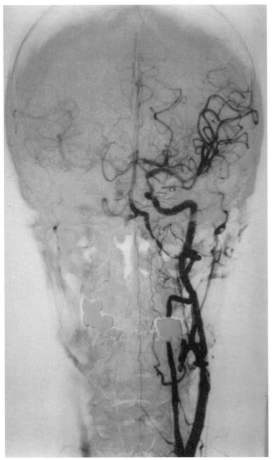

A

Figure 18.3 A. Arteriogram in patient with giant-cell arteritis who had brain stem infarction. The proximal left vertebral artery is segmentally narrowed. Several more segmentally narrowed areas of the distal left vertebral artery are also visible. B. Magnetic resonance imaging angiogram of same patient showing similar narrowing of distal vertebral arteries near formation of the basilar artery.

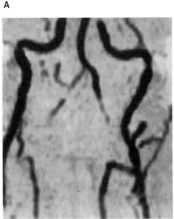

B

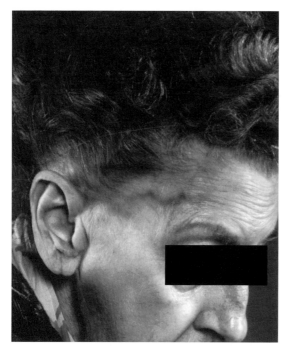

Figure 18.4   Intensely inflamed temporal artery in a patient with giant-cell arteritis.

NONPAINFUL CRANIAL SYNDROMES CAUSED BY GIANT-CELL ARTERITIS

The following complications may accompany the headache of GCA and are important features of the disease that the headache may portend.

Optic Neuropathy

Optic neuropathy is the most feared complication of GCA. Amaurosis fugax occurs in 10–12% of patents with GCA,[2,34] and permanent loss of vision due to anterior ischemic optic neuropathy (AION) occurs in 8%[2] to 23%.[35] Prior to the advent and widespread use of corticosteroid therapy, however, most series reported that patients with transient loss of vision went on to develop permanent, bilateral loss of vision due to AION.[1,23,24,28] Following monocular onset, the second eye became affected within days.[28,36] The combination of prompt diagnosis and effective corticosteroid therapy has drastically reduced the number of patients with permanent loss of vision due to GCA.[37]

AION results most commonly from vasculitis of the posterior ciliary artery, and less commonly from central retinal artery occlusion.[1,28] In the acute phase, ophthalmoscopy shows sludging of blood in retinal arterioles, which can be orthostatically sensitive.[38] Loss of vision precedes the funduscopic changes by roughly 36 hours,[28] although optic neuropathy is occasionally entirely retrobulbar without acute funduscopic changes.[28] In the acute phase, the disk is pale with blurred disk margins due to papilledema.[28] As AION evolves, the absolute amount of disk elevation tends to be modest (< 3 diopters in most cases), with infrequent areas of disk hemorrhage.[27] Edema resolves within 10 days or so, and within 2–4 weeks it is replaced by optic atrophy, even in retrobulbar cases.[28] Residual visual field defects are usually altitudinal.[28] Central retinal artery occlusion causes pallor and edema of the entire retina and optic disk, together with a macular cherry-red spot.[1]

Ocular Motility Disorders

Diplopia occurs in roughly 2%[2] to 14%[1,34] of patients with GCA, and it may fluctuate daily.[1,24,38] Any level of the oculomotor apparatus can be involved, including the extraocular muscles, nerves,[39] and brain stem,[40] but the extraocular muscles are the most common site.[24,27] Ptosis and miosis may occur together (Horner's syndrome) or separately, as well as in conjunction with other oculomotor disturbances.[39,40]

Neuro-Otologic Disorders

GCA is one of several vasculitides that can lead to acute auditory nerve infarction, but it is a rare occurrence.[1,2] Acute unilateral hearing loss is a more suggestive symptom than vertigo, but we have seen GCA patients with vertigo that resolved with corticosteroid therapy.[2]

Encephalopathy

The differential diagnosis of encephalopathy in the GCA patient is extensive. Corticosteroid therapy may be related primarily (steroid psychosis) or secondarily (steroid-induced metabolic abnormalities, systemic and central nervous system infections, including those that occur in immunocompromised hosts). Many unrelated causes are also prevalent in the elderly, including degenerative dementia, chronic subdural hematoma, and sedating medications. Finally, acute encephalopathy may be caused by GCA itself as a result of cerebral infarction.[7,11,20,24,26,41,42] Cognitive changes may result from thalamic, mesial temporal, and mesencephalic involvement in some cases, and in such cases computed tomography or preferably magnetic resonance imaging (which images these structures better than computed tomography) should be performed. Acute encephalopathy has been a poor prognostic sign, and many such patients have progressed to coma and died.[7,11,20,24,26] With appropriate corticosteroid therapy, some patients stabilize and over time may experience some recovery.[41,42] One comatose patent had triphasic waves on the electroencephalogram, and corticosteroid treatment led to complete recovery.[42] Recurrent episodes of acute encephalopathy with progressive cognitive impairment can lead to a more chronic multi-infarct dementia due to cervicocephalic arterial involvement by GCA.[41] We have found that encephalopathy and dementia are rare occurrences,[2,41] though earlier literature suggested that they were common complications.[43,44]

Although there is no evidence that GCA directly causes seizures, seizures may complicate the clinical course of the disease in any patient who has sustained a cortical infarction, whether or not the underlying mechanism was related to GCA. Seizures may also complicate the clinical course of GCA in patients with encephalopathy related primarily or secondarily to corticosteroids, so there are various reasons seizures may occur in the encephalopathic patient with GCA.

OTHER NEUROLOGIC FEATURES OF GIANT-CELL ARTERITIS

Peripheral Neuropathic Syndromes

When GCA affects large peripheral arteries and their branches,[12] sometimes the nutrient arteries of peripheral nerves[2] are included, resulting in mononeuropathies or mononeuritis multiplex.[24,30,45–52] The incidence of acute ischemic mononeuropathies in GCA patients is difficult to estimate but is probably around 2%.[30] Prognosis for neurologic recovery with corticosteroid treatment is good, provided that vascular compromise does not lead to loss of the affected limb.[30] Essentially all named peripheral nerves can be involved as ischemic mononeuropathies. Among spinal nerves, the fifth cervical has been reported to be susceptible to GCA by several authors.[30,47,50,51]

Patients with GCA also can develop mononeuropathies that occur at common compression sites, unrelated to vasculitis. For example, approximately 5% have carpal tunnel syndrome.[30] Some of these cases may be related to median nerve compression by synovitis related to PMR.

Mild abnormalities of nerve conduction studies and electromyography are common in elderly patients. Although such findings may suggest a peripheral neuropathy, the relationship of such neuropathies to GCA is uncertain. In other patients, however, antecedent ischemic mononeuropathies may accrue and eventually resemble a "diffuse," severe, peripheral neuropathy.[30,46,52]

GCA does not cause an inflammatory myopathy, although there are rare examples of localized inflammation in muscle.[15] PMR may falsely lead to the clinical suspicion of a myopathy, and corticosteroid therapy commonly causes a mild, noninflammatory myopathy ("steroid myopathy"). In typical cases of PMR without vasculitic involvement of the peripheral nervous system, electromyographic results are normal.[30]

On rare occasion, GCA may cause an acute cervical myelopathy.[2,26,53,54] The vasculitis presumably extends to the anterior spinal artery from the vertebral arteries.[26] Myelopathic involvement may presage a fatal outcome,[26] although prompt treatment with corticosteroids may permit neurologic stabilization[2] and improvement.[53]

Cerebrovascular Disease

Arterial Bruits

Clinically auscultable bruits reflect the topographic distribution of GCA. Carotid bruits occur in 10–20% of all GCA patents and are often bilateral.[2,16] Among patients with bilateral carotid bruits, 60% also have upper limb bruits or claudication or both.[2] Approximately 40% of GCA patients with carotid bruits sustain some type of ischemic eye or brain complication (amaurosis fugax, transient ischemic attack, permanent visual loss, or stroke), although permanent deficits (permanent visual loss and stroke) do not occur more often than in GCA patients without carotid bruits.[2]

Transient Ischemic Attack and Stroke

The known propensity of GCA to affect carotid and vertebral arteries should be considered in GCA patients with transient ischemic attacks (TIAs) and cerebral infarction,[2,41] even though atherosclerosis, hypertension, and cardiac disease remain the most important causes of cerebral infarction in the elderly with or without GCA.[34] Approximately 4% of GCA patients experience a TIA or stroke at some point during their illness.[2] A relatively greater proportion of TIAs and infarctions occur in the vertebrobasilar territory versus the carotid territory in GCA patients, as compared with the general population.[2] There are few clinical features that reliably distinguish a vasculitic from an atheromatous cause, though in rare instances atheroembolic material has been observed funduscopically or angiographically in the setting of active GCA.[2,38] Lacunar infarction syndromes specifically due to hypertensive small vessel disease would not be expected to result from a cervicocephalic arteritis, but it may be difficult to reliably distinguish a small from a large vessel stroke syndrome without neuroimaging.

LABORATORY EVALUATION

Blood Tests

Erythrocyte sedimentation rate should be measured. Though nonspecific, the combination of headache and an elevated ESR in an elderly patient should alert the clinician to the possibility of GCA. The ESR is elevated in approximately 97% of patients with GCA who are not taking corticosteroids. The mean value is 85 (standard deviation, 32) mm in 1 hour (Westergren's method).[31] Other acute-phase reactant proteins are also increased.

Complete blood counts typically reveal a normochromic microcytic anemia (mean hemoglobin value, 11.7 g per dl; standard deviation, 1.6) and thrombocytosis (mean platelet count, 427×10^3 per μl, standard deviation 116×10^3).[31]

Mild elevation of serum transaminases and alkaline phosphatase occurs in 15%, and elevation of plasma alpha-2 globulins occurs in 72%.[31]

Temporal Artery Biopsy

Confirmation by temporal artery biopsy (TAB) should be considered in every patient thought to have GCA. Glucocorticoids can be started before TAB if necessary, but in that case, TAB should be performed as soon as possible to avoid corticosteroid-induced histologic suppression or alteration of vasculitis in the TAB specimen, which would make diagnosis more problematic. However, occasional patients may continue to show histologic evidence of GCA even if TAB is performed as long as 6 weeks after the institution of corticosteroids with clinical resolution of symptoms.[55,56] When a TAB specimen is not obviously abnormal, we obtain a 5-cm specimen from the most symptomatic side, and if frozen sections are negative, we obtain bilateral specimens.[57] Histologic features include intimal proliferation with luminal stenosis, disruption of the internal elastic lamina by a mononuclear cell infiltrate, invasion and necrosis of the media progressing to panarteritic involvement by mononuclear cells, giant-cell formation with granulomata within the mononuclear cell infiltrate, and, variably, intraluminal thrombosis (see Figure 18.1). Involvement of the affected artery is often patchy (skip lesions).[37,58] If the TAB segment is long (4–6 cm), and multiple histologic sections are taken, 86% of cases will be correctly diagnosed by unilateral biopsy.[58]

Aortic Arch and Cerebral Angiography

Although they are not advised as routine diagnostic tests for GCA, some patients with GCA undergo aortic arch or cerebral angiography for stroke-related symptoms. Vertebral and external carotid arteries, including the superficial temporal artery, may show vasculitic changes of alternating stenotic segments[2] or occlusion[41] (see Figure 18.3), although superficial temporal artery angiography is less reliable than TAB for establishing a diagnosis. Internal carotid arteries may be occluded[2,17,41,59] but rarely have a characteristic vasculitic pattern. Subclavian, axillary, and proximal brachial arterial involvement produces a characteristic angiographic pattern of vasculitis consisting of long smooth stenotic segments alternating with nonstenotic segments and tapered occlusions[11–18] in patients undergoing aortic arch angiography (see Figure 18.2).

TREATMENT AND PROGNOSIS

Oral corticosteroids are the mainstay of treatment. Most patients require prednisone for 1–2 years with initial doses of 40–60 mg daily. If a patient presents with an acute neurologic syndrome or rapidly worsening neurologic status, whether it be visual loss, mononeuritis multiplex, or acute encephalopathy, treatment may begin with an intravenous pulse over several days (1,000 mg methylprednisolone per day), or with a high oral dose of corticosteroids (up to 120 mg prednisone), although no controlled study has compared the efficacy and safety of this more aggressive regimen to conventional therapy. The starting dose is then tapered over a few weeks so that by the end of the first month of therapy, most patients are taking about 40 mg of prednisone daily. Subsequent reductions by 2.5- to 5.0-mg increments may be made every 1–3 weeks as tolerated. A patient with GCA who has a relapse may require only a modest increase in the dose to control the flare of symptoms.

Following initiation of treatment, headache usually resolves within days. The ESR may drop within days and become normal in a week or two. Neurologic deficits can improve, but irreversible end-organ infarction may preclude clinically significant gains in some patients. Occasionally, mild headache may persist for 2–4 weeks even though the disease is adequately treated. Jaw claudication may also persist for several weeks in a mild form before resolving completely. Neurovascular complications may occur during initial tapering of corticosteroid dosage—often around 1 month after beginning treatment[2]—underscoring the need for ESR monitoring and the importance of small decrements in steroid dosage.

The frequent and potentially serious consequences of long-term corticosteroid therapy (such as diabetes mellitus, vertebral compression fractures, steroid myopathy, steroid psychosis, and immunosuppression-related infections) have led many to question the long-standing therapeutic strategy of high doses and prolonged duration. Some studies have suggested that much lower doses and more rapid tapering schedules are sufficient. One such study advocated initiating treatment with 20 mg of prednisolone daily and tapering it to 10 mg daily within 3 months.[60] Although many patients may respond to this regimen with symptomatic improvement of headache, PMR, and reduction of ESR, a substantial number of patients experience worsening of symptoms.[60] Headache and PMR, the most common symptoms of GCA, are not the reason these patients are treated with high-dose steroids. Higher doses are required to prevent irreversible ischemic ophthalmologic and neurologic complications, which may be an early manifestation or, less commonly, may develop during a flare.[2]

Other immunosuppressant drugs, including azathioprine,[61] methotrexate,[62] cyclophosphamide,[63] and dapsone,[64] have been tried for their corticosteroid-sparing effects. Corticosteroid dosages have been successfully lowered in some patients on each of these drugs, but results have been inconsistent. Toxicity can be a significant problem, particularly with dapsone and cyclophosphamide. Azathioprine has no immediate effect, and its corticosteroid-sparing effects may not be evident for a year.[61] Limited experience suggests that cyclophosphamide may be the most consistently effective immunosuppressant other than corticosteroids,[57,64] and that it may permit more rapid steroid tapering when instituted following a relapse.

REFERENCES

1. Hollenhorst RW, Brown JR, Wagener HP, et al. Neurologic aspects of temporal arteritis. Neurology 1960;10:490.
2. Caselli RJ, Hunder GG, Whisnant JP. Neurologic disease in giant cell (temporal) arteritis. Neurology 1988;38:352.
3. Banks PM, Cohen MD, Ginsburg WW, Hunder GG. Immunohistologic and cytochemical studies of temporal arteritis. Arthritis Rheum 1983;26:1201.
4. Weyand CM, Hicok KC, Hunder GG, Goronzy JJ. Tissue cytokine patterns in patients with polymyalgia rheumatica and giant cell arteritis. Ann Intern Med 1994;121:484.
5. Shiiki H, Shimokama T, Watanabe T. Temporal arteritis: Cell composition and the possible pathogenetic role of cell-mediated immunity. Hum Pathol 1989;20:1057.
6. Wawryk SO, Ayberk H, Boyd AW, Rode J. Analysis of adhesion molecules in the immunopathogenesis of giant cell arteritis. J Clin Pathol 1991;44:497.
7. Wilkinson IMS, Russell RWR. Arteries of the head and neck in giant cell arteritis: A pathological study to show the pattern of arterial involvement. Arch Neurol 1972;27:378.
8. Hunder GG, Lie JT, Goronzy JJ, Weyand CM. Pathogenesis of giant cell arteritis. Arthritis Rheum 1993;36:757.

9. Hellman DB. Immunopathogenesis, diagnosis, and treatment of giant cell arteritis, temporal arteritis, polymyalgia rheumatica, and Takayasu's arteritis. Curr Opin Rheumatol 1993;5:25.
10. Cardell BS, Hanley T. A fatal case of giant-cell or temporal arteritis. J Pathol Bacteriol 1951;63:587.
11. Heptinstall RH, Porter KA, Barkley H. Giant-cell (temporal) arteritis. J Pathol Bacteriol 1954;67:507.
12. Klein RG, Hunder GG, Stanson AW, et al. Large artery involvement in giant cell (temporal) arteritis. Ann Intern Med 1975;83:806.
13. Östberg G. Morphological changes in the large arteries in polymyalgia arteritica. Acta Med Scand 1972;533(Suppl):135.
14. Evans JM, O'Fallon MO, Hunder GG. Increased incidence of aortic aneurysm and dissection in giant cell (temporal) arteritis: A population-based study. Ann Intern Med 1995;122:502.
15. Andrews JM. Giant-cell ("temporal") arteritis: A disease with variable clinical manifestations. Neurology 1966;16:963.
16. Hamrin B, Jonsson N, Landberg T. Involvement of large vessels in polymyalgia arteritica. Lancet 1965;1:1193.
17. Howard GF III, Ho SU, Kim KS, et al. Bilateral carotid artery occlusion resulting from giant cell arteritis. Ann Neurol 1984;15:204.
18. Pollock M, Blennerhassett JB, Clarke AM. Giant cell arteritis and the subclavian steal syndrome. Neurology 1973;23:653.
19. Bruk MI. Articular and vascular manifestations of polymyalgia rheumatica. Ann Rheum Dis 1967;26:103.
20. Cooke WT, Cloake PCP, Govan ADT, et al. Temporal arteritis: A generalized vascular disease. QJM 1946;15:47.
21. Crompton MR. The visual changes in temporal (giant-cell) arteritis: Report of a case with autopsy findings. Brain 1959;82:377.
22. Graham E, Holland A, Avery A, et al. Prognosis in giant-cell arteritis. BMJ 1981;282:269.
23. Mowat AG, Hazleman BL. Polymyalgia rheumatica: A clinical study with particular reference to arterial disease. J Rheumatol 1974;1:190.
24. Russell RWR. Giant-cell arteritis: A review of 35 cases. QJM 1959;28:471.
25. Whitfield AGW, Bateman M, Cooke WT. Temporal arteritis. Br J Ophthalmol 1963:47:555.
26. Gibb WRG, Urry PA, Lees AJ. Giant cell arteritis with spinal cord infarction and basilar artery thrombosis. J Neurol Neurosurg Psychiatry 1985;48:945.
27. Barricks ME, Traviesa DB, Glaser JS, et al. Ophthalmoplegia in cranial arteritis. Brain 1977;100:209.
28. Wagener HP, Hollenhorst RW. The ocular lesions of temporal arteritis. Am J Ophthalmol 1958;45:617.
29. Evans JM, Bowles CA, Bjornsson J, et al. Thoracic aneurysm and rupture in giant cell arteritis. Arthritis Rheum 1994;37:1539.
30. Caselli RJ, Daube JR, Hunder GG, et al. Peripheral neuropathic syndromes in giant cell (temporal) arteritis. Neurology 1988;38:685.
31. Campbell JK, Caselli RJ. Headache and Other Craniofacial Pain. In WG Bradley, RB Daroff, GM Fenichel, CD Marsden (eds), Neurology in Clinical Practice: Principles of Diagnosis and Management. Boston: Butterworth, 1991;1507.
32. Kinmont PDC, McCallum DI. Skin manifestations of giant-cell arteritis. Br J Dermatol 1964;76:299.
33. Das AK, Laskin DM. Temporal arteritis of the facial artery. J Oral Surg 1966;24:226.
34. Huston KA, Hunder GG, Lie JT, et al. Temporal arteritis: A 25-year epidemiologic, clinical, and pathologic study. Ann Intern Med 1978;88:162.
35. Koorey DJ. Cranial arteritis: A twenty-year review of cases. Aust N Z J Med 1984;14:143.
36. Calamia KT, Hunder GG. Clinical manifestations of giant cell (temporal) arteritis. Clin Rheum Dis 1980;6:389.
37. Hall S, Persellin S, Lie JT, et al. The therapeutic impact of temporal artery biopsy. Lancet 1983;2:1217.
38. Hollenhorst RW. Effect of posture of retinal ischemia from temporal arteritis. Arch Ophthalmol 1967;7:569.
39. Dimant J, Grob D, Brunner NG. Ophthalmoplegia, ptosis, and miosis in temporal arteritis. Neurology 1980;30:1054.
40. Monteiro MLR, Coppeto JR, Greco P. Giant cell arteritis of the posterior cerebral circulation presenting with ataxia and ophthalmoplegia. Arch Ophthalmol 1984;102:407.
41. Caselli RJ. Giant cell (temporal) arteritis: A treatable cause of multi-infarct dementia. Neurology 1990;40:753.
42. Tomer Y, Neufeld MY, Shoenfeld Y. Coma with triphasic wave pattern in EEG as a complication of temporal arteritis. Neurology 1992;42:439.

43. Paulley JW, Hughes JP. Giant-cell arteritis, or arteritis of the aged. BMJ 1960;2:1562.
44. Vereker R. The psychiatric aspects of temporal arteritis. J Ment Sci 1952;98:280.
45. Dux S, Pithk S, Rosenfeld JB. Popliteal neuritis complicating temporal arteritis. Harefuah 1981;101:291.
46. Feigal DW, Robbins DL, Leek JC. Giant cell arteritis associated with mononeuritis multiplex and complement-activating 19S IgM rheumatoid factor. Am J Med 1985;79:495.
47. Fryer DG, Singer RS. Giant-cell arteritis with cervical radiculopathy. Bull Mason Clinic 1971;25:143.
48. Massey EW, Weed T. Sciatic neuropathy with giant-cell arteritis [letter]. N Engl J Med 1978;298:917.
49. Meneely JK Jr, Bigelow NH. Temporal arteritis: A critical evaluation of this disorder and a report of three cases. Am J Med 1953;14:46.
50. Sánchez MC, Arenillas JLC, Gutierrez DA, et al. Cervical radiculopathy: A rare symptom of giant cell arteritis. Arthritis Rheum 1983;26:207.
51. Shapiro L, Medsger TA Jr, Nicholas JJ. Brachial plexitis mimicking C5 radiculopathy: A presentation of giant cell arteritis [letter]. J Rheumatol 1983;10:670.
52. Warrell DA, Godfrey S, Olsen EGJ. Giant-cell arteritis with peripheral neuropathy. Lancet 1968;1:1010.
53. Brennan MJW, Sandyk R. Reversible quadriplegia in a patient with giant-cell arteritis. S Afr Med J 1982;62:81.
54. Cloake PCP. Temporal arteritis. Proc R Soc Med 1951;44:847.
55. Achkar AA, Lie JT, Hunder GG, O'Fallon WW, et al. How does previous corticosteroid treatment affect the biopsy findings in giant cell (temporal) arteritis? Ann Intern Med 1994;120:987.
56. Evans JM, Batts KP, Hunder GG. Persistent giant cell arteritis despite corticosteroid treatment. Mayo Clin Proc 1994;69:1060.
57. Caselli RJ, Hunder GG. Giant Cell (Temporal) Arteritis and Cerebral Vasculitis. In RT Johnson, JW Griffin (eds), Current Therapy in Neurologic Disease (4th ed). St. Louis: Decker, 1993;196.
58. Hall S, Hunder GG. Is temporal artery biopsy prudent? Mayo Clin Proc 1984;59:793.
59. Cull RE. Internal carotid artery occlusion caused by giant cell arteritis. J Neurol Neurosurg Psychiatry 1979;42:1066.
60. Lundberg I, Hedfors E. Restricted dose and duration of corticosteroid treatment in patients with polymyalgia rheumatica and temporal arteritis. J Rheumatol 1990;17:1340.
61. De Silva M, Hazleman BL. Azathioprine in giant cell arteritis/polymyalgia rheumatica: A double-blind study. Ann Rheum Dis 1986;45:136.
62. Krall PL, Mazenec DJ, Wilke WS. Methotrexate for corticosteroid-resistant polymyalgia rheumatica and giant cell arteritis. Cleve Clin J Med 1989;56:253.
63. DeVita S, Tavoni A, Jeraitano G, et al. Treatment of giant cell arteritis with cyclophosphamide pulses [letter]. J Intern Med 1992;232:373.
64. Demaziere A. Dapsone in the long-term treatment of temporal arteritis [letter]. Am J Med 1989;87:3.

19
Brain Tumors and Other Space-Occupying Lesions

John Edmeads

Many patients with headaches worry, at one time or another, about whether they harbor brain tumors. As physicians, we know that those concerns are almost always groundless. The vast majority of headaches are caused by benign dysfunctional disorders such as migraine and tension-type headaches, and only the smallest minority are symptoms of ominous disease. Nevertheless, sooner or later we encounter patients whose headaches are caused by brain tumors or other space-occupying lesions such as subdural hematoma and brain abscess. Our task is to recognize them.

To do so, we must consider the following questions: (1) How many people with brain tumors or other space-occupying lesions have headache? (2) What are the mechanisms that produce such headaches? (3) Are specific types of space-occupying lesions, or lesions in specific locations, more likely to cause headaches? (4) What are the characteristics of headaches associated with space-occupying lesions? (5) What features of a patient with headache suggest the possibility of a brain tumor or other space-occupying lesion and the need for special investigations?

PREVALENCE OF HEADACHE AMONG PATIENTS WITH TUMORS AND OTHER SPACE-OCCUPYING LESIONS

Our medical ancestors, living before the era of statistics and epidemiology, seldom wrote about their experiences in any quantitative way, but it is clear that they perceived headache as a major feature of patients with brain tumor. Gowers, in 1888,[1] wrote of brain tumors, "Of the general symptoms, headache is the most constant, absent only in very rare cases." Cushing, in 1908,[2] drew on his extensive personal experience of brain tumors to write that "some degree of headache . . . is usual." Gowers and Cushing, though skilled and perceptive clinicians, had no technology that would allow them to diagnose brain tumor early, before increased intracranial pressure declared itself. Access to specialized health care was limited by socioeconomic and geographic factors. Therefore, it is likely that they were seeing a preponderance of patients with large, and perhaps end-stage, lesions. Gowers's statement that "optic neuritis [papilledema] occurs in a large proportion, probably about four-fifths, of the cases of intracranial tumor, whatever be the seat or nature of the growth" reinforces this notion, because nowadays, when more patients have access to neurologists and neurosurgeons early in the course of their symptoms, and imaging procedures permit detection of even small lesions, papilledema is found in only 10%[3] to 50%[4] of patients with cerebral tumors (and most clinicians would be more accepting of the lower figure).

Kunkle et al.,[5] in 1942, were among the first to present their experience with brain tumors in a quantitative fashion. Their results likely mirror their medical times: Of their 72 patients with brain tumor seen at the New York Hospital, 90% had headaches. Fewer than half of their patients with supratentorial lesions had headache as their first symptom, whereas most people with posterior fossa tumors experienced headache as their earliest symptom. The more recent (1962) Mayo Clinic series of Rushton and Rooke,[6] compiled in an era of angiography and brain scanning, reported that 60% of their brain tumor patients had headaches. The 1987 series of Iversen et al.,[7] with modern neuroimaging available to assist early diagnosis, revealed a headache prevalence of 53% in their patients with brain tumor; in 16% of their patients, headache was the first symptom, especially if the tumor was located in the posterior fossa. Forsyth and Posner,[8] in 1993, reported 111 consecutive patients at the Memorial Sloan-Kettering Cancer Center who had had brain tumors detected by computed tomography (CT) or magnetic resonance imaging (MRI) scans; 48% had headaches. Of these 111 patients with brain tumors, only 30 were imaged primarily because of their headaches. Vazquez-Barquero et al.,[9] in 1994, noted that only 8% of 183 adults with brain tumors presented with headaches and no other features. About one-third of their series had headaches in association with other features such as weakness or seizures, and the remainder had no significant headaches.

It seems, therefore, that as modern neuroimaging techniques have allowed the earlier detection of brain tumors, before they grow to a large size, the prevalence of headache as a significant symptom of tumor has fallen to approximatley 50%. The 1994 study of Suwanwela et al.,[10] which documented a 71% prevalence of headache in their 171 patients with brain tumor, appears to contradict this, but this unusually high prevalence might be attributable to the lack of early access to technology for some of the population in their area, and to the inclusion in the study of pediatric patients, whose higher incidence of posterior fossa tumors would produce more headaches (see next two sections).

There are some significant differences between adults and children in terms of the headaches that may result from brain tumors. Posterior fossa tumors are more common in childhood, and because posterior fossa mass lesions are more likely to cause headaches than supratentorial ones, "tumor headaches" are generally encountered more often in children than in adults. Honig and Charney, in 1982,[11] reported that among 105 children with brain tumors, 72 had headaches. In the majority of these, headache preceded other symptoms, but within a short time most became associated with demonstrable neurologic abnormalities—reflecting the fact that, in contradistinction to the large "silent areas" in the supratentorial compartment, the posterior fossa is a clinically eloquent area that complains early when attacked by disease. Seventy-eight percent of these children with tumor headache had vomiting, two-thirds had papilledema, and two-thirds had precipitation of headache by maneuvers that altered intracranial pressure (coughing, sneezing, straining, and recumbency), as opposed to the 32–48% incidence of these features in adults with brain tumors.[6,8] This reflects the proclivity of posterior fossa mass lesions to produce, early in their course, increased intracranial pressure by obstructing the egress of cerebrospinal fluid (CSF) from the ventricular system. In the more recent series of Kennedy and Nathwani,[12] headache was the presenting symptom in 53% of the children with brain tumors, but the great majority of these had other symptoms and signs as well, and 46% had papilledema. The median duration of headache before tumor diagnosis in these children was 5 months (ranging from 3 months to 5 years), testimony to the difficulty sometimes encountered in diagnosing headaches in children.[13] Kennedy and Nathwani commented on the ability of brain tumor headaches in children to mimic migraine or tension-type headaches, sometimes for years.

In space-occupying lesions other than brain tumors, notably subdural hematomas and brain abscesses, headache is a more frequent and earlier symptom. McKissock[14] reported that 81% of his 216 patients with chronic subdural hematoma had headache, with a lesser prevalence in acute (11%) and subacute (53%) subdural hematomas. The difference in prevalence of headache between tumor and subdural hematoma is believed to be attributable to the (usually) more rapid evolution and greater extent of the hematomas (see next section on Mechanisms of Headache Production); and the lesser occurrence of headache in acute and subacute subdural hematomas compared with chronic subdural hematoma may be due to the underlying traumatic cerebral changes in the former, obtunding consciousness early and making it difficult to elicit a history of headache.

In brain abscesses, "the most common symptom . . . is a progressively severe headache which is intractable to symptomatic therapy. In published clinical series, headache was present in 70% to 90% of patients."[15] Again, the higher prevalence of headache in abscess, compared with tumor, may be due to the generally faster evolution of abscesses and to the not infrequent meningeal reaction and occasional low-grade fever that may accompany abscess.

Other conditions, such as hydrocephalus, cerebral edema, and large arteriovenous malformations, may behave like space-occupying lesions and cause headache. These are discussed in other chapters of this volume.

MECHANISMS OF HEADACHE PRODUCTION IN SPACE-OCCUPYING LESIONS

Space-occupying lesions cause headache by directly or indirectly distorting pain-sensitive intracranial structures (such headaches are known as traction headaches). These structures are[16] (1) the large arteries at the base of the brain (the circle of Willis) and the first few centimeters of their immediate branches; (2) the meningeal (dural) arteries; (3) the large venous channels of the brain and dura; (4) some portions of the dura, particularly those adjacent to blood vessels, including the tentorium and the diaphragma sellae; and (5) the cranial nerves that carry pain fibers (V, VII, IX, and X). The parenchyma of the brain is not sensitive to pain (see Chapter 1).

Mass lesions can produce headaches by pressing directly on a pain-sensitive structure (local traction). For example, a meningioma of the convexity may distort the immediately adjacent middle meningeal artery, causing pain that may be felt in the ipsilateral frontotemporal region. A posterior fossa tumor, such as a dermoid, may press on the seventh cranial nerve, producing headache that is felt behind the ipsilateral ear (which is the cutaneous distribution of the seventh nerve). Pain arising from the intracranial cavity is visceral pain and, like all visceral pain, is not perceived as emanating directly from the affected tissue, but rather is referred to more superficial structures; the referral may be fairly local, as with the convexity meningioma, or may be somewhat distant, as with the posterior fossa tumor. As a rule, lateralized lesions refer pain ipsilaterally, supratentorial lesions refer pain frontally, and posterior fossa lesions refer pain to the back of the head.

Sometimes a mass lesion distorts more remote pain-sensitive structures, causing pain that may be referred deceptively. An example of such "distant traction" is a large glioma of the right frontal lobe, which, because of its size, displaces the brain stem downward, stretching the pain-sensitive lower cranial nerves in the posterior fossa or the upper two cervical nerves, thereby producing pain referred to the back of the head. Another example of distant traction is the posterior fossa tumor that compresses either the aqueduct of Sylvius or the fourth ventricle, resulting in hydrocephalus. The distended anterior horns of the lateral ventricles stretch pain-sensitive supratentorial structures (likely the veins draining into the superior sagittal sinus) leading to bifrontal headache.

In both these examples of distant traction, it is possible, and perhaps likely, that careful questioning might elicit a history of an earlier, more appropriately located headache from local traction that was subsequently superseded or overshadowed by the headaches caused by distant traction.

It is evident that distant traction usually embodies a significant element of increased intracranial pressure. There is no consensus about whether increased intracranial pressure alone can cause headache or whether it must be accompanied by shifts or distortion of intracranial contents (Figure 19.1). Schumacher and Wolff[17] produced increased intracranial pressure in volunteers by intrathecal infusion of saline and found that headache seldom resulted; but Sorensen and Corbett[18] reported that "artificial production of elevated spinal fluid pressure using saline infusion usually produces frontal and temporal headaches but may be associated with unilateral or holocranial head pain of any sort. Some patients sense no pain despite rapid rises in CSF pressure during the infusion test."

There are some unusual mechanisms through which brain tumors may produce headache. When metastatic tumor involves the meninges diffusely (meningeal carcinomatosis), the generalized headache that results is due to meningeal irritation and may be associated with physical signs of that irritation, such as a stiff neck. Even less commonly, brain tumors may produce headaches that closely resemble migraine, sometimes even to the extent of incorporating a migrainous visual aura.[19–23] Some of these tumors were located in the parietal or occipital regions (Figure 19.2), which makes intuitive sense, but others were either intraventricular or sited in the interhemispheric frontal fissure, areas not traditionally incriminated in the genesis of migraine. To further complicate the issue, Shuper et al.[24] have reported that following successful combined wholebrain radiotherapy and chemotherapy of their posterior fossa or pineal tumors (actually 14–32 months after termination of therapy), four children developed

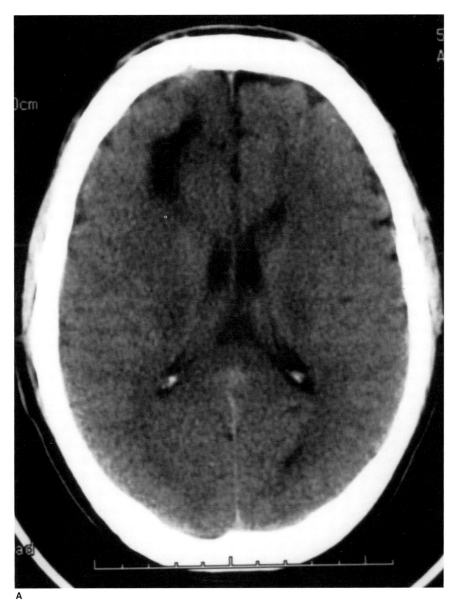

A

Figure 19.1   A. This 53-year-old man has a 7-year history of seizures. Unenhanced computed tomography of head shows a hypodense lesion, presumed to be a low-grade glioma, in the right frontal subcortical region, without any significant displacement of intracranial structures. No headaches at this time.

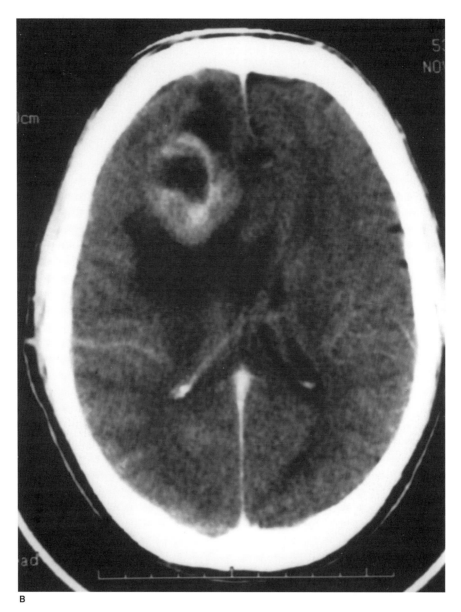

B

Figure 19.1   B. Four months later the patient developed increasingly frequent and severe right frontal headaches. Repeat computed tomographic scan with enhancement shows growth of tumor, severe edema, and marked midline shift. Biopsy revealed glioblastoma multiforme.

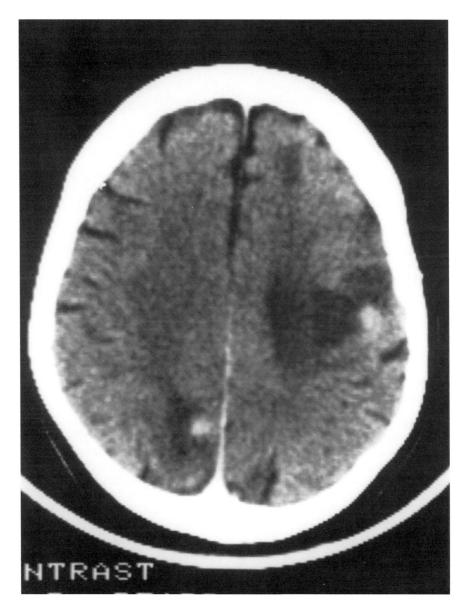

NTRAST

Figure 19.2 At the age of 52 years, this woman, for the first time in her life, developed recurrent episodes of obscuration of vision by bright zigzag lines, followed by transient diffuse headaches. Examination revealed mild weakness and hyperreflexia of her right upper limb. Note enhancing lesions in right occipital and posterior left frontal regions. Four years earlier she had had a lumpectomy for breast carcinoma.

episodic severe hemicranial headaches associated with nausea and transient visual loss, hemisensory deficit, dysphasia, or hemiparesis. These children had no prior history of similar headaches, no family history of migraine, and no evidence of tumor recurrence. The mechanism by which these migrainous manifestations were produced is obscure. Shuper et al. suspect transient vascular instability related to the radiotherapy. From a practical standpoint, it is important to be aware that occurrence of headaches in treated brain tumor patients does not necessarily signify tumor recurrence.

EFFECTS OF NATURE AND LOCATION OF LESIONS ON HEADACHE PRODUCTION

As a rule, slowly growing supratentorial tumors of the brain parenchyma produce headaches less frequently than do more rapidly growing tumors. The extent of this difference is controversial. Forsyth and Posner,[25] from their neuro-oncologic perspective, noted that in slowly growing cerebral tumors such as low-grade astrocytomas, gangliogliomas, etc., seizures were far more common than headaches; when gliomas grew faster, the incidence of headaches increased to about 50%. Salcman's surgical review,[4] on the other hand, noted that "headache is the initial symptom in almost 40% of patients with glioblastoma multiforme, and in more than 35% of all patients with cerebral gliomas"; 71% of glioma patients had headaches at some time in their course, and 77% of those with glioblastoma multiformes. Consonant with the concept that slower growing supratentorial tumors were less likely to cause headache, Salcman noted that only 23% of oligodendrogliomas produced headache.

Meningiomas are usually indolently progressive, and they produce headaches significantly less frequently than do gliomas. Most authors[8,26] note the occurrence of headache in about one-third of patients with supratentorial meningiomas. In the series of Cushing and Eisenhardt,[27] headache was a common presenting symptom of supratentorial meningiomas, but given that papilledema was almost always associated, it is reasonable to conclude that these tumors were referred late, after increased intracranial pressure had supervened. The more recent series,[8,26] compiled with the aid of more sensitive neuroimaging procedures, indicate that headache is an uncommon presenting feature of supratentorial meningiomas.

Metastatic tumors are rapidly progressive and, as expected, are frequently associated with headache. In one series[28] it was noted that "headache is the initial complaint in 50% to 60% of patients." Most authors,[25] however, have found an overall (i.e., including both early and late) incidence of headache in about 50% of patients with metastatic brain tumor. The precise incidence varies with the location of the metastases; posterior fossa lesions are much more likely to produce headaches.

The principle that posterior fossa tumors are more likely to cause headaches, and cause them earlier in the clinical course, is exemplified in all series from the time of Cushing to the present. Location appears to be a more important determinant of headache than tumor type, probably because posterior fossa lesions impinge early on the CSF pathways and lead to increased intracranial pressure. Forsyth and Posner's[8] experience that 82% of their posterior fossa tumors were associated with headache is representative. Lavyne and Patterson[26] reported that headache was the first symptom of brain tumor in most patients with posterior fossa tumors, except for those with cerebellopontine angle tumors. Many cerebellopontine angle tumors are acoustic schwannomas, which are now usually detected as the result of otoneurologic investigation of hearing loss, etc., long before they reach the size necessary to produce headache.

Tumors of the sellar and parasellar regions, such as pituitary adenomas and craniopharyngiomas, do not often present headache as the initial symptom,[29] even though the diaphragma sellae is pain sensitive, because the visual and endocrine symptoms (e.g., amenorrhea, infertility) are usually more obvious to the patients (at least to adult patients; in children with tumors of the sellar region, headache usually is the earliest symptom because they often are unaware of the endocrine and visual manifestations). However, once the tumor attains sufficient bulk either to distort the markedly pain-sensitive vessels at the base of the brain or to cause increased intracranial pressure by obstructing the third ventricle, headache supervenes. Very rapid increase in the size of a sellar lesion, as in pituitary apoplexy, causes catastrophic headache, and of course other acute symptoms such as visual impairment and obtundation.[30]

Some principles emerge from consideration of the relationships between certain types and locations of lesions and the headaches they may produce: (1) Rapidly growing lesions produce headache earlier than more slowly progressing ones. (2) Posterior fossa lesions, even slowly growing ones, are more likely to cause headaches than supratentorial ones because they are positioned to obstruct CSF drainage and cause increased intracranial pressure. (3) Headache may not be an early or prominent manifestation of a mass lesion if that lesion is situated to involve, before pain-sensitive structures, more eloquently symptomatic intracranial functions such as the special senses or the endocrine status.

Individual sensitivity may play a role in determining whether an individual with a specific type of tumor in a specific location is more or less likely than someone else in a similar situation to experience headache. Forsyth and Posner[25] have made the intriguing observation that those brain tumor patients with a past history of benign dysfunctional headaches are more likely to experience headaches with their tumors than those with no such prior headache history. A parallel observation on the sensitizing effect of previous benign dysfunctional headaches (notably migraine) has been made about patients with ischemic cerebrovascular disease who experience headaches as a symptom of actual or incipient cerebral infarction.[31] It seems that those with a history of migraine or other benign dysfunctional headaches may be particularly likely to develop headaches as a symptom of lesions. A clinical corollary is that these constitutionally headache-prone individuals could be at special risk of having their new headaches written off as simply a slight worsening of their migraine.

CHARACTERISTICS OF HEADACHES CAUSED BY MASS LESIONS

Is there such a thing as a "brain tumor headache"? Certainly our medical ancestors thought so. Gowers,[1] in 1888, described the headaches of brain tumors as "constant, with paroxysmal exacerbations . . . with severity usually such that sleep is more or less disturbed by it, and in the acute paroxysms the mind may be unhinged by the intense agony. It is usually increased by whatever causes passive congestion of the brain, as a cough, or muscular effort . . . the locality of the pain does not always correspond to the locality of the disease." He noted the concurrence of "optic neuritis" (papilledema) in about four-fifths of brain tumor patients, and commented on the association with vomiting, particularly when the tumor was located within the posterior fossa.

While acknowledging the variability of headaches in brain tumor, Cushing, in 1908,[2] emphasized the tendency of headaches to occur particularly in the morning hours. He found the location to be of little diagnostic value, unless it was always in the same spot and associated with local tenderness of the skull, in which case it indicated, most likely, an underlying meningioma. He noted that "intracranial pain . . . is rarely absent; it may be insufferable." He pointed out that headache "may figure as the only symptom until late in the disease," but suggested that it was more usual for the headache to be accompanied by nausea and vomiting and "choked disk" (papilledema). Interestingly, given Cushing's eponymous association with the response, he commented that "pressure symptoms which characterise acute lesions (namely, rise in blood pressure, slow vagus pulse, and Cheyne-Stokes respiration) are conspicuous by their absence" in brain tumors.

Perhaps because of their access to technology that permits the identification of intracranial mass lesions at earlier stages, modern authorities seem not to encounter these classic presentations with the same frequency as did Gowers and Cushing. The early morning accentuation of brain tumor headaches is no longer usual; Dalessio[32] noted that if connected to the time of day the headache of brain tumor is more severe in the early part of the day, though not in the early hours of the morning, and Forsyth and Posner[8] reported that onset of headache in the morning occurred in only 17% of their brain tumor patients who had headaches, and morning worsening of the headaches occurred in only one-third. Nor are brain tumor headaches now regarded as among the most severe head pains. Dalessio[32] and Lavyne and Patterson[26] commented that migraine headache is usually much more intense than brain tumor headache. Dalessio singles out the headache of subdural hematoma, however, as being "usually intense," which may relate to the usually brisk evolution of this lesion and its association with increased intracranial pressure. Forsyth and Posner[8,25] describe most brain tumor headaches as "moderate to severe" in intensity, though less than half of their patients with brain tumor headaches considered the headaches to be the worst part of their illnesses; headache disturbed sleep in only about one-third of their patients, and headache could be relieved by simple analgesics in about half (in the presence of increased intracranial pressure, however, headache relief with simple analgesics became uncommon).

Coughing, straining, sudden head movements, jolting of the head, and sudden changes in posture are still reported by modern authors as triggers and exacerbators of brain tumor (and other intracranial mass lesion) headaches,[8,25,26,32] but they make the point that migraine headaches may also be worsened noticeably by the same maneuvers. It has been remarked[24] that brain tumor headache is "commonly aggravated by fever," which can also be seen in migraine. Forsyth and Posner,[8,25] among their patients with brain tumor headaches, found none whose pain was precipitated (as opposed to worsened) by changes in posture, coughing, or exertion; in only one-third of their patients were headaches worsened by bending over, and in only one-fourth were they aggravated by Valsalva's maneuver.

Rushton and Rooke[6] encountered nausea or vomiting in 46% of their brain tumor patients but found no clear relationship between those associated symptoms and increased intracranial pressure. Forsyth and Posner[8,25] found that 48% of their brain tumor patients had nausea or vomiting and that those symptoms tended to be related to increased intracranial pressure. Other neurologic features, such as seizures or weakness, accompany brain tumor headaches in the majority of cases. Of Forsyth and Posner's 111 patients with brain tumors,[8,25] only 30 (27%) were imaged primarily because of headache; in only 16% of brain tumor patients of Iversen et al.[7] were headaches the first symptom; in a study by Vazquez-Barquero et al.,[9] only 8% of adult patients with brain tumors had headaches and no other neurologic symptoms. Thus, although headache is not an uncommon symptom of brain tumors, it seldom walks alone.

In summarizing their experience with brain tumor headaches, Forsyth and Posner[8,25] stressed that classic brain tumor headaches were uncommon, that most of the headaches suffered by their tumor patients had characteristics consistent with tension-type headaches, and that a few of their patients' headaches seemed migrainous (though the migrainous headaches all displayed some atypical features). Silberstein and Marcelis[33] reached the same conclusion, noting, based on their review of the literature, that "there is a significant overlap between the headache of brain tumor and migraine and tension-type headache."

IDENTIFYING BRAIN TUMOR HEADACHES

Clearly, when a patient presents with a "classic" brain tumor headache (recent onset; morning occurrence; progressive worsening; triggering or exacerbation by sudden head movements, changes in posture, or straining; and association with nausea, vomiting, or neurologic symptoms) diagnosis is easy, and the need for imaging (CT or MRI) is evident. However, a full house is as rare in medicine as it is in poker. The majority of brain tumor headaches do not exhibit these classic features; they are nondescript, resembling mundane tension-type headaches and sometimes even migraine. How, then, are we to suspect that an ominous lesion underlies them?

The following features are danger signals that suggest that a patient's headaches are not simply tension-type or migraine headaches. The first two are "soft" signs that warrant consideration of investigation; the others are "hard" evidence of something amiss, and demand imaging. (1) Recent onset, especially in or after middle age. The majority of benign dysfunctional headaches (migraine and tension-type headaches) begin between childhood and young adulthood; headaches with later onset may be ominous. (2) Change in an established headache pattern, including increased frequency or intensity, refractoriness to medication, or the development of new features. (3) The association of other symptoms, especially if they occur or persist between headaches. (4) Any abnormal physical sign on neurologic examination.

MRI is more sensitive than CT scanning in detecting intracranial mass lesions,[34] but CT still suffices to demonstrate the vast majority of brain tumors, subdural hematomas, and brain abscesses. CT or MRI is indicated whenever there is a reasonable suspicion, clinically, that headache may be due to an intracranial mass lesion. That clinical suspicion must rest, now as in the time of Gowers and Cushing, on a careful history and a careful physical examination—for which technology is no substitute.

Why not simply do CT or MRI on all patients who present with headaches? In these days of managed care, indiscriminate imaging of headaches is not cost effective. The Quality Standards Subcommittee of the American Academy of Neurology reported that of 897 CT and MRI scans performed in patients with clear-cut migraine and normal physical examinations, only 4 (or 0.4%) were abnormal, revealing three intracranial tumors and one arteriovenous malformation.[35] The patient with the arteriovenous malformation and one of the tumor patients also had seizures and would have had imaging in any case. The second tumor, a papilloma of the choroid plexus, was clearly incidental. The third tumor was a glioblastoma. Commenting on this series, Frishberg[36] maintained that in adults with recurrent migraine, with no recent change in pattern, no seizures, and no focal symptoms or signs, the routine use of neuroimaging is unwarranted.

In patients with nonmigrainous headaches and with normal neurologic examinations, the yield is somewhat better. In the American Academy of Neurology series,[35] 1,825 imaging procedures on patients with nonmigrainous headaches and normal examinations yielded 21 tumors, 6 arteriovenous malformations, 3 aneurysms, 5 subdural hematomas, and 8 cases of hydrocephalus—a total of 2.4% abnormal conditions. One might argue that this yield, though small, is sufficient to justify widespread screening of nonmigrainous headaches through neuroimaging. A useful counterpoint is the study of Dumas et al.[37] In their series of 373 patients with chronic headaches (longer than 6 months' duration), with no neurologic abnormalities on examination, who were referred because of increased severity of headaches, change in headache pattern, resistance to treatment, or family history of intracranial lesions, 402 CT scans (mostly enhanced) were done. Fourteen scans showed mild and irrelevant abnormalities such as cerebral atrophy or old infarcts. Four showed lesions deemed significant: two osteomas, one low-grade glioma, and one aneurysm. Only the aneurysm was treated. The authors' conclusion that the price of discovering this single treatable lesion, in terms of imaging costs, was $72,243 is perhaps contrived. One might argue that by using a 6-month duration of headache as an entry criterion they biased their series toward patients not very likely to have progressive lesions. The brain tumor headache patients of Forsyth and Posner[8,25] had a mean duration of symptoms, prior to diagnosis, of 3.5 weeks (though the range was from a few days to a year). Nevertheless, it is difficult to escape the conclusion that routine scanning of patients with headaches, no other symptoms, and normal neurologic examinations is not cost effective.

SUMMARY

Only a tiny minority of headaches are due to brain tumors or other intracranial mass lesions, but recognition of those few is critical. About 50% of adults with brain tumors have headaches as a significant symptom of their disease. This figure is higher in children (50–70%). With other mass lesions, such as subdural hematoma and brain abscess, headaches are more often encountered (in 80–90%), perhaps because of the more rapid evolution of hematomas and abscesses compared with most neoplasms.

Factors that determine whether or not a mass lesion will produce headache include (1) its rate of growth: rapidly expanding lesions are more likely to produce headache; (2) its location: posterior fossa lesions, more prone than supratentorial lesions to cause increased intracranial pressure, are more likely to cause headache; and (3) the patient's history of benign dysfunctional headaches, such as migraine: such a history may sensitize the patient so that he or she is more likely to develop headache as a symptom of a mass lesion.

The headaches produced by brain tumors and other mass lesions seldom appear as isolated symptoms. Only about 8–12% of adults and children with brain tumors had headaches as their only symptom, and among those, most also had abnormal neurologic examinations.

The "classic" brain tumor headache—occurring in the morning, precipitated by maneuvers that increase intracranial pressure, and accompanied by vomiting— is unusual. Brain tumors in both adults and children are likely to produce headaches that can mimic tension-type and even migraine headaches.

Routine neuroimaging (CT or MRI) of all headaches is not a cost-effective way to diagnose intracranial lesions. The keys to diagnosis, as always, are thorough history taking and careful examination. If these steps reveal a patient with recent onset of a headache that does not conform to the profile of migraine, or a recent change in a headache pattern, then neuroimaging should be considered. If they reveal the presence of other symptoms, particularly between headaches, or the presence of any physical abnormality, then imaging is essential. A careful clinician is the best instrument for detecting brain tumors in patients with headaches.

REFERENCES

1. Gowers WR. A Manual of Diseases of the Nervous System. American Edition. Philadelphia: Blakiston, 1888;884.
2. Cushing H. Surgery of the Head. In WW Keen (ed), Surgery: Its Principles and Practice. 1908. Published in facsimile by the Classics of Neurology and Neurosurgery Library. Birmingham, AL: Gryphon Editions, 1983;222.
3. Galicich JH, Sundaresan N. Metastatic Brain Tumors. In RH Wilkins, SS Rengachary (eds), Neurosurgery. New York: McGraw-Hill, 1985;600.
4. Salcman S. Supratentorial Gliomas: Clinical Features and Surgical Therapy. In RH Wilkins, SS Rengachary (eds), Neurosurgery. New York: McGraw-Hill, 1985;581.
5. Kunkle EC, Ray BS, Wolff HG. Studies on headache: The mechanisms and significance of the headache associated with brain tumor. Bull NY Acad Med 1942;18:400.
6. Rushton JG, Rooke ED. Brain tumor headache. Headache 1962;2:147.
7. Iversen HK, Strange P, Sommer W, Tyalve E. Brain tumor headache related to tumor size, histology, and location. Cephalalgia 1987;7(Suppl 6):394.
8. Forsyth PA, Posner JB. Headaches in patients with brain tumors: A study of 111 patients. Neurology 1993;43:1678.
9. Vazquez-Barquero A, Ibanez FJ, Herrera S, et al. Isolated headache as the presenting clinical manifestation of intracranial tumor: A prospective study. Cephalalgia 1994;14:270.
10. Suwanwela N, Phanthumchinda K, Kaoropthum S. Headache in brain tumor: A cross-sectional study. Headache 1994;34:435.

11. Honig PJ, Charney EB. Children with brain tumor headaches. Am J Dis Child 1982;136:121.
12. Kennedy CR, Nathwani A. Headache as a presenting feature of brain tumours in children. Cephalalgia 1995;15(Suppl 16):15.
13. Hockaday JM. Headaches in Children. In FC Rose (ed), Handbook of Clinical Neurology (Vol. 4): Headache. Amsterdam: Elsevier, 1986;31.
14. McKissock W. Subdural hematoma: A review of 389 cases. Lancet 1960;1:1365.
15. Britt RH. Brain Abscess. In RH Wilkins, SS Rengachary (eds), Neurosurgery. New York: McGraw-Hill, 1985;1928.
16. Ray BS, Wolff HG. Experimental studies on headache: Pain-sensitive structures of the head and their significance in headache. Arch Surg 1940;41:813.
17. Schumacher GA, Wolff HG. Experimental studies on headache. Arch Neurol Psychiatry 1941;45:199.
18. Sorensen PS, Corbett JJ. High Cerebrospinal Fluid Pressure. In J Olesen, P Tfelt-Hansen, KMA Welch (eds), The Headaches. New York: Raven, 1993;679.
19. Pepin EP. Cerebral metastasis presenting as migraine with aura. Lancet 1990;336:127.
20. Greulich W. Migrane un epilepsie bei zerebralem menineom. Fortschr Neurol Psychiatr 1988;56:44.
21. Pearce JM, Foster JB. An investigation of complicated migraine. Neurology 1965;15:333.
22. Debryne J, Crevits L, van der Eecken H. Migraine-like headache in intraventricular tumors. Clin Neurol Neurosurg 1982;84:51.
23. Schlake HP, Grotemeyer KH, Husstedt IW, et al. Symptomatic migraine: Intracranial lesions mimicking migrainous headache: A report of three cases. Headache 1991;31:661.
24. Shuper A, Packer RJ, Vezina LG, et al. Complicated migraine-like episodes in children following cranial irradiation and chemotherapy. Neurology 1995;45:1837.
25. Forsyth PA, Posner JB. Intracranial Neoplasms. In J Olesen, P Tfelt-Hansen, KMA Welch (eds), The Headaches. New York: Raven, 1993;705.
26. Lavyne MH, Patterson RH. Headache Associated with Brain Tumor. In DJ Dalessio (ed), Wolff's Headache and Other Head Pain (5th ed). New York: Oxford University Press, 1987;343.
27. Cushing H, Eisenhardt L. Meningiomas: Their Classification, Regional Behaviour, Life History, and Surgical End Results. Springfield, IL: Thomas, 1938;56.
28. Takakura K, Sano K, Hojo S. Hirano A. Metastatic Tumors of the Central Nervous System. Tokyo: Igaku, 1982;28.
29. Carmel PW. Craniopharyngiomas. In RH Wilkins, SS Rengachary (eds), Neurosurgery. New York: McGraw-Hill, 1985;905.
30. Wakai S, Fukushima T, Teramoto A, Sano K. Pituitary apoplexy: Its incidence and clinical significance. J Neurosurg 1981;55:187.
31. Portenoy RK, Abissi CJ, Lipton RB, et al. Headache in cerebrovascular disease. Stroke 1984;15:1009.
32. Dalessio DJ. Clinical Observations on Headache. In DJ Dalessio (ed), Wolff's Headache and Other Head Pain (5th ed). New York: Oxford University Press, 1987;407.
33. Silberstein SD, Marcelis J. Headache associated with changes in intracranial pressure. Headache 1992;32:84.
34. Lear J, Weston P. CT scanning and pseudotumor cerebri [letter]. Lancet 1994;343:1638.
35. Alter M, Daube JR, Franklin G, et al. Practice parameter: The utility of neuroimaging in the evaluation of patients with normal neurological examinations. Neurology 1994;44:1353.
36. Frishberg BM. The utility of neuroimaging in the evaluation of headache in patients with normal neurological examinations. Neurology 1994;44:1191.
37. Dumas MD, Pexman JHW, Kreeft JH. Computed tomography evaluation of patients with chronic headache. Can Med Assoc J 1994;151:1447.

20
Headache in Spontaneous Carotid and Vertebral Artery Dissections

Bahram Mokri

In the past two decades, much progress has been made in recognizing the clinical features, angiographic and imaging characteristics, outcome, incidence, and rate of recurrence of spontaneous carotid and vertebral artery dissections.[1,2] Among the cervicocephalic arterial dissections, the most commonly involved vessel is the extracranial internal carotid artery (ICA), followed by dissections of the vertebral arteries (VA). VA dissections may extend to the intracranial segment of the artery or may be entirely intracranial. ICA dissections only infrequently extend intracranially. Other intracranial dissections are rare and show far less specific angiographic and imaging features. Intracranial dissections carry the risk of subarachnoid hemorrhage. This chapter addresses the headaches associated with spontaneous VA and extracranial ICA dissections.

INCIDENCE

Spontaneous ICA and VA dissections are well-recognized causes of stroke in young and middle-aged adults,[3] although many of the VA dissections and most ICA dissections do not cause strokes.[4,5] A study of the population of Rochester, MN, determined an annual incidence rate of 2.6 per 100,000 for symptomatic spontaneous ICA dissections.[6] Because some dissections are asymptomatic or are only minimally symptomatic (and therefore not recognized), the true incidence of ICA dissections is undoubtedly somewhat higher. In our practice, the frequency of VA dissections is about one-third that of ICA dissections. It is therefore reasonable to assume that the combined true annual incidence of spontaneous ICA and VA dissections is approximately 4–5 per 100,000 population.

PATHOLOGY AND PATHOGENESIS

Cervicocephalic arterial dissections occur as the result of penetration of circulating blood through an intimal tear into the wall of the artery. The penetrated blood subsequently extends for varying distances along the vessel. The penetration of blood is typically within the media. It would be quite unusual to note subintimal or subadventitial penetration of blood in spontaneous dissections of the extracranial segments of the ICA and VA (B. Mokri, D. G. Piepgras, unpublished data).

When the blood penetrates through the arterial wall, one of the following may occur:

1. An elongated intramural hematoma may be formed, pushing the lumen to one side and thus creating an elongated narrowing of the true lumen (Figure 20.1A). Angiographically, this appears as a long segment of stenosis, frequently with irregular borders and sometimes quite tight and resembling a string (the "string sign"). The stenosis often begins at about 1–2 cm above the bifurcation and usually, although not invariably, extends to the carotid canal. Here, as demonstrated by angiography, often a fairly abrupt distal reconstitution of the lumen occurs (Figure 20.1B).
2. The intramural hematoma may become large enough to completely compress and occlude the true lumen of the vessel (Figure 20.2A). When angiogram is carried out, a tapered, flamelike occlusion of the ICA is noted, usually about 1–2 cm above the bifurcation (Figure 20.2B).
3. The intramural hematoma may find its way back into the true lumen distally, in which case two parallel channels of circulation are noted, similar to a double-barreled gun. One lumen is the original true lumen, and the other one is the false lumen created by the dissection (Figure 20.3).
4. Sometimes the intramural hematoma may expand toward the adventitia and create an aneurysmal dilatation—a "dissecting aneurysm" (Figure 20.4). Sometimes these aneurysms may contain thrombi and cause distal embolization (Figure 20.5).
5. Any combination of the above might be encountered. Particularly noted is the occurrence of stenosis and one or even more dissecting aneurysms in the same vessel.

ETIOLOGY

Despite the name "spontaneous" dissections—meaning no report of an overt trauma—sometimes a trivial or mild trauma is reported, such as coughing, blowing the nose, turning the head, sleeping in the wrong position, sports activities, etc. The etiologic factors in spontaneous ICA dissections can be classified in two major groups, the *extrinsic* and *intrinsic* factors. The extrinsic factors mostly relate to the role of trivial trauma. Flexion and extension or rotation of the neck have been implicated as possible mechanisms of trauma to the ICA and VA.[7–9] The intrinsic factors pertain to a number of arterial diseases that may predispose the vessel to the development of dissection. Angiographic changes of fibromuscular dysplasia have been noted in the ICAs, VAs, or renal arteries in approximately 12–15% of the patients with ICA dissections.[1,2,10–15] Carotid and VA dissections have been reported in Marfan's syndrome[16–18] and in Ehlers-Danlos syndrome.[19,20] Cystic medial necrosis[21–25] has been noted in a number of

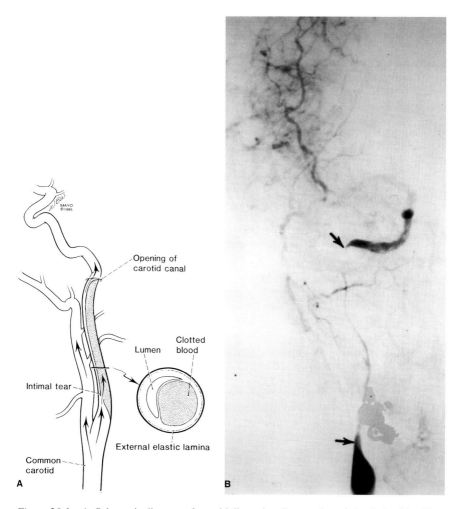

Figure 20.1 A. Schematic diagram of carotid dissection. Penetration of circulating blood has resulted in an elongated intramural hematoma, which in turn has compressed the true lumen, resulting in an elongated narrowing of the true lumen. (Modified with permission from TM Sundt Jr, BW Pearson, DG Piepgras, et al. Surgical management of aneurysms of the distal extracranial internal carotid artery. J Neurosurg 1986;64:169.) B. Carotid angiogram demonstrating the elongated stenosis as marked between the two arrows ("string sign"). Note the fairly abrupt reconstitution of the lumen at about the carotid canal (upper arrow).

patients with ICA dissections. The occurrence of multivessel cervicocephalic and visceral dissections,[26,27] the higher incidence of intracranial aneurysms in patients with spontaneous cervicocephalic dissections,[28] the familial association of intracranial aneurysms and cervicocephalic dissections,[29] the familial occurrence of arterial dissections and congenitally bicuspid aortic valve,[30] and the familial occurrence of carotid and VA dissections[31] all point to the presence of

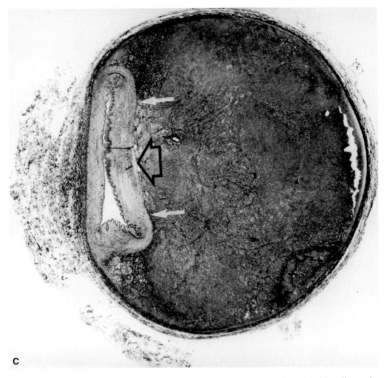

c

Figure 20.1 continued   C. Cross section of internal carotid artery involved by dissection. The intramural hematoma has compressed (arrows) and narrowed the true lumen of the vessel.

an underlying primary arterial disease, sometimes familial, that may predispose the arteries to the development of dissection. Using monoclonal antibody technique, abnormalities of elastin and fibrillin have been noted in cultured dermal fibroblasts in a significant percentage of patients with spontaneous ICA and VA dissections.[32,33] In patients with ICA dissections, hypertension is more common than in the general population.[4] Migraine has been considered a risk factor by some.[34] The role of smoking and contraceptives is less clear.

AGE AND SEX

Spontaneous ICA and VA dissections usually occur in middle-aged or younger persons. Overall, more than 70% of the patients are younger than 50 years. In our experience the mean age has been approximately 45. The disease is slightly more common in women, and the female patients are somewhat younger than the male patients. Furthermore, the patients with VA dissections are somewhat younger than those with ICA dissections (mean age, 40.5 versus 46.5 years).

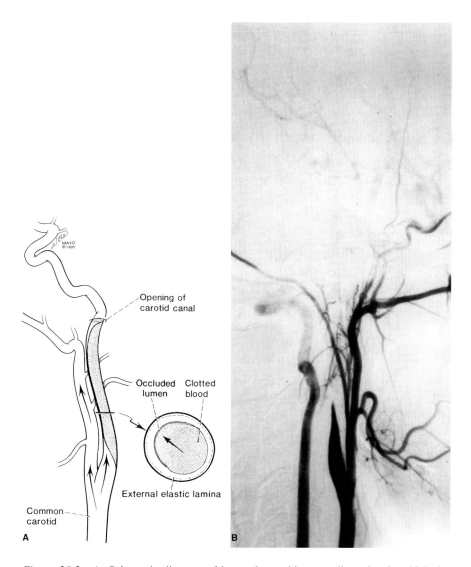

Figure 20.2   A. Schematic diagram of internal carotid artery dissection in which the intramural hematoma has become so large that it has squeezed the true lumen to complete occlusion. (Reprinted with permission of the Mayo Foundation.) B. On angiography the occlusion has a tapered, flamelike appearance. (Reprinted with permission from B Mokri. Dissections of Cervicocephalic Arteries. In FB Meyer [ed], Sundt's Occlusive Cerebrovascular Disease [2nd ed]. Philadelphia: Saunders, 1994;45; with permission of the Mayo Foundation.)

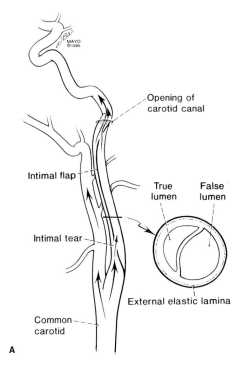

Figure 20.3   A. Schematic diagram of internal carotid artery dissection. Here the intramural hematoma has reopened distally to the true lumen and therefore a double lumen is created. (Reprinted with permission of the Mayo Foundation.) B. Carotid angiogram in a patient with internal carotid artery dissection and double lumen. The two lumens are separated by a long intimal flap (arrows). (Reprinted with permission from B Mokri, TM Sundt Jr, OW Houser, DG Piepgras. Spontaneous dissection of the cervical internal carotid artery. Ann Neurol 1986;19:126, with permission of Little, Brown.)

CLINICAL MANIFESTATIONS

Internal Carotid Artery Dissections

In most patients the initial manifestation of an ICA dissection is pain (headache, face pain, or neck pain), usually ipsilateral to the site of the dissection. In a smaller percentage of patients, cerebral ischemic symptoms may be the initial presenting manifestation. Symptoms and signs in spontaneous ICA dissections are listed in Table 20.1 in decreasing order of frequency. Overall, the common clinical syndromes with which the patients present include (1) a syndrome of hemicrania plus an ipsilateral oculosympathetic palsy, (2) a syndrome of hemicrania and delayed focal cerebral ischemic symptoms (stroke or transient ischemic attacks [TIAs]), and less commonly (3) a syndrome of lower cranial nerve palsies usually associated with ipsilateral headache or face pain.[1,4,35–39]

Sometimes these syndromes, particularly the first two, coexist, and one dominates the clinical picture. Additional manifestations, such as neck pain, amaurosis fugax, subjective or objective bruits, dysgeusia, ocular motor palsy or fifth-nerve palsy, or scintillating scotomas, may occur. Spontaneous dissections of the ICA may be asymptomatic or may present monosymptomatically as bruit only, oculosympathetic palsy only, headache only, hemilingual palsy only, or ocular motor palsy only. However, such modes of manifestation are quite uncommon.

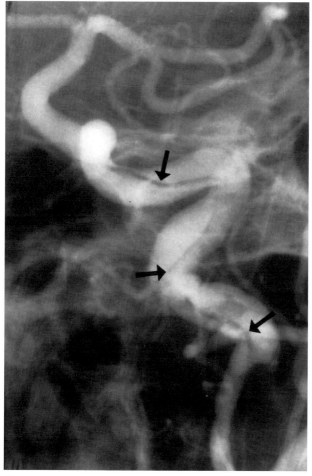

B

Vertebral Artery Dissections

The most common symptom of VA dissection is headache and neck pain.[1,2,11,14,40,41] The most common clinical syndrome is a posterior headache, with or without neck pain, followed after a period of delay by stroke or TIAs in vertebral basilar distribution. Less frequently, patients may present with vertebral basilar TIAs or stroke only or with only headache, neck pain, or both; in an occasional patient the VA dissection may occur asymptomatically (Table 20.2). Dissections of the intracranial segment of the vertebral arteries sometimes present as subarachnoid hemorrhage. Some of the rare and unusual modes of presentation of VA dissections include vertigo and upside-down vision,[42] hemifacial spasm,[43] pain in upper extremity,[44] sometimes mimicking myocardial infarction,[45] acute cervical epidural hemorrhage (B. Mokri, unpublished data), bilateral distal upper limb amyotrophy,[46] intermittent left upper limb pain mimicking myocardial infarction, respiratory arrest,[47] and

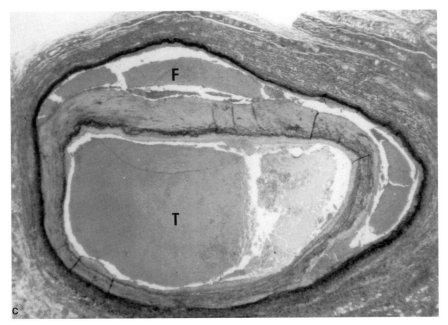

Figure 20.3 continued   C. On cross section, the true lumen (T) and the false lumen (F) can be seen (elastin van Gieson's stain).

transient amnesia.[48] The most common presentation, however, is headache, neck pain, or both, followed after a period of delay by a lateral medullary syndrome (Wallenberg's syndrome) with or without additional manifestations. Occurrence of lateral medullary syndrome in a young person, especially when preceded by a posterior headache or neck pain, should strongly suggest VA dissection.

Angiographic Features

The most common angiographic features of ICA and VA dissections include stenosis, often irregular and tapered (Figure 20.1B and Figure 20.6), aneurysms (Figure 20.4B), intimal flaps (Figure 20.3B), and occlusion (Figure 20.2B).[1,2,5,11,24,36,37,49,50] Sometimes distal branch occlusions are seen, especially in ICA dissections, indicating distal embolization (Figure 20.5). Also with tight stenoses of ICA, slow flow in ICA–middle cerebral artery circulation may be demonstrated. The angiographic features of the ICA and VA dissections are listed in Tables 20.3 and 20.4 in decreasing order of frequency.

Magnetic Resonance Imaging and Angiography

Magnetic resonance imaging (MRI) and magnetic resonance angiography (MRA) have demonstrated increasing usefulness in the diagnosis of ICA and

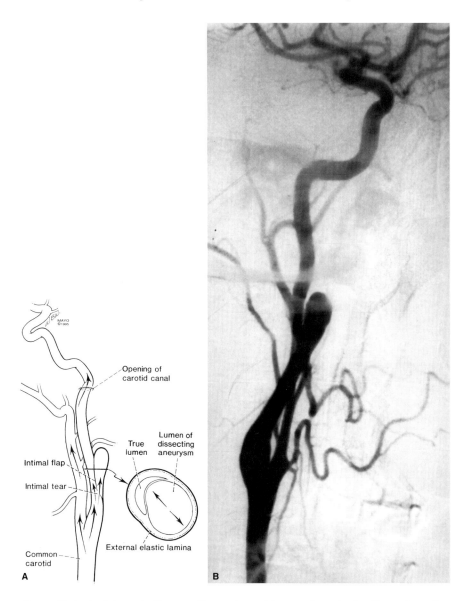

Figure 20.4   A. Schematic diagram of internal carotid artery dissection leading to formation of a dissecting aneurysm. (Reprinted with permission of the Mayo Foundation.) B. Carotid angiography demonstrating a dissecting aneurysm. (Reprinted with permission from B Mokri. Dissections of Cervicocephalic Arteries. In FB Meyer [ed], Sundt's Occlusive Cerebrovascular Disease [2nd ed]. Philadelphia: Saunders, 1994;45; with permission of the Mayo Foundation.)

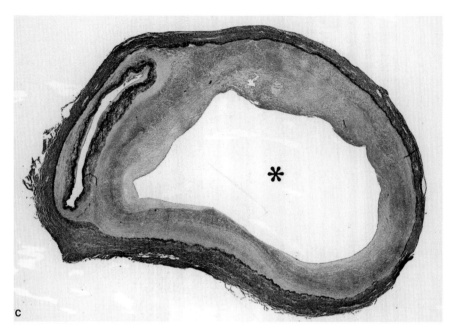

Figure 20.4 continued   C. Cross section through a dissecting aneurysm demonstrating the aneurysmal sac (asterisk) next to the true lumen of the internal carotid artery, both surrounded by the external elastic lamina (elastin van Gieson's stain). (Reprinted with permission from B Mokri. Dissections of Cervicocephalic Arteries. In FB Meyer [ed], Sundt's Occlusive Cerebrovascular Disease [2nd ed]. Philadelphia: Saunders, 1994;45; with permission of the Mayo Foundation.)

VA dissections.[51–55] In cross-sectional imaging of the artery at the involved level, not only the lumen but also the intramural hematoma can be seen—the lumen as a dark circle of flow void smaller than the normal caliber of the original vessel, and the intramural clot as a hyperintense and bright crescent or circle (in both T1 and T2 images) surrounding the flow void circle (Figure 20.7). MRA can demonstrate arterial stenosis and many of the aneurysms. MRI and MRA likely will evolve into the imaging modalities of choice for most cases of ICA and VA dissections. With the current techniques, however, tight stenoses may appear as signal void, many of the intimal irregularities may be missed, and the smaller aneurysms may not be demonstrated. Even now, one can document the presence of dissection by MRI or MRA in many patients and avoid subjecting them to invasive angiography, though some of the more subtle changes that may provide etiologic clues may be missed. Close to one-half of VA dissections and 20% of ICA dissections occur bilaterally. Concomitant spontaneous dissections of the ICAs and VAs are not rare.

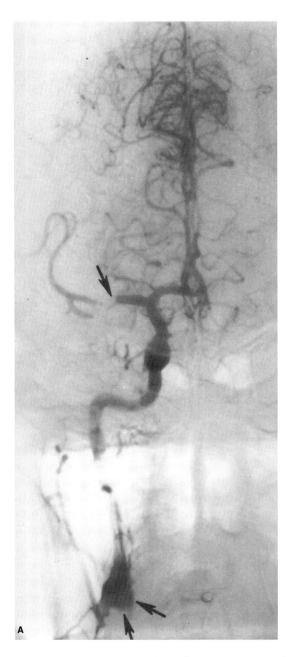

Figure 20.5 A. Carotid angiogram demonstrating a dissecting aneurysm (lower two arrows) with an embolus lodged in the origin of the right middle cerebral artery (upper arrow).

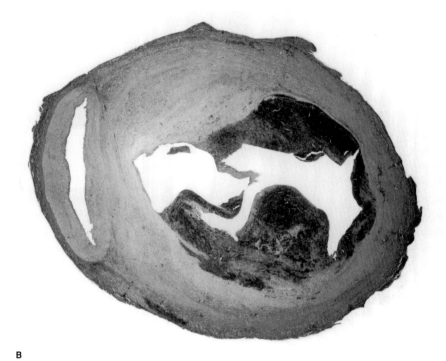

B

Figure 20.5 continued   B. Cross section of the right internal carotid artery at the level of the aneurysm. Aneurysmal sac is located within the media and contains organized thrombus. The lumen of the internal carotid artery is clearly seen next to the sac of the aneurysm (hematoxylin and eosin stain). (Reprinted with permission from B Mokri, DE Piepgras, TM Sundt Jr, BW Pearson. Extracranial internal carotid artery aneuryms. Mayo Clin Proc 1982;57:310, with permission of the Mayo Foundation.)

Doppler Sonography

Doppler sonography is a simple, noninvasive method that can be helpful in diagnosis of ICA dissection and in monitoring its evolution and resolution.[56–59] The test is less helpful in VA dissections.[60]

TREATMENT

The treatment of ICA and VA dissections has not been studied prospectively, although a European trial comparing antiplatelet and anticoagulant therapy in acute ICA dissection has been initiated.[61] Many patients do well regardless of treatment or lack of it, although some may end up with stroke. The mechanism of stroke is likely hemodynamic in a significant minority and embolic in the

Table 20.1   Frequency of symptoms and signs in 70 patients with spontaneous dissections of extracranial internal carotid artery

Symptom or sign	Number of patients	Percentage
Headache	59	84
Focal cerebral ischemic symptoms	43	61
TIAs	24	—
Stroke	13	—
TIAs and stroke	6	—
Oculosympathetic paresis	37	53
Bruits (subjective, objective, or both)	32	46
Neck pain	16	23
Light-headedness	15	21
Syncope	8	—
Amaurosis fugax	8	—
Scalp tenderness	5	—
Neck swelling	3	—
Dysgeusia	2	—
Lower cranial nerve palsies	2	—
Asymptomatic*	1	—
Sensation of pulsation in neck	1	—

*Symptoms related to a concomitant vertebral artery dissection.
TIA = transient ischemic attack.
Source: Reprinted with permission from B Mokri. Traumatic and spontaneous extracranial internal carotid artery dissections. J Neurol 1990;237:356.

Table 20.2   Clinical manifestations in 25 patients with spontaneous vertebral artery dissections

Symptoms and signs	Number of patients
Headache with or without neck pain, with delayed (5 hours to 2 weeks) vertebrobasilar ischemic symptoms	13
Brain stem stroke (especially lateral medullary syndrome)	10
Vertebrobasilar transient ischemic attack	3
Vertebrobasilar ischemic symptoms associated with or followed by headache with or without neck pain	3
Vertebrobasilar ischemic symptoms alone	4
Other	
Focal unilateral headache	1
Severe occipital headache and neck stiffness (subarachnoid hemorrhage)	1
Asymptomatic (symptoms related to internal carotid artery dissection)	3

Source: Reprinted with permission from B Mokri, OW Houser, BA Sandok, DG Piepgras. Spontaneous dissections of the vertebral arteries. Neurology 1988;38:880.

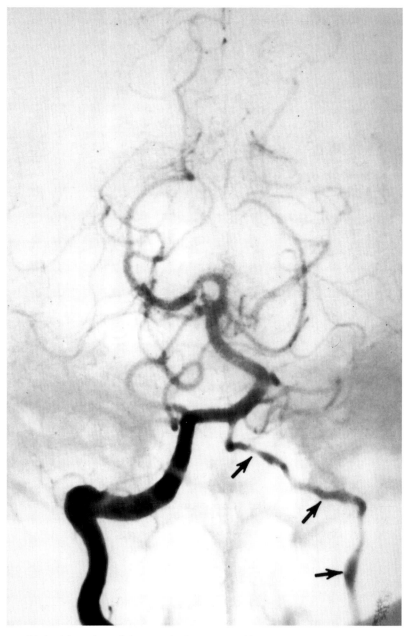

Figure 20.6   Dissection of the vertebral artery manifested by an elongated segment of irregular stenosis (arrows). (Reprinted with permission from B Mokri. Dissections of Cervicocephalic Arteries. In FB Meyer [ed], Sundt's Occlusive Cerebrovascular Disease [2nd ed]. Philadelphia: Saunders, 1994;45; with permission of the Mayo Foundation.)

Table 20.3 Angiographic findings in 70 patients with spontaneous internal carotid artery dissections (involving 90 arteries)

Angiographic findings	Number	Percentage
Luminal stenosis	69	77
Aneurysm	35	39
Intimal flaps	25	28
Slow internal carotid artery–middle cerebral artery flow	22	24
Occlusion	15	17
Distal branch occlusions (emboli)	11	12

Source: Reprinted with permission from B Mokri. Traumatic and spontaneous extracranial internal carotid artery dissections. J Neurol 1990;237:356.

Table 20.4 Initial angiographic findings in 25 patients with spontaneous vertebral artery dissections (involving 35 arteries)

Angiographic findings	Number	Percentage
Stenosis (often irregular and tapered)	28	80
Aneurysm	5	14
Occlusion	4	11
Intimal flap only	1	—

Source: Reprinted with permission from B Mokri, OW Houser, BA Sandok, DG Piepgras. Spontaneous dissections of the vertebral arteries. Neurology 1988;38:880.

majority. Because it is virtually impossible to predict with certainty the likelihood of occurrence of embolic stroke in each patient, one common practice (in the absence of medical contraindications to anticoagulant therapy) has been to treat the patients with anticoagulant medication (warfarin, or in urgent cases, heparin with a subsequent switch to warfarin) for about 3 months, followed by antiplatelet treatment for a similar length of time. Anticoagulation is not advised if a massive cerebral infarction has already occurred or if there is hemorrhagic infarction.[62] In dissections that are extended intracranially, great caution should be exercised. A cerebrospinal fluid examination is recommended prior to commencement of anticoagulant treatment. Obviously, subarachnoid hemorrhage is a contraindication to anticoagulant therapy. Resection of a residual dissecting aneurysm that has been a source of embolization should be considered if technically possible.[4] In patients with subarachnoid hemorrhage due to leaking intracranial dissections, surgery should be considered when possible. Occasional patients with tight stenosis of the ICA who present with hemodynamic ischemic symptoms may benefit from STA–middle cerebral artery bypass.[63,64]

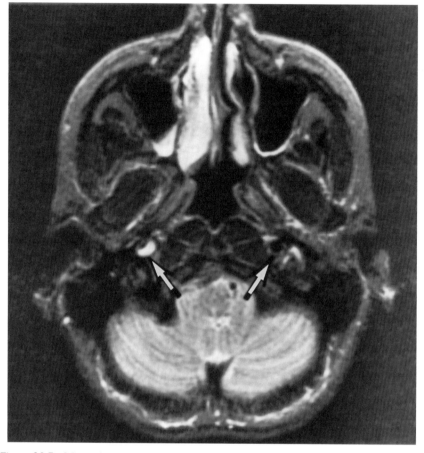

Figure 20.7   Magnetic resonance imaging of the head in a patient with unilateral internal carotid artery dissection. The two arrows point to the internal carotid arteries. On the right, the normal-sized, dark, round area of flow void is seen. On the left, the region of the flow void is much smaller, reflecting the narrowed lumen of the vessel. The region of flow void is surrounded by a bright crescent reflecting the intramural hematoma.

RATE OF RECURRENCE AND OUTCOME

Recurrence of dissection in a previously dissected and healed vessel is exceedingly rare. In a patient who has developed dissection of an ICA or VA, the development of dissection in the uninvolved ICAs or VAs is uncommon but not rare. The recurrence rate for such dissections is 2% for the first month and much less frequent from then on (1% per year for all age groups, but somewhat more frequent for the younger patients and somewhat less frequent for the older patients).[64]

The majority of the patients with spontaneous ICA or VA dissections experience excellent clinical and angiographic recovery.[4,37] A complete or excellent clinical recovery occurs in about 85% of the patients with spontaneous

ICA dissections. Angiographically, stenotic lesions either completely resolve or markedly improve in about 85% of the involved vessels. About 60% of the dissecting aneurysms resolve or diminish in size. For VA dissections, the rate of clinical recovery is about the same in that more than 85% of the patients make complete or very good recoveries, although the prognosis for those with subarachnoid hemorrhage is more guarded. Angiographically, more than 75% of the nonoccluded vessels involved by dissection either significantly improve or return to normal[5,37] (Figure 20.8). Death from massive infarct and edema may occur, but fortunately is quite uncommon (< 5%). Studies that have drawn their cases from acute stroke registries have reported significantly higher death and disability rates.[65] These, however, do not represent the usual profile of the disease.

HEADACHE IN INTERNAL CAROTID ARTERY AND VERTEBRAL ARTERY DISSECTIONS

Cephalic pain is a cardinal manifestation of ICA and VA dissections. Some patients (about one-fourth) also have neck pain, more commonly with VA dissections (about one-half) than with ICA dissections. Generally speaking, pain (headache, face pain, neck pain) by far is the most frequent feature of the clinical syndromes with which ICA and VA dissections present, and it is the initial manifestation of ICA dissections in about 80% of the symptomatic cases (Table 20.5). The headaches and face pains of ICA and VA dissections are usually focal and unilateral (Table 20.6).

Data from Silbert et al.,[66] based on the study of 135 patients with symptomatic ICA dissection and 26 patients with symptomatic VA dissection (VAD), show the presence of pain in 79% of the patients with ICA dissections (ICAD) and in 88% of the patients with VAD (Table 20.7). In their series, in those patients with dissections who did have headaches, the headache was the initial manifestation in 47% for the ICAD group and in 33% for the VAD group. Other investigators have also reported high incidence of headaches in such patients.[1,2,67–69] Orbital or facial pain is also quite common in ICA dissections, but not in VA dissections. In Silbert's series, orbital or facial pain without associated headache was noted in 10% of the patients with ICAD, and an additional 53% had orbital and facial pain plus headaches. None of the patients with VAD had orbital or facial pain. Neck pain was more common in VAD (46%) than in ICAD (26%). The features of headaches in ICAD and VAD are listed in Table 20.8. The pain of ICAD is typically unilateral and mostly distributed over the anterior head and orbital and facial area. The pain of VAD is typically distributed over the posterior head regions. It can be unilateral or bilateral (Figure 20.9). When unilateral, the pain is always ipsilateral to the symptomatic dissection.

In ICA dissections, headaches, when present, precede other manifestations (occurring as the initial symptom) in about one-half of the cases. In about 10% of the patients, the headaches follow other clinical manifestations of the disease, whereas in about 40% they occur along with other manifestations of the disease. In VA dissections, headaches, when present, occur as the initial manifestation in one-third of the patients; only in a small number of patients do they follow other

344

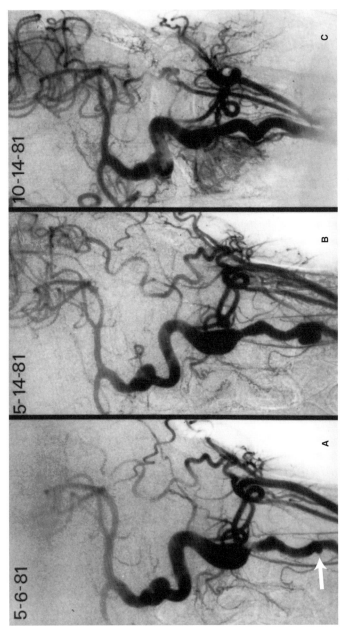

5-6-81   5-14-81   10-14-81

A   B   C

Figure 20.8   Cerebral angiograms demonstrating evolution and resolution of dissecting aneurysm and reflecting dynamic nature of the angiographic changes of dissections. A. Dissection of cervical segment of internal carotid artery manifested by elongated, irregular narrowing. A tiny expansion is noted in the stenotic area (arrow). B. Within 8 days the tiny expansion (in retrospect, a small dissecting aneurysm) has evolved into a definite dissecting aneurysm. The stenosis persists. C. Five months later both the stenosis and the aneurysm have completely resolved. (Reprinted with permission from B Mokri. Dissections of Cervicocephalic Arteries. In FB Meyer [ed], Sundt's Occlusive Cerebrovascular Disease [2nd ed]. Philadelphia: Saunders, 1994;45; with permission of the Mayo Foundation.)

Table 20.5 Initial manifestation in 65 patients with spontaneous dissection of the internal carotid artery

Manifestation	Number of patients
Headache	47 (80%)
Neck pain	5
Transient ischemic attack or stroke	8
Amaurosis fugax	3
Syncope	2
Total	65

Source: B Mokri, TM Sundt Jr, EA Shuster, et al. Unpublished data.

Table 20.6 Location of headache in 33 patients with spontaneous dissection of the internal carotid artery

Location	Number of patients
Diffuse, bilateral	2
Diffuse, unilateral	3
Focal, unilateral	28
Orbital, periorbital	20
Ear, mastoid process	13
Frontal	12
Temporal	9
Angle of mandible	4
Face	3
Occipital	3

Source: Reprinted with permission from B Mokri, TM Sundt Jr, OW Houser, et al. Spontaneous dissection of the cervical internal carotid artery. Ann Neurol 1986;19:126.

Table 20.7 Frequency of pain associated with symptomatic spontaneous internal carotid artery and vertebral artery dissections

	Internal carotid artery dissections (n = 135)	Vertebral artery dissections (n = 26)
Headache	92 (68%)	18 (69%)
Additional orbital, facial pain, or both	71 (53%)	0
Orbital or facial pain alone	13 (10%)	0
Neck pain	35 (26%)	12 (46%)
Without other pain	2	5 (19%)
Overall frequency of pain (head, face, or neck)	107 (79%)	23 (88%)

Source: Data from PL Silbert, B Mokri, WI Schievink. Headache and neck pain in spontaneous internal carotid and vertebral artery dissections. Neurology 1995;45:1517.

Table 20.8   Features of headache of spontaneous internal carotid artery (n = 135 patients) and vertebral artery (n = 26 patients) dissections

	Headache of internal carotid artery dissections (n = 92)	Headache of vertebral artery dissections (n = 18)
Onset		
Preceding other manifestations (as the initial symptom)	43 (47%)	6 (33%)
With other manifestations	40 (43%)	11 (61%)
Following other manifestations	9 (10%)	1 (6%)
Mode of onset		
Gradual	78 (85%)	13 (72%)
Abrupt	13 (14%)	4 (22%)
Gradual/abrupt	1	1
Location		
Unilateral frontal/frontotemporal	56 (61%)	1
Unilateral occipital/parieto-occipital	8	10 (56%)
Hemicranial	21 (23%)	1
Generalized	7	1
Bioccipital	0	5 (28%)
Ipsilateral*	84 (91%)	12 (67%)
Character		
Constant	67 (73%)	10 (56%)
Pulsating	23 (25%)	8 (44%)

*When headache is unilateral, it is *always* at the same side on the dissection.

Source: Data from PL Silbert, B Mokri, WI Schievink. Headache and neck pain in spontaneous internal carotid and vertebral artery dissections. Neurology 1995;45:1517.

manifestations of the disease; and in the majority (more than 60%) they occur along with the manifestations of disease, which usually consist of ischemic events (stroke or TIAs) in vertebrobasilar distribution (see Table 20.8). When the headaches of dissection precede other clinical manifestations, the interval between the onset of the headache and other manifestations may vary from hours to many days; the median delay is 96 hours (mean delay, 8.8 days) for ICA dissections and 14.5 hours (mean delay, 3.7 days) for VA dissections.

In about three-fourths of the patients with ICA and VA dissections, the onset of headache is gradual. More than 10% of the patients with ICA dissections and more than 20% of the patients with VA dissections who have headaches say that onset of the headache is severe, sudden, and "thunderclap." When such headaches are the initial manifestation of the disease, a diagnosis of subarachnoid hemorrhage is often entertained. Some of the patients with intracranial VA dissections or intracranial extensions of extracranial VA dissections may present with subarachnoid hemorrhage and such headaches. However, in most of the patients with carotid or VA dissections who present with sudden severe headaches, fortunately a concomitant subarachnoid hemorrhage does not exist.

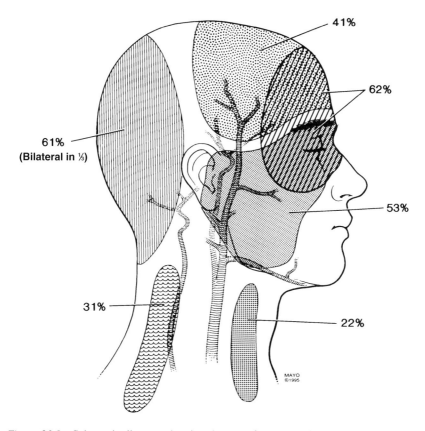

Figure 20.9   Schematic diagram showing the most frequent regions of headache and neck pain in internal carotid artery and vertebral artery dissections. Note that for internal carotid artery dissection, the most common site of pain is frontal, orbital, and periorbital, with the neck pain mostly in the anterolateral aspect of the neck. For vertebral artery dissections, the most frequent location of the headache is occipital, with the neck pain in the posterolateral aspect of the neck. (Based on data from PL Silbert, B Mokri, WI Schievink. Headache and neck pain in spontaneous internal carotid and vertebral artery dissections. Neurology 1995;45:1517; Reprinted with permission of the Mayo Foundation.)

   The headache of dissection is throbbing only in less than one-fourth of ICA dissections and in somewhat more than 40% of the patients with VA dissections. The majority of the patients, however, have nonthrobbing headaches, described as constant, steady aching or steady sharp pain.
   Facial and orbital pains are quite common in ICAD but are rare in VAD. In Silbert's series, facial pain (including ear pain) was noted in one-third of the patients with ICAD, and orbital and eye pain in more than 42% of those patients. None of the patients with VAD reported facial or orbital pain. Orbital and facial pains are always ipsilateral to the ICA involved by dissection.

Table 20.9   Neck pain in symptomatic spontaneous internal carotid artery (n = 135 patients) and vertebral artery (n = 26 patients) dissections

	Internal carotid artery dissections	Vertebral artery dissections
Frequency	35 (26%)	12 (46%)
Onset		
Preceding other manifestations (as the initial symptom)	9	5
With other manifestations	25	7
After other manifestations	1	0
Location		
Anterolateral	30/35 (86%)	0
Posterolateral	1/35 (3%)	8/12 (67%)
Posterior bilateral	0	4/12 (33%)
Anterior midline	4/35 (11%)	0

Source: Reprinted with permission from PL Silbert, B Mokri, WI Schievink. Headache and neck pain in spontaneous internal carotid and vertebral artery dissections. Neurology 1995;45:1517.

Neck pain occurs in about one-fourth of patients with ICAD and slightly fewer than half of patients with VAD. Neck pain can be the initial manifestation of VAD in about 20% of cases, whereas in ICAD, the neck pain may be the initial manifestation in only 6% or 7%. In ICAD, the neck pain is located in the anterolateral aspect of the neck in more than 86% of cases; in VAD, it is located in the posterolateral aspect of the neck in practically all of the patients and is unilateral in about two-thirds and bilateral in about one-third of the cases (Table 20.9).

One question that might arise is what effect carotid or VA dissection would have on preexisting headache, as well as how likely would be the development of new headaches after such dissections. In the cohort of 161 patients studied by Silbert et al., about 30% of the patients with ICA and VA dissections reported no prior history of headache (Table 20.10). About 19% of the patients had a history of migraine, and about half had a history of muscle contraction headaches. Following dissection, about one-third of the patients who had a history of migraines reported either resolution or decrease in their migraine headaches. Of 121 patients who did not have a history of migraines, only three reported new development of migraine-type headaches (< 2.5%). Therefore, more patients reported having obtained some relief from their migraine headaches than reported having developed new migraine headaches following their dissections. It is possible that long-term use of aspirin as an antiplatelet agent had a role in relief of migraine headaches in some of these patients. A small percentage of patients with ICA dissection (8%) reported a decrease in or resolution of their muscle contraction tension headaches after the dissection, and 14% reported having developed muscle contraction headaches following the dissection. A small percentage of patients with ICA dissections may end up with chronic daily headaches or chronic dissection headaches that may linger for months or even a few years (Table 20.11). Chronic dissection headaches are headaches, often different from headaches previously experienced by the patients, that develop with the onset of the dissection.

Table 20.10   History of headache in symptomatic spontaneous internal carotid artery and vertebral artery dissections

	Internal carotid artery dissections (n = 135)	Vertebral artery dissections (n = 26)
Migraine	24 (18%)	6 (23%)
Without aura	11	5
With aura	12	1
Acephalgic	1	—
Muscle contraction headache	69[a] (51%)	11 (42%)
Other headaches		
Mixed vascular-tension	7	3
Cluster	3	—
Miscellaneous[b]	9	—
No prior headache history	40 (30%)	8 (31%)

[a]Including eight patients who also had history of migraine.
[b]Related to menstruation, sinus disease, or unclassified.
Source: Data from PL Silbert, B Mokri, WI Schievink. Headache and neck pain in spontaneous internal carotid and vertebral artery dissections. Neurology 1995;45:1517.

Table 20.11   Postdissection headache

	Internal carotid artery dissections	Vertebral artery dissections
Migraine		
Decreased or resolved	6/23 (26%)	2/6 (33%)
Developed	3/111 (3%)	0/20
Muscle contraction headaches		
Decreased or resolved	10/69 (8%)	0/11
Developed	5/66 (14%)	0/15
Chronic daily headaches developed	4/135 (3%)	0/26
Chronic dissection headache developed	4/135 (3%)	0/26

Source: Data from PL Silbert, B Mokri, WI Schievink. Headache and neck pain in spontaneous internal carotid and vertebral artery dissections. Neurology 1995;45:1517.

Instead of resolving within a period of days or weeks, they may persist steadily, with a fluctuating intensity, or intermittently for months or even a few years.

About 60% of the patients with ICA dissections and 50% of the patients with VA dissections who have headaches point to the uniqueness of their headaches; i.e., the headaches have features never experienced by them previously.

Although the pathology in the ICA dissection is typically in the cervical segment of the vessel, the occurrence of neck pain is far less common than that of headache or face pain, consistent with the observation that stimulation of the carotid artery bifurcation can produce frontal, orbital, periorbital, and facial

Table 20.12   Migraine prevalence in the general population and in patients with internal carotid artery and vertebral artery dissections

Population	Male (%)	Female (%)
U.S. population[a]		
All ages	5.7	17.6
Age of maximum prevalence (35–45 years)	8	27
ICAD and VAD cohort[b] (aged 30–50 years)	10.2	31
ICAD and VAD cohort[c]		
Cohort	40 (20/50)	
Control	24 (24/100)	

[a]Data from WF Stewart, RB Lipton, DD Celentano, ML Reed. Prevalence of migraine headache in the United States: Relation to age, income, race, and other sociodemographic factors. JAMA 1992;267:64.
[b]Data from PL Silbert, B Mokri, WI Schievink. Headache and neck pain in spontaneous internal carotid and vertebral artery dissections. Neurology 1995;45:1517.
[c]Data from J D'Anglejan-Chatillon, V Ribeiro, JL Mas, BD Youl, et al. Migraine: A risk factor for dissection of cervical arteries. Headache 1989;29:560.
ICAD = internal carotid artery dissection; VAD = vertebral artery dissection.

pain.[70] The headache of VAD is typically occipital and may be explained by the fact that upper cervical nerves innervate the vasculature of the posterior fossa.[71] Electrical stimulation of vertebrobasilar arteries can cause pain in the neck and occipital area. Balloon inflation of distal internal carotid arteries and middle cerebral arteries can cause focal pain in ipsilateral temporal, orbital, and frontal areas,[72] and balloon inflation of vertebrobasilar arteries can cause ipsilateral focal pain primarily in the occipital area and posterolateral neck and shoulder.[73]

MIGRAINE AND CAROTID ARTERY DISSECTION

The relationship of migraine to carotid artery dissection presents a number of issues. First, carotid or VA dissection may present a clinical picture similar to migraine or may masquerade as a migraine stroke.[74–76] Second, occasionally patients may report onset of migraine headaches after a bout of ICA dissection. Third, after dissection more patients get relief from their migraines than develop migraine headaches.[67,77] Fourth, migraines have been implicated as one of the predisposing factors for cervical artery dissection. D'Anglejan-Chatillon et al., in a prospective study, recorded a history of migraines in 40% of the patients with ICA and VA dissections (male and female patients combined) but in only 24% of the controls.[34] Silbert, in the study of a cohort of patients with ICA and VA dissections, found a history of migraine in 10.2% of the males and 31% of the females aged 30–50 years. Stewart's data on prevalence of migraine in the U.S. population[78] showed a rate of 8% in the men and 27% in the women aged 35–45 years (the age range of maximum prevalence). These data are summarized in Table 20.12. Silbert's data, when compared with Stewart's prevalence data, suggest that any increased prevalence of migraine in patients with ICA or VA dissection is minimal. However, the prevalence of migraine in patients with dissection may be underestimated in retrospective studies. Past history of migraine does not seem to increase the likelihood of strokes in patients with ICA and VA dissections. Data from Biousse et al.[68] suggest that in patients with extracranial ICA dissection, when there is history of migraine the dissection is more likely to be associated with pain. Silbert's data did not demonstrate that history of migraine had any significant influence on the frequency of pain in ICA or VA dissections. However, it was noted that the headache of ICA and VA dissections tended to be more pulsatile in patients who have a history of migraine.

REFERENCES

1. Hart RG, Easton JD. Dissections of cervical and cerebral arteries. Neurol Clin 1983;1:155.
2. Mokri B. Dissections of Cervicocephalic Arteries. In FB Meyer (ed), Sundt's Occlusive Cerebrovascular Disease (2nd ed). Philadelphia: Saunders, 1994;45.
3. Bogousslavsky J, Regli F. Ischemic stroke in adults younger than 30 years of age: Cause and prognosis. Arch Neurol 1987;44:479.
4. Mokri B, Sundt TM Jr, Houser OW, Piepgras DG. Spontaneous dissection of the cervical internal carotid artery. Ann Neurol 1986;19:126.
5. Mokri B, Houser OW, Sandok BA, Piepgras DG. Spontaneous dissections of the vertebral arteries. Neurology 1988;38:880.
6. Schievink WI, Mokri B, Whisnant JP. Internal carotid artery dissection in a community: Rochester, Minnesota, 1987–1992. Stroke 1993;24:1678.
7. Barnett HJM. Progress towards stroke prevention: Robert Wartenberg Lecture. Neurology 1980;30:1212.
8. Stringer WL, Kelly DL Jr. Traumatic dissection of the extracranial internal carotid artery. Neurosurgery 1980;6:123.
9. Zelenock GB, Kazmers A, Whitehouse WM Jr, et al. Extracranial internal carotid artery dissections: Noniatrogenic traumatic lesions. Arch Surg 1982;117:425.
10. Andersen CA, Collins GJ Jr, Rich NM, et al. Spontaneous dissection of the internal carotid artery associated with fibromuscular dysplasia. Am Surg 1980;46:263.
11. Chiras J, Marciano S, Vega Molina J, Touboul J, et al. Spontaneous dissecting aneurysm of the extracranial vertebral artery (20 cases). Neuroradiology 1985;27:327.
12. Garcia-Merino JA, Gutierrez JA, Lopez-Lozano JJ, et al. Double lumen dissecting aneurysms of the internal carotid artery in fibromuscular dysplasia: Case report. Stroke 1983;14:815.
13. Kramer W. Hyperplasie fibromusclaire et anévrisme extracranien de la carotide interne avec syndrome parapharyngien typique. Rev Neurol (Paris) 1969;120:239.
14. Mas JL, Bousser MG, Hasboun D, Laplane D. Extracranial vertebral artery dissections: A review of 13 cases. Stroke 1987;18:1037.
15. Ringel SP, Harrison SH, Norenberg MD, et al. Fibromuscular dysplasia: Multiple "spontaneous" dissecting aneurysms of the major cervical arteries. Ann Neurol 1977;1:301.
16. Mokri B, Okazaki H. Cystic medial necrosis and internal carotid artery dissection in a Marfan's sibling: Partial expression of Marfan's syndrome. J Stroke Cerebrovasc Dis 1992;2:100.
17. Austin MG, Schaefer RF. Marfan's syndrome, with unusual blood vessel manifestations. Arch Pathol 1957;64:205.
18. Youl BD, Coutellier A, Dubois B, Leger JM, et al. Three cases of spontaneous extracranial vertebral artery dissection. Stroke 1990;21:618.
19. Lach B, Nair SG, Russell NA, Benoit BG. Spontaneous carotid-cavernous fistula and multiple arterial dissections in type IV Ehlers-Danlos syndrome: Case report. J Neurosurg 1987;66:462.
20. Schievink WI, Limburg M, Oorthuys JWE, Fleury P, et al. Cerebrovascular disease in Ehlers-Danlos syndrome type IV. Stroke 1990;21:626.
21. Boström K, Liliequist B. Primary dissecting aneurysm of the extracranial part of the internal carotid and vertebral arteries: A report of three cases. Neurology 1967;17:179.

22. Brice JG, Crompton MR. Spontaneous dissecting aneurysms of the cervical internal carotid artery. BMJ 1964;2:790.
23. Liliequist B. The roentgenologic appearance of spontaneous dissecting aneurysm of the cervical internal carotid artery: Report of a case. Vasc Surg 1968;2:223.
24. Luken MG III, Ascherl GF Jr, Correll JW, et al. Spontaneous dissecting aneurysms of the extracranial internal carotid artery. Clin Neurosurg 1979;26:353.
25. Thapedi IM, Ashenhurst EM, Rozdilsky B. Spontaneous dissecting aneurysm of the internal carotid artery in the neck: Report of a case and review of the literature. Arch Neurol 1970;23:549.
26. Mokri B, Stanson AW, Houser OW. Spontaneous dissections of the renal arteries in a patient with previous spontaneous dissections of the internal carotid arteries. Stroke 1985;16:959.
27. Mokri B, Houser OW, Stanson AW. Multivessel cervicocephalic and visceral arterial dissections: Pathogenic role of primary arterial disease in cervicocephalic arterial dissections. J Stroke Cerebrovasc Dis 1991;1:117.
28. Schievink WI, Mokri B, Piepgras DG. Angiographic frequency of saccular intracranial aneurysms in patients with spontaneous cervical artery dissection. J Neurosurg 1992;76:62.
29. Schievink WI, Mokri B, Michels VV, et al. Familial association of intracranial aneurysms and cervical artery dissections. Stroke 1991;22:1426.
30. Schievink WI, Mokri B. Familial arterial dissections and congenitally bicuspid aortic valve. Stroke 1995;26:1935.
31. Mokri B, Piepgras DG, Wiebers DO, et al. Familial occurrence of spontaneous dissection of the internal carotid artery. Stroke 1987;18:246.
32. Mokri B, Roche PC, O'Brien JF, Schievink WI, et al. Abnormalities of elastin in spontaneous internal carotid and vertebral artery dissections. Ann Neurol 1994;36:263.
33. Mokri B, Roche PC, O'Brien JF. Fibrillin and elastin abnormalities in spontaneous internal carotid (ICA) and vertebral artery (VA) dissections. J Neurol 1995;242:S66.
34. D'Anglejan-Chatillon J, Ribeiro V, Mas JL, Youl BD, et al. Migraine: A risk factor for dissection of cervical arteries. Headache 1989;29:560.
35. D'Anglejan Chatillon J, Ribeiro V, Mas JL, et al. Dissection de l'artère carotide interne extracranienne: Soixante-deux observations. Presse Med 1990;19:661.
36. Fisher CM, Ojemann RG, Roberson GH. Spontaneous dissection of cervico-cerebral arteries. Can J Neurol Sci 1978;5:9.
37. Mokri B. Traumatic and spontaneous extracranial internal carotid artery dissections. J Neurol 1990;237:356.
38. Mokri B, Silbert P, Schievink W, Piepgras D. Cranial nerve palsies in spontaneous dissections of internal carotid arteries. Neurology 1996;46:356.
39. Mokri B, Schievink WI, Olsen KD, Piepgras DG. Spontaneous dissection of the cervical internal carotid artery: Presentation with lower cranial nerve palsies. Arch Otolaryngol Head Neck Surg 1992;118:431.
40. Caplan LR, Baquis GD, Pessin MS, et al. Dissection of the intracranial vertebral artery. Neurology 1988;38:868.
41. Caplan LR, Zarins CK, Hemmati M. Spontaneous dissection of the extracranial vertebral arteries. Stroke 1985;16:1030.
42. Charles N, Froment C, Rode G, et al. Vertigo and upside down vision due to an infarct in the territory of medial branch of the posterior inferior cerebellar artery caused by dissection of a vertebral artery. J Neurol Neurosurg Psychiatry 1992;53:188.
43. Matsumoto K, Toshikazu S, Hideyuki K. Hemifacial spasm caused by spontaneous dissecting aneurysm of the vertebral artery. J Neurosurg 1991;74:650.
44. Giroud M, Gras P, Dumas R, et al. Spontaneous vertebral artery dissection initially revealed by a pain in one upper arm. Stroke 1993;24:480.
45. Linden D, Steinke W, Schwartz A, et al. Spontaneous vertebral artery dissection initially mimicking myocardial infarction. Stroke 1992;23:1021.
46. Pullicino P. Bilateral distal upper limb amyotrophy and watershed infarcts from vertebral dissection. Stroke 1994;25:1870.
47. Roos KL, Harris T. Vertebral artery dissection manifested by respiratory arrest. J Neuroimaging 1992;2:161.
48. Laterra J, Gebarski S, Sackellares JC. Transient amnesia resulting from vertebral artery dissection. Stroke 1988;19:98.
49. Ehrenfeld WK, Wylie EJ. Spontaneous dissection of the internal carotid artery. Arch Surg 1976;111:1294.

50. Houser OW, Mokri B, Sundt TM Jr, et al. Spontaneous cervical cephalic arterial dissection and its residuum: Angiographic spectrum. AJNR 1984;5:27.
51. Quint DJ, Spickler EM. Magnetic resonance demonstration of vertebral artery dissection: Report of two cases. J Neurosurg 1990;72:964.
52. Goldberg HI, Grossman RI, Gomori JM, et al. Cervical internal carotid artery dissecting hemorrhage: Diagnosis using MR. Radiology 1986;158:157.
53. Bui LN, Brant-Zawadzki M, Verghese P. Magnetic resonance angiography of cervicocranial dissection. Stroke 1993;24:126.
54. Kitanka C, Tanaka JI, Kuwahara M, et al. Magnetic resonance imaging study of intracranial vertebrobasilar artery dissections. Stroke 1994;28:571.
55. Zuber M, Meary E, Meder JF, et al. Magnetic resonance imaging and dynamic CT scan in cervical artery dissections. Stroke 1994;25:576.
56. Steinke W, Rautenberg W, Schwartz A, et al. Noninvasive monitoring of internal carotid artery dissection. Stroke 1994;25:998.
57. Rothrock JF, Lim V, Press G, et al. Serial magnetic resonance and carotid duplex examinations in the management of carotid dissection. Neurology 1989;39:686.
58. Ley-Pozo J, Ringelstein EB. Noninvasive detection of occlusive disease of the carotid siphon and middle cerebral artery. Ann Neurol 1990;28:640.
59. Müllges W, Ringelstein EB, Leibold M. Noninvasive diagnosis of internal carotid artery dissections. J Neurol Neurosurg Psychiatry 1992;55:98.
60. Sturzenegger M, Mattle HP, Rivoir A, Rihs F, et al. Ultrasound findings in spontaneous extracranial vertebral artery dissection. Stroke 1993;24:1910.
61. Krämer G. Anticoagulation versus acetyl salicylic acid in carotid dissection [abstract]. J Neurol 1992;239:3.
62. Saver JL, Easton JD, Hart RG. Dissections and Trauma of Cervicocerebral Arteries. In HJM Barnett, JP Mohr, BM Stein, FM Yatsu (eds), Stroke: Pathophysiology, Diagnosis, and Management (2nd ed). New York: Churchill Livingstone, 1992;671.
63. Sundt TM Jr, Pearson BW, Piepgras DG, et al. Surgical management of aneurysms of the distal extracranial internal carotid artery. J Neurosurg 1986;64:169.
64. Mokri B, Piepgras DG, Houser OW. Traumatic dissections of the extracranial internal carotid artery. J Neurosurg 1988;68:189.
65. Schievink WI, Mokri B, O'Fallon WM. Rate of recurrence of cervical arterial dissection stroke. N Engl J Med 1994;330:393.
66. Silbert PL, Mokri B, Schievink WI. Headache and neck pain in spontaneous internal carotid and vertebral artery dissections. Neurology 1995;45:1517.
67. Fisher CM. The headache and pain of spontaneous carotid artery dissection. Headache 1982;22:60.
68. Biousse V, D'Anglejan J, Touboui PJ, Evrard SA, et al. Headache in 67 patients with extracranial internal carotid artery dissection. Cephalalgia 1991;11:232.
69. Sturzenegger M. Headache and neck pain: The warning symptoms of vertebral artery dissection. Headache 1994;34:187.
70. Fay T. Atypical facial neuralgia: Syndrome of vascular pain. Ann Otol Rhinol Laryngol 1932;41:1030.
71. Moskowitz MA, Buzzi MG, Sakas DE, Linnik MD. Pain mechanisms underlying vascular headaches: Progress report 1989. Rev Neurol (Paris) 1989;145:181.
72. Nichols FT, Mawad M, Mohr JP, et al. Focal headache during balloon inflation in the internal carotid and middle cerebral arteries. Stroke 1990;21:555.
73. Nichols FT, Mawad M, Mohr JP. Focal headache during balloon inflation in vertebral and basilar arteries. Headache 1993;33:87.
74. Bousser MG, Baron JC, Chiras J. Ischemic strokes and migraine. Neuroradiology 1985;27:583.
75. Shuaib A. Stroke from other etiologies masquerading as migraine-stroke. Stroke 1991;22:1068.
76. Young G, Humphrey P. Vertebral artery dissection mimicking migraine. J Neurol Neurosurg Psychiatry 1995;59:340.
77. Leys D, Moulion TH, Stojkovic T, et al. Follow-up of patients with history of cervical artery dissection. Cerebrovasc Dis 1995;5:43.
78. Stewart WF, Lipton RB, Celentano DD, Reed ML. Prevalence of migraine headache in the United States: Relation to age, income, race, and other sociodemographic factors. JAMA 1992;267:64.

21

Low Cerebrospinal Fluid Pressure Headache

Christine L. Lay, J. Keith Campbell, and Bahram Mokri

The production, absorption, and flow of cerebrospinal fluid (CSF) play key roles in the dynamics of intracranial pressure. Alterations in CSF pressure lead to neurologic symptoms, and the most common clinical manifestation is headache. Intracranial hypotension (ICH) occurs when there is decreased production of CSF, increased absorption of CSF, or leakage of CSF from a meningeal tear or defect.

Low CSF pressure headache is a familiar and distinct syndrome, seen most frequently after a lumbar puncture (LP). Patients describe an orthostatic headache, which develops in the upright position and is relieved with recumbency. Normal intracranial pressure is 70–200 mm H_2O, and symptoms of ICH typically develop with pressures below 50–90 mm H_2O. Although only 30–80% of patients with increased intracranial pressure develop headache, most patients with decreased intracranial pressure experience headache.[1] Marshall,[2] however, notes that not all individuals with low CSF pressure develop headache.

In the intact craniospinal vault, the brain is supported by the CSF, such that a brain weight of 1,500 g in air is only 48 g in CSF.[3] As the CSF pressure decreases, there is a reduction in the buoyancy of the brain's supportive cushion. As the brain "sags" in the cranial cavity, there is traction on the anchoring and supporting structures of the brain.[4–7] In fact, recent studies have shown that a "descent of the brain" can be seen on magnetic resonance imaging (MRI).[3,8–10] MRIs are obtained with the patient supine; it is likely that this descent of the brain would appear even more pronounced if the MRIs were to be obtained with the patient in an upright posture. Traction on pain-sensitive intracranial and meningeal structures, particularly cranial nerves V, IX, and X, the upper three cervical nerves, and bridging veins, is thought to cause headache and some of the associated symptoms.[6,11] In the upright position this traction is exaggerated, hence the postural component of the headache. Secondary vasodilatation of the cerebral vessels to compensate for the low CSF pressure may contribute to the vascular component of the headache by increasing brain volume.[5,12–14] Because jugular venous compression increases headache severity, it seems likely that venodilatation is a contributing factor in the headache.[11]

The International Headache Society[15] classifies a low CSF pressure headache as one that "occurs or worsens less than 15 minutes after assuming the upright position and disappears or improves less than 30 minutes after resuming the recumbent position." Classification may be further based on etiology,[1,16,17] for which categories include (1) post-LP (diagnostic, with myelography or spinal anesthesia), (2) spontaneous, (3) traumatic (with or without clinically obvious CSF leak), (4) postoperative (following craniotomy, spinal surgery, ventricular shunting), and (5) associated with other medical conditions (severe dehydration, diabetic coma, uremia, hyperpnea, meningoencephalitis, severe systemic infection). The orthostatic headaches seen most often are those of the post-LP, spontaneous, and CSF shunt overdrainage syndromes.

CLINICAL HISTORY AND EXAMINATION

The headache caused by ICH may be of sudden or gradual onset. Often it is described as an intense, severe, throbbing, or dull pain that may be generalized or focal.[16,18–22] Frontal pain is described by patients as often as is occipital and diffuse pain.[23] Exacerbating factors include erect posture, head movement, coughing, straining, or sneezing, and jugular venous compression.[1,18,23,24] Relief is typically obtained with recumbency, usually within minutes. The headache is rarely relieved with analgesics.[5] Interestingly, Schievink[17] described a patient who experienced some relief from headache during menses. Depending on the underlying etiology, the headache may spontaneously resolve within 2 weeks; but in some cases it may last months[25,26] or, in the experience of the present authors, years.

In 1825, Magendie described vertigo and unsteadiness in a patient following the removal of CSF.[24] Today the list of reported associated symptoms is varied and extensive. Commonly, patients may experience nausea, vomiting, anorexia, vertigo, dizziness, diaphoresis, neck stiffness, blurred vision, and photophobia.[4,5,7,17,18,24,25,27–30] Others have also reported the occurrence of tinnitus,[1,7,16,18,23,29,31] bilateral hyperacusis,[7,8] unsteadiness or staggering gait,[13,16] diplopia,[3,31,32] transient visual obscurations,[3] hiccups, and dysgeusia. Horton[3] recommends specifically asking the patient whether the asthenopia is improved with recumbency. In a review of 73 cases of ICH,[3] 17 (23%) experienced visual symptoms with their postural headaches. Yamamoto[33] described a case of severe postural headache associated with nausea and galactorrhea, which was thought to be due to compromised pituitary function secondary to compression of the pituitary stalk.

Neurologic examination is typically normal. Frequently, mild neck stiffness is noted.[34] Unilateral or bilateral abducens palsies have been reported,[3,31] as have visual field defects.[3,8] A slow pulse, or vagus pulse, has also been described.[5]

ETIOLOGY

Post–Lumbar Puncture Headache

In 1891 Quinke introduced the LP,[1] and in 1898 Bier suffered and was the first to report post-LP headache.[23] He proposed that ongoing leakage of CSF through the dural puncture site was the cause of the headache. This belief is maintained today; it is supposed that leakage of CSF through the dural rent made by the LP needle exceeds the rate of CSF production, resulting in low CSF pressure.[13,35]

The most common complication of an LP is headache.[36,37] The reported incidence ranges from 10–30%.[13,23,36–38] DiGiovanni[39] reports a range of 0.50–60.0%, stating that the incidence is dependent on the type of procedure. The incidence is 13% for surgical LP, 18% for obstetric, and 32% for LP done for diagnostic purposes. The lower incidence in surgical patients may be related to the prolonged time of recumbency after the surgical procedure. The typical individual who experiences a post-LP headache is a young woman with a low body mass index.[35,38] The incidence in women is twice that in men.[23,36,37,40] Children younger than 13 years and adults older than 60 are less likely to experience a post-LP headache.[41,42] Iqbal,[43] in an MRI study of 11 patients, found that the volume of CSF leakage after an LP did not correlate with the occurrence of a post-LP headache. The amount of CSF removed at the time of LP has also been shown not to influence the occurrence of headache.[38] Continued leakage of CSF has been shown to occur, whether or not headache develops.[44]

Onset of the headache may be within minutes or after up to 12 days[36]; however, more commonly it occurs within 12–24 hours of the LP.[30,45] Without treatment, the headache typically lasts 2–14 days (an average of 4–8 days).[1] Dripps[36] reported that 72% of cases resolved in less than 7 days and 96% resolved within 6 months.[46] Glass[47] reported an incapacitating postmyelogram headache that persisted for 18 weeks and resolved only after surgical repair of the puncture site. Vilming[40] reports that the more severe the post-LP headache, the more likely it is to be associated with other symptoms.

A number of different methods have been proposed to reduce the incidence of post-LP headache, including having patients lie supine or prone after the procedure, use of small-gauge needles (22 gauge or smaller), removal of the needle with the patient in the prone position, and hydration of the patient.[37] However, the only proven method is the use of small-gauge needles, which in many cases is not practical.[20,23,42,48–50] Raskin[23] comments on personal success with the method of removing the needle while the patient lies in the prone position.

Spontaneous Low Cerebrospinal Fluid Pressure

The clinical syndrome of spontaneous low CSF pressure headache or spontaneous ICH has been recognized for more than 55 years, but its etiology remains a matter of speculation. The syndrome was first proposed by Schaltenbrand in 1938,[51,52] who termed it *aliquorrhea* and described a headache syndrome virtually identical to that following LP. He proposed three pathophysiologic mechanisms to explain the symptoms: (1) decreased CSF production by the choroid plexus, due to a reversible disturbance of vasomotor function of the choroid plexus; (2) increased CSF absorption; and (3) CSF leakage through small tears.[4,19,47] Since that time, some authors have offered support for the decreased CSF production mechanism.[16,18,33,53] Yamamoto et al.[33] proposed that decreased production of CSF leads to brain sagging with compression of the pituitary-hypothalamic axis and consequently to further reduction in CSF production. Murros and Fogelholm[54] noted slit-like ventricles and tight basilar cisterns on computed tomographic (CT) scan in an individual with spontaneous ICH, and speculated whether the tight ventricles contributed to decreased CSF production by the choroid plexus. However, small ventricles are likely a consequence of a CSF leak rather than a cause of decreased CSF production.

A more accepted theory is that of CSF leakage, which may occur in the context of rupture of an arachnoid membrane.[27] It is believed that although the syndrome is considered spontaneous, careful questioning often elicits a history of minor trauma or an inciting event. In a review of 39 cases seen at the Mayo Clinic, 52% were associated with a history of minor trauma or an inciting event. Contributing factors may involve a fall onto the buttocks,[16,30] a sudden twist or stretch,[3,27] sexual intercourse or orgasm,[55] a sudden sneeze or paroxysm of coughing,[19] vigorous exercise,[7] strenuous brachial effort during racket sports,[32] or "trivial trauma."[56] These relatively minor events may cause rupture of spinal epidural cysts (formed during fetal development) or of perineural (Tarlov) cysts or a tear in a dural nerve sheath,[8,25,27,30,32,57,58] with resultant cryptic CSF leakage. Leakage of CSF into the petrous or ethmoidal regions[13] or through the cribriform plate can also occur, and although overt CSF otorrhea and CSF rhinorrhea may result, it is not uncommon for the patient to swallow the fluid and be unaware of the leak. Raskin[59] proposes that small CSF leaks are likely to be missed.

Hyperabsorption has also been proposed to explain low CSF pressure headache.[21,22,60,61] However, Rando and Fishman[25] suggest that in the absence of high intracranial pressure there are no known physiologic mechanisms to explain increased CSF absorption, and they propose that the findings of hyperabsorption are also consistent with those of CSF leakage.

Recently, a fourth mechanism has been recognized in the development of postural headache. Patients who have had CSF shunts placed (for various neurosurgical indications) may develop a headache syndrome essentially identical to that of spontaneous low CSF pressure headache.[62]

Although some reports suggest a female predominance of the spontaneous syndrome,[3,16,18,22] a review of our case series of 39 patients shows an equal representation of men and women. Because the majority of reports are based on small case series or on review of previously reported cases, the incidence of spontaneous low CSF pressure headache is unknown. Headache is a common ailment, and ICH patients typically present with a normal neurologic examination; thus the syndrome is probably underrecognized. Of course, other causes of spontaneous positional headache, such as a colloid cyst of the third ventricle, must be ruled out.[57]

As previously noted, there is often a history of minor trauma. Frequently the symptoms are delayed in relation to the inciting incident (by hours to months),[63] and indeed the trauma may be so minor as to be forgotten by the patient. Typically, the headache resolves in 2–4 weeks,[25] but it may take 16 weeks[26] or longer in some cases. In general, recurrences are rare.[16,18,27]

INVESTIGATIONS

Cerebrospinal Fluid Analysis

In cases of post-LP headache, the clinical history usually suffices for diagnosis; however, an LP may be necessary to document low CSF pressure, especially in suspected cases of spontaneous low CSF pressure.[12] To obtain an accurate measurement of the opening pressure, it is recommended that the measurement be performed with the patient in the lateral decubitus position. To ascertain correct placement of the spinal needle, CSF flow should be observed either spontaneously, with gentle aspiration,[16,51] or with Valsalva's maneuver.[1] LPs on these patients are not uncommonly recorded as difficult; sometimes repeated attempts are made; and traumatic blood-tinged fluids are not rare. So-called dry taps may sometimes be encountered, and in some patients, cisternal taps have been done to collect the fluid. In rare instances when the CSF pressure is negative (below that of atmospheric pressure), a sucking noise may be heard when the stylet is removed from the LP needle, and subsequently on radiography, air may be visible within the lateral ventricles.[16] An opening pressure consistent with a diagnosis of ICH has been reported to range from 0–70 mm H_2O.[4,5,16,19,26] However, in our series of 39 patients with proven spontaneous ICH, the opening pressure was sometimes in the range of normal, especially if the measurement was made after a period of recumbency.

In general, CSF analysis proves relatively benign in low pressure headache. Common abnormalities include a moderate pleocytosis, the presence of red blood cells, and elevated protein. Schaltenbrand originally postulated that hyperemia of the brain and meninges occurred with ICH and resulted in diapedesis of red blood cells into the subarachnoid space.[19,51] The elevated protein may be related to lowered CSF pressure leading to disruption of normal hydrostatic and oncotic pressure across the venous sinus and arachnoid villi, resulting in the passage of serum protein into the CSF.[12,25,29] Pleocytosis also likely reflects a reactive phenomenon secondary to hydrostatic pressure changes.[25,28] Additionally, there may be disruption of bridging cortical veins, which could lead to the observed abnormalities.[9]

Radioisotope Cisternography

A study particularly useful for identifying CSF leaks is radioisotope cisternography.[64] Placement of numbered cotton pledgets in the nose for subsequent detection of radioactivity aids in detection and localization of CSF leakage through the paranasal sinuses. A radioactive tracer is injected into the lumbar subarachnoid space, followed by gamma camera scanning of the entire neuraxis at 4, 8, and 24 hours (and sometimes longer) to observe the pattern of distribution of radioactivity. Normal CSF flow involves cephalad migration from the site of injection to the cerebral convexities and the sylvian fissures.[5] It is advisable to look for early accumulation within the bladder and kidneys, or leakage of isotope outside of the normal confines of the subarachnoid space (Figure 21.1). Numerous studies have concluded, based on results of cisternography, that CSF hyperabsorption, demonstrated by early appearance of tracer in the bladder or CSF leakage, explained examples of ICH.[21,22,61] However, this early appearance of tracer in the bladder may be a product of a leak and not necessarily a marker for hyperabsorption.[25] Water-soluble myelography and CT myelography have also been used to help localize the site or sites of CSF leakage (Figure 21.2), and still some leaks may be missed. Although CT myelography has a somewhat higher yield, the yield of both tests may be suboptimal.[13]

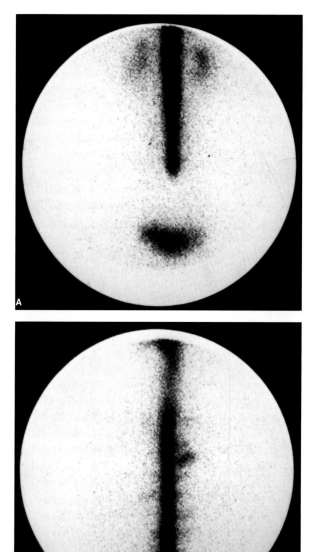

Figure 21.1 A. Posterior view scintiscan showing early accumulation of isotope in the kidneys and bladder after intrathecal administration. B. Extra-arachnoid leakage in the midthoracic region.

Neuroimaging

Both CT and MRI have been useful in evaluating low pressure headache. Like CSF analysis, these imaging studies are generally not done in cases of post-LP headache, where the diagnosis is more obvious. Murros and Fogelholm[54]

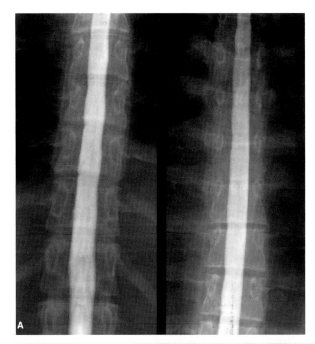

Figure 21.2 A. Oil-based pantopaque myelogram with sub-arachnoid placement of dye. B. Small extravasation of dye at T2 on the right and increasing subdural collection of dye through the ruptured root sleeve.

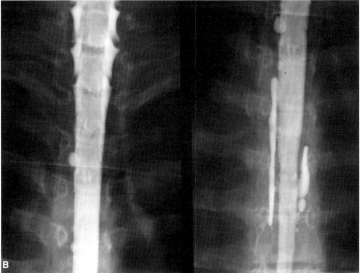

reported on the CT findings in a patient with spontaneous ICH. The ventricles were slit-shaped, with associated tight basal cisterns and scant CSF over the cortex. These changes resolved after resolution of the headache and were believed to be secondary to brain edema, perhaps itself secondary to venous dilatation.

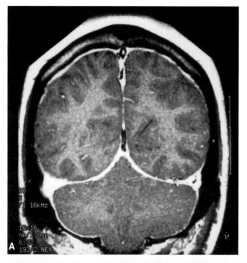

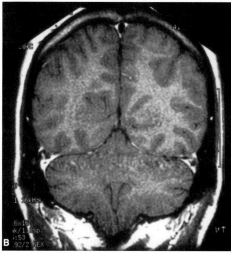

Figure 21.3   A. Magnetic resonance imaging coronal views demonstrating contiguous meningeal enhancement involving the convexity, falx, and tentorium. B. Resolution of meningeal enhancement following surgical repair of a lumbar cerebrospinal fluid leak.

Subdural hematomas or hygromas have been observed on both CT and MRI in association with low intracranial pressure syndromes.[3,10,25,26,29,56] The cause of the subdural hematomas is presumably rupture of the bridging veins as the CSF volume decreases and the brain sags, pulling away from the dura.[25] Grant et al.[65] measured CSF volume by MRI in 20 patients and found that the majority of reduced CSF volume could be explained by loss of fluid over the cortical sulci; thus, Grant et al. proposed such fluid loss as an explanation for the subdural hematomas seen in ICH.

In recent years, interesting findings have been noted on MRIs enhanced with gadolinium in patients with spontaneous ICH. Diffuse meningeal enhancement (DME) was first noted by Mokri et al.,[28] and it has subsequently been seen in many cases, including many in our own series[10,63,66] (Figure 21.3). Before DME was a recognized feature of spontaneous ICH, patients were often subjected to extensive testing to rule out other causes of DME such as meningeal carcinomatosis, meningitis, subarachnoid hemorrhage, neuroborreliosis, and neurosarcoidosis.[28,66] Meningeal enhancement has been observed to be contiguous (without skip areas) and involves both supratentorial and infratentorial compartments. The enhancement is pachymeningeal, without abnormal enhancement in the depth of the cortical sulci or around the brain stem.[10] Bourekas et al.,[48] in reporting on MRI findings in a post-LP headache patient, noted DME. The DME is believed to be secondary to vascular dilatation; in keeping with the Monro-Kellie doctrine, CSF volume fluctuates reciprocally with changes in the volume of other intracranial contents in an intact skull.[8,25,66,67] Venous engorgement results in a greater concentration of gadolinium in the dural vasculature and interstitial fluid of the dura, because the latter lacks tight junctions.[25] Others have attributed the DME to inflammation of the pachymeninges,[63,66,68] based on results of meningeal biopsy, and still others have found normal results on meningeal biopsy.[10] Meningeal biopsies in nine patients in our series have not shown any inflammatory changes. Debate continues as to the exact etiology of the DME, but Fishman and Dillon[8] have proposed that the meningeal fibrosis seen on biopsy was a late manifestation of chronic venous congestion. DME has been observed to improve or resolve with resolution of the headache.[8,10,28,31,66]

A second finding of interest is downward displacement of the brain.[8–10] Findings include cerebellar tonsilar herniation, descent of the brain stem, flattening of the basis pontis, and bowing of the optic chiasm over the pituitary gland, all of which are believed to contribute to the associated symptoms of low pressure headache. The authors note that the descent of the brain structures might have been worse if the scans had been performed with the patient in an upright position. These abnormalities diminish or resolve when the patient is asymptomatic.[10] Kasner et al.[69] described a case of spontaneous ICH associated with the radiographic appearance of a Chiari type I malformation, which resolved with resolution of the headache. A similar case is included in our series (Figure 21.4).

MANAGEMENT

Given enough time, a low pressure headache may resolve without treatment. However, in many instances intervention not only helps to speed recovery but may be necessary for a full recovery. Unfortunately, few scientific clinical trials have evaluated the effectiveness of the various treatment strategies employed. The most conservative treatment is avoidance of the upright position, with strict bed rest and the possible addition of analgesics. Frequently, however, patients are unable to comply with strict bed rest, and analgesics provide little relief.[4,5,20–22] Use of an abdominal binder has also been proposed.[5,70] Beyond these simple methods, treatment is aimed at increasing CSF volume either through fluid restoration or elimination of leakage. Strategies employed in an effort to restore CSF volume, and possibly to temporarily increase production above normal, include increased intravenous or oral fluid intake, increased salt intake, carbon dioxide inhalation, and corticosteroid therapy.[18,20,35,54,60] Theophylline[23] has also been used with some success to treat post-LP headache. Intravenous and oral caf-

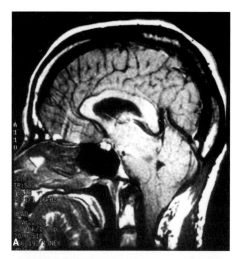

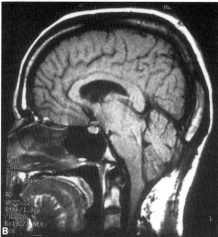

Figure 21.4   A. Same patient as shown in Figure 21.3. Magnetic resonance imaging sagittal view demonstrating descent of brain with crowding of the posterior fossa structures, resembling a Chiari type I malformation. B. Return to normal posterior fossa appearance with ascent of brain, following surgical repair of the cerebrospinal fluid leak.

feine have similarly been held to be beneficial in the treatment of low pressure headache.[5,7,13,18,23] It has been proposed that both theophylline and caffeine produce intracerebral arterial constriction via blockade of the adenosine receptors in the brain, leading to increased CSF pressure and reduction in headache.[71] A rather successful method of restoring the intracranial CSF volume, and thereby reducing headache, is a continuous epidural infusion of saline[7,56,72] or dextran.[73]

Epidural blood patching (EBP) was first introduced by Gormley in 1960 and involves the infusion of 10–20 ml of autologous blood into the epidural space.[5] In the treatment of post-LP headache, it has a success rate of 96.8%[12] and is 85–100% effective in the treatment of spontaneous low pressure headache,[19,20] even in headache of over 2 years' duration.[74] The mechanism that accounts for the success of EBP is not completely understood. Presumably, it works by tamponade of a dural leak, followed by fibrin deposition and eventual scar formation in 3 weeks' time,[5] but our experience has shown that lumbar placement of the EBP can be effective even when the site of the leakage is unknown or is above the site of the patch. Raskin proposes that, as with epidural infusions, introduction of the blood leads to an increase in CSF pressure (by compression of the dural sac), which antagonizes adenosine receptors and results in headache relief.[23] Surgical repair of a CSF leak may be required in some cases, particularly if more conservative measures fail.[9] Additionally, surgical treatment of subdural hematoma may be necessary. It has been noted that some headaches are relieved after myelography or cisternography, perhaps secondary to irritation and eventual healing of the leak.[30]

CONCLUSION

Low CSF pressure headache following an LP rarely creates a clinical dilemma; however, spontaneous onset, if not considered as a cause of new onset headache, may result in extensive and unnecessary clinical investigation. The diagnosis is suggested by positional headache, with or without associated symptoms, perhaps in the setting of minor trauma. Although low opening CSF pressure is likely to be confirmed by LP, in some cases the pressure may at times be normal. It is reasonable to obtain a head imaging study and to hold off on further workup unless the headache persists despite conservative treatment or EBP. If the MRI changes described previously are seen and if an adequate trial of bed rest and EBP have failed, radioisotope cisternography or water-soluble myelography and CT myelography should be considered. With radioisotope cisternography, the nasal pledget technique of seeking cryptic CSF rhinorrhea should be used. These procedures also offer an opportunity to examine the spinal fluid. Repeated EBP, continuous epidural saline infusion for 24–48 hours, and, rarely, surgical repair of the defect may be needed.

The condition of low CSF pressure is relatively benign, is self-limiting, and often carries an excellent prognosis. It is recognized with increasing frequency, and as it becomes more familiar, clinicians will gain more facility with its diagnosis and treatment.

REFERENCES

1. Silberstein SD, Marcelis J. Headache associated with changes in intracranial pressure. Headache 1992;32:84.
2. Marshall J. Lumbar-puncture headache. J Neurol Neurosurg Psychiatry 1950;13:71.
3. Horton JC, Fishman RA. Neurovisual findings in the syndrome of spontaneous intracranial hypotension from dural cerebrospinal fluid leak. Ophthalmology 1994;101:244.
4. Lipman IJ. Primary intracranial hypotension: The syndrome of spontaneous low cerebrospinal fluid pressure with traction headache. Dis Nerv Syst 1977;38:212.
5. Marcelis J, Silberstein SD. Spontaneous low cerebrospinal fluid pressure headache. Headache 1990;30:192.
6. Campbell JK, Caselli RJ. Headache and Other Craniofacial Pain. In WG Bradley, RB Daroff, GM Fenichel, CD Marsden (eds), Neurology in Clinical Practice. Stoneham, MA: Butterworth, 1991;1511.

7. Capobianco DJ, Kuczler FJ. Case report: Primary intracranial hypotension. Mil Med 1990;155:64.
8. Fishman RA, Dillon WP. Dural enhancement and cerebral displacement secondary to intracranial hypotension. Neurology 1993;43:609.
9. Jacobs MB, Wasserstein PH. Spontaneous intracranial hypotension: An uncommon and underrecognized cause of headache. West J Med 1991;155:178.
10. Pannullo S, Reich JB, Krol G, et al. MRI changes in intracranial hypotension. Neurology 1993;43:919.
11. Kunkle EC, Ray BS, Wolff HG. Experimental studies on headache: Analysis of the headache associated with changes in intracranial pressure. Arch Neurol Psychiatry 1943;49:323.
12. Cass W, Edelist G. Postspinal headache. JAMA 1974;227:786.
13. Fernandez E. Headaches associated with low spinal fluid pressure. Headache 1990;30:122.
14. Alksne JF. Headache Associated with Changes in Intracranial Pressure. In D Dalessio (ed), Wolff's Headache and Other Head Pain (4th ed). New York: Oxford University Press, 1980;301.
15. Headache Classification Committee of the International Headache Society. Classification and diagnostic criteria for headache disorders, cranial neuralgias, and facial pain. Cephalalgia 1988;8(Suppl 7):51.
16. Bell WE, Joynt RJ, Sahs AL. Low spinal fluid pressure syndromes. Neurology 1958;8:157.
17. Schievink WI, Reimer R, Folger WN. Surgical treatment of spontaneous intracranial hypotension associated with a spinal arachnoid diverticulum. J Neurosurg 1994;80:736.
18. Teng P, Papatheodorou C. Primary cerebrospinal fluid hypotension. Los Angeles Neurol Soc 1968;33:121.
19. Baker CC. Headache due to spontaneous low spinal fluid pressure. Minn Med 1983;66:325.
20. Gaukroger PB, Brownridge P. Epidural blood patch in the treatment of spontaneous low CSF pressure headache. Pain 1987;29:199.
21. Labadie EL, van Antwerp J, Bamford CR. Abnormal lumbar isotope cisternography in an unusual case of spontaneous hypoliquorrheic headache. Neurology 1976;26:135.
22. Molins A, Alvarez J, Sumalla J, et al. Cisternographic pattern of spontaneous liquoral hypotension. Cephalalgia 1990;10:59.
23. Raskin NH. Lumbar puncture headache: A review. Headache 1990;30:197.
24. Page F. Intracranial hypotension. Lancet 1953;2:6749.
25. Rando TA, Fishman RA. Spontaneous intracranial hypotension: Report of two cases and review of the literature. Neurology 1992;42:481.
26. Diamond S, Baltes BJ. Headache associated with low spinal fluid pressure syndrome (primary intracranial hypotension). Illinois Medical Journal 1973;144:560.
27. Lasater GM. Primary intracranial hypotension. Headache 1970;10:63.
28. Mokri B, Krueger BR, Miller GM, Piepgras DG. Meningeal gadolinium enhancement in low-pressure headaches. J Neuroimaging 1993;3:11.
29. Sipe JC, Zyroff J, Waltz TA. Primary intracranial hypotension and bilateral isodense subdural hematomas. Neurology 1981;31:334.
30. Nosik WA. Intracranial hypotension secondary to lumbar nerve sleeve tear. JAMA 1955;157:1110.
31. Berlit P, Berg-Dammer E, Kuehne D. Abducens nerve palsy in spontaneous intracranial hypotension [scientific note]. Neurology 1994;44:1552.
32. Garcia-Albea E, Cabrera F, Tejeiro J, et al. Delayed postexertional headache, intracranial hypotension, and racket sports [letter]. J Neurol Neurosurg Psychiatry 1992;55:975.
33. Yamamoto M, Suehiro T, Nakata H, et al. Primary low cerebrospinal fluid pressure syndrome associated with galactorrhea. Intern Med 1993;32:228.
34. Shenkin HA, Finneson BE. Clinical significance of low cerebral spinal fluid pressure. Neurology 1958;8:157.
35. Dana C. Puncture headache. JAMA 1917;68:1017.
36. Dripps RD, Vandam LD. Long-term follow-up of patients who received 10,098 spinal anesthetics. JAMA 1954;156:1486.
37. Tourtellotte WW, Haerer AF, Heller GL, et al. Post–lumbar puncture headaches. Springfield, IL: Thomas, 1964.
38. Kuntz KM, Kokmen E, Stevens JC, et al. Post–Lumbar Puncture Headaches: Experience in 501 consecutive procedures. Neurology 1992;42:1884.
39. DiGiovanni AJ, Dunbar BS. Epidural injections of autologous blood for post–lumbar puncture headache. Anesth Analg 1970;49:268.
40. Vilming ST, Schrader H, Monstad I. The significance of age, sex, and cerebrospinal fluid pressure in post–lumbar puncture headache. Cephalalgia 1989;9:99.
41. Tourtellotte WW. A randomized double-blind clinical trial comparing the 22 versus 26 gauge needle in the production of post–lumbar puncture syndrome in normal individuals. Headache 1972;12:73.

42. Bolder PM. Post–lumbar puncture headache in pediatric oncology patients. Anesthesiology 1986;65:696.
43. Iqbal J, Davis LE, Orrison WW. An MRI study of lumbar puncture headaches. Headache 1995;35:420.
44. Pool JL. Myeloscopy: Intraspinal endoscopy. Surgery 1942;11:169.
45. Crawford JS. The prevention of headache consequent upon dural puncture. Br J Anaesth 1972;44:598.
46. Vandam L. Neurological sequelae of spinal and epidural anesthesia. Int Anesthesiol Clin 1986;24:231.
47. Glass H, Goldstein AS, Ruskin R, et al. Chronic postmyelogram headache. Arch Neurol 1971;25:168.
48. Bourekas EC, Jonathan SL, Lanzieri CF. Postcontrast meningeal MR enhancement secondary to intracranial hypotension caused by lumbar puncture. J Comput Assist Tomogr 1995;19:299.
49. Rasmussen BS, Blom L, Hansen P, et al. Postspinal headache in young and elderly patients. Anesthesiology 1989;44:571.
50. Geurts JW, Haanschoten MC, Van Wijk, et al. Post-dural headache in young patients. Acta Anaesthesiol Scand 1990;34:350.
51. Schaltenbrand G. Neuere Anschauugen zur Pathophysiologie der Liquorzirkulation. Zentralbl Neurochir 1938;3:290.
52. Schaltenbrand G. Normal and pathological physiology of the cerebrospinal fluid circulation. Lancet 1953;1:805.
53. Huber M. Spontaneous hypoliquorrhea: Seven observations. Schweiz Arch Neurol Neurochir Psychiatr 1970;106:9.
54. Murros K, Fogelholm R. Spontaneous intracranial hypotension with slit ventricles. J Neurol Neurosurg Psychiatry 1983;46:1149.
55. Paulson GW, Klawans HL. Benign orgasmic cephalgia. Headache 1974;13:181.
56. Gibson BE, Wedel DJ, Faust RJ, et al. Continuous epidural saline infusion for the treatment of low CSF pressure headache. Anesthesiology 1988;68:789.
57. Ferraraccio BE. Positional headache due to spontaneous intracranial hypotension [letter]. South Med J 1992;85:57.
58. Lake AP, Minckler J, Scanlan RL. Spinal epidural cyst: Theories of pathogenesis. J Neurosurg 1974;40:774.
59. Raskin NH. Headache. New York: Churchill Livingstone, 1988;290.
60. Kraemar G, Hopf HC, Eissner D. CSF hyperabsorption: A cause of spontaneous low CSF pressure headache. Neurology 1987;37(Suppl):230.
61. Weber WE, Heidendal GA, de Krom MC. Primary intracranial hypotension and abnormal radionuclide cisternography: Report of a case and review of the literature. Clin Neurol Neurosurg 1991;93:55.
62. Major O, Fedorcsak I, Sipos L, et al. Slit-ventricle syndrome in shunt operated children. Acta Neruchirurgica 1994;127:69.
63. Sable SG, Ramadan NM. Meningeal enhancement and low CSF pressure headache. Cephalalgia 1991;11:275.
64. Vilming ST, Titus F. Low Cerebrospinal Fluid Pressure. In J Olesen, P Tfelt-Hansen, KMA Welch (eds), The Headaches. New York: Raven, 1993;687.
65. Grant R, Condon B, Hart I, et al. Changes in intracranial CSF volume after lumbar puncture and their relationship to post-LP headache. J Neurol Neurosurg Psychiatry 1991;54:440.
66. Hochman MS, Naidich TP, Kobetz SA, et al. Spontaneous intracranial hypotension with pachymeningeal enhancement on MRI. Neurology 1992;42:1628.
67. Fishman RA. Intracranial hypotension [letter]. Neurology 1994;44:1981.
68. Good DC, Ghobrial M. Pathologic changes associated with intracranial hypotension and meningeal enhancement on MRI. Neurology 1993;43:2698.
69. Kasner SE, Rosenfeld J, Farber RE. Spontaneous intracranial hypotension: Headache with a reversible Arnold-Chiari malformation. Headache 1995;35:557.
70. Rice GG, Dabbs CH. The use of peridural and subarachnoid injections of saline solutions in the treatment of severe postspinal headache. Anesthesiology 1950;11:17.
71. Phillis JW, Delong RE. An involvement of adenosine in cerebral blood flow regulation during hypercapnia. Gen Pharmacol 1987;18:133.
72. Petersen RC, Freeman DP, Know CA, et al. Successful treatment of spontaneous low cerebrospinal fluid pressure headache [Abstract]. Ann Neurol 1987;22:148.
73. Aldrete JA. Persistent post-dural-puncture headache treated with epidural infusion of dextran. Headache 1993;33:265.
74. Parris WC. Use of the epidural blood patch in the treatment of chronic headache [letter]. Anesthesiology 1986;65:344.

22
Headache and the Neck

Nikolai Bogduk

Of all the headaches, headache of cervical origin is the least well accepted and the most often disputed. Yet, paradoxically, it is arguably the best understood in terms of its anatomy and physiology. What is controversial is not whether cervical headaches occur, but how often they occur and how they can be reliably distinguished from other entities.

Headache of cervical origin is pain stemming from the cervical spine that is referred to the head. In this regard, it is analogous to back pain referred to the buttocks or lower limbs. It is for this reason that experts on cervical headache are more likely to be found among spinal physicians, and among pain specialists who deal with spinal pain in general, than among neurologists.

Terminology presents some difficulty. The term *cervical headache* is convenient because it is succinct; it also combines the two critical elements—the patient has headache but it is cervical in origin. However, the term is also intrinsically misleading, in that it implies that the headache is in the neck. The better term would be *cervicogenic headache,* but that term has been captured and identified with one group of researchers who have used a particular, idiosyncratic approach to this entity.[1–3] This leaves *cervical headache* as the only available generic term that encompasses all manner of headaches of cervical origin.[4]

NEUROANATOMY

Central to the mechanisms of cervical headache is the trigeminocervical nucleus, the column of gray matter formed by the pars caudalis of the spinal nucleus of the trigeminal nerve and the gray matter of the upper three cervical spinal cord segments.[5–8] To this column relay nociceptive afferents from the trigeminal nerve and from the first three cervical spinal nerves.[7] The trigeminal and spinal afferents each form multiple collateral terminals, and within the trigeminocervical nucleus these terminals overlap and converge on common second-order neurons. This convergence constitutes the basis for referred pain.

Convergence between cervical afferents can result in referral of pain from one cervical receptive field to another. An example might be pain from neck muscles that is perceived in the distribution of the greater occipital nerve. Convergence between trigeminal and cervical afferents may result in cervical pain being perceived in the territory of the trigeminal nerve. In this regard, it is the first division of the trigeminal nerve that exhibits the greatest overlap with terminals of cervical nerves. Consequently, cervical pain is most commonly referred to the territory of the first division of the trigeminal nerve.

A variety of clinical experiments have demonstrated these patterns of referral. Electrical stimulation of the C1 dorsal roots produces pain in the forehead, orbit, and vertex.[9] Stimulation of the posterior neck muscles with injections of hypertonic saline and other agents produces a variety of patterns of referred pain to the head.[10–13] Distension of the C2–3 zygapophyseal joint with injections of contrast medium produces occipital headache in normal volunteers,[14] as does distension of the atlanto-occipital or atlantoaxial joints.[15]

PERIPHERAL ANATOMY

The neuroanatomy of the trigeminocervical nucleus dictates that afferents from the upper three cervical nerves are the most likely to converge with trigeminal afferents. Consequently, any of the structures innervated by the first three cervical nerves would be potential sources of referred head pain. These include the joints and ligaments of the median atlantoaxial joint,[16] the atlanto-occipital[17] and lateral atlantoaxial joints,[17,18] the C2–3 zygapophyseal joint,[19] the suboccipital and upper posterior neck muscles,[19] the upper prevertebral muscles,[20] the spinal dura mater,[16] the vertebral artery,[21–23] the C2–3 intervertebral disk,[24,25] and the trapezius and sternocleidomastoid.[20]

HISTORICAL PERSPECTIVE

Gordon Holmes[26] is perhaps the earliest prominent physician to have recognized that headaches could arise from the neck. He addressed headaches associated with tender nodules in the posterior neck muscles, which were ascribed to fibrositis. This gave rise to the notion of "rheumatic" headache, an idea shared by his contemporaries.[27,28]

In time this notion was resurrected[29] or replaced by views that headaches could be caused by trigger points[30,31] or weakened fibro-osseous insertions.[32,33] The problem that besets this literature is that it is declarative but not scientific. Signs of tenderness were declared as the cardinal diagnostic criterion, and treatment was recommended in the form of injections of local anesthetics or sclerosants. However, at no time has the pathology of the alleged lesion been demonstrated; nor have the diagnostic tests or recommended treatments ever been subjected to controlled studies.

Indeed, it has been shown that tender areas occur in various neck and head muscles in many forms of headache, including migraine.[34–37] They are not necessarily indicative of the cause of the headache and may simply be secondary features or epiphenomena. Furthermore, recent studies have cast doubt on the ability of expert observers to agree on the presence of a trigger point.[38] Consequently, it is questionable whether such tender areas represent primary areas of muscle pathology.

Nevertheless, the notion of a tender-spot headache still attracts adherents, who seem unperturbed by the lack of compelling clinical and therapeutic data and are satisfied that their alleged experience of success in treating such headaches vindicates the notion.

A major milestone in the history of cervical headache was the announcement by Hunter and Mayfield[39] in 1949 that occipital neuralgia could be caused by compression of the greater occipital nerve between the posterior arch of the atlas and C2. By 1955, however, Mayfield[40] was more reserved about his earlier success in the treatment of the condition by greater occipital neurectomy.

That report, however, did not prevent the beginning and persistence of a fashion for greater occipital nerve blocks and greater occipital neurectomy for the treatment of occipital headache.[41–45] The practice of greater occipital neurectomy has been challenged,[46,47] and it has been shown[48] that the greater occipital nerve cannot be damaged in the way proposed by Hunter and Mayfield.[39] The alternate view has been proposed that occipital headache probably represents referred pain from upper cervical synovial joints.[47,49–53] The fashion for greater occipital nerve blocks, however, has not waned; and their use remains a contemporary issue.

A parallel stream of thought was initiated by Barré.[54] He proposed that headaches could be caused by irritation of the vertebral nerve by arthritis of the cervical spine. Others adopted or endorsed that contention and added that a whole host of cervical lesions could cause headache in the same way.[55–60] By most of these authors, however, the mechanism of headache has not been more explicitly defined than as "irritation of the vertebral nerve." Only Pawl[60] ventured to state that irritation of the vertebral nerve by cervical disk lesions or other lesions produces an autonomic barrage that results in spasm of the vertebrobasilar system, which produces head pain by causing ischemia of the vessel walls.

In both humans and the monkeys the so-called vertebral nerve consists of no more than gray rami communicantes accompanying the vertebral artery, and moreover, stimulation of these nerves, or of the cervical sympathetic trunk, in the monkey, failed to influence vertebral blood flow.[22] Thus, neither anatomic nor physiologic evidence was found that could support the vertebral nerve irritation theory. These experimental findings supported clinical opinion that there was no basis for belief in the Barré syndrome, otherwise known as migraine cervicale.[61,62]

Another explanation has been that headaches are caused by cervical spondylosis. This belief, however, has never been supported by appropriate epidemiologic data, particularly in view of the fact that cervical spondylosis is just as common in asymptomatic individuals as in patients with neck pain.[63]

The notion that occipital headache arises in cervical spondylosis because of spasm of the posterior neck muscles that attach to the occiput[60,64–67] has never been verified, electromyographically or otherwise. Treatment of lower cervical spondylosis by anterior cervical fusion can relieve the associated headache, but not in all cases.[60,66,67] Other authorities[68,69] consider arthrosis of the upper cervical synovial joints to be the source of headache in cervical spondylosis. Because these joints are innervated by the C1–3 spinal nerves, they have direct access to the neuroanatomic pathways that mediate referred pain to the head. For this reason, studies of the upper cervical joints remain an unresolved issue in cervical headache.

CONTEMPORARY ISSUES

The modern era is characterized by a shift away from reliance on declarations based on clinical experience and toward evidence-based medicine. Consonant with this shift have been studies that have pursued the mechanism and cause of cervical headache according to scientific principles as opposed to enthusiastic polemic. Gradually, the notions of the earlier part of this century are being replaced by systematic studies and data.

Cervicogenic Headache

An entity proposed by Sjaastad et al.,[1] cervicogenic headache has captured the attention of other European groups.[70] It is defined by clinical features, cardinal among them unilaterality, provocation of headache by neck movements or by pressure over points in the neck, neck pain, and reduced range of motion of the neck.[3] The headache is said to be characterized by nonclustering episodes, varying duration, and pain of a nonthrobbing nature emanating from the neck and spreading into the oculofrontotemporal regions of the head; the headaches may be accompanied by nausea, vomiting, dizziness, phonophobia, photophobia, blurred vision, and difficulty swallowing.[3]

Studies of cervicogenic headache have focused on distinguishing it from cluster headache with respect to forehead sweating[71] and pupillometry,[72] and on looking for radiographic features, of which none have been found.[70,73] Otherwise, it has been argued[1,74] that cervicogenic headache may previously have been described by Barré[54] and by Hunter and Mayfield.[39]

The frailty of this entity is that its definition and diagnosis rely on a constellation of clinical features; however, none of those features—nor any combination of them—is unique to headaches of cervical origin. The same features can occur in migraine and in tension-type headache, and even in cluster headache and chronic paroxysmal hemicrania. The features that are said to indicate a cervical source are weak and nonspecific.

As discussed previously, tenderness in the posterior neck muscles is not specific to any particular cause of headache. Reduced neck motion is difficult to quantify and to identify reliably, and does not necessarily imply a pain-producing lesion in the cervical spine.

One available distinguishing criterion is that blockade of cervical structures or cervical nerves should relieve headache of cervical origin.[75] Following initial observations in this regard,[76] others explored it in subsequent studies and found that many, but not all, patients diagnosed clinically as having cervicogenic headache could be temporarily relieved of their pain by blocking of the greater occipital nerve or the C2 spinal nerve.[70,77] Response to such diagnostic blocks, however, has not been incorporated as an essential diagnostic criterion for cervicogenic headache[3] but without such a discriminating criterion, the entity will remain a contentious issue among physicians intent on defining headache purely on clinical features and clinical patterns.

Neck-Tongue Syndrome

Neck-tongue syndrome is a disorder characterized by acute unilateral occipital pain precipitated by sudden movement of the head, usually rotation, and accompanied by a sensation of numbness in the ipsilateral half of the tongue.[78] The pain appears to be caused by temporary subluxation of a lateral atlantoaxial joint, whereas the numbness of the tongue arises because of impingement, or stretching, of the C2 ventral ramus against the edge of the subluxated articular process.[79] The numbness occurs because proprioceptive afferents from the tongue pass from the ansa hypoglossi into the C2 ventral ramus.[78]

Neck-tongue syndrome can occur in patients with rheumatoid arthritis or with congenital joint laxity.[80] Hypomobility in the contralateral lateral atlantoaxial joint may predispose one to the condition.[80]

Some investigators have found immobilization by a soft collar to be adequate therapy[81]; others have resorted to atlantoaxial fusion[80] or resection of the C2 spinal nerves.[82] Surgical findings have confirmed that the syndrome involves compression of the C2 spinal nerves by the lateral atlantoaxial joint.[82]

C2 Neuralgia

A characteristic form of headache can be caused by lesions affecting the C2 spinal nerve. The C2 nerve runs behind the lateral atlantoaxial joint, resting on its capsule.[18,79] Inflammatory or other disorders of the joint may cause the nerve to become incorporated in the fibrotic changes of chronic inflammation.[83,84] Release of the nerve relieves the symptoms. Otherwise, the C2 spinal nerve and its roots are surrounded by a sleeve of dura mater and a plexus of epiradicular veins, lesions of which can compromise the nerve. These include meningioma,[85] neurinoma,[83] and anomalous vertebral arteries,[86] but the majority of reported cases have involved venous abnormalities, ranging from single to densely interwoven dilated veins surrounding the C2 spinal nerve and its roots[87] to U-shaped arterial loops or angiomas compressing the C2 dorsal root ganglion.[83,87,88]

Nerves affected by vascular abnormalities exhibit a variety of features indicative of neuropathy, such as myelin breakdown, chronic hemorrhage, axon degeneration and regeneration, and increased endoneurial and pericapsular connective tissue.[87] It is not clear, however, whether the vascular abnormality causes the neuropathic changes or is only coincident with them.

C2 neuralgia is characterized by intermittent, lancinating pain in the occipital region associated with lacrimation and ciliary injection. The pain typically occurs in association with a background of dull occipital pain and dull, referred pain in the temporal, frontal, and orbital regions. Most often, this latter pain is focused on the fronto-orbital region, but when severe it encompasses all three regions. However, the distinguishing feature of C2 neuralgia is a cutting or tearing sensation in the occipital region, which is the hallmark of its neurogenic basis.

The frequency of attacks varies from four to five per day to two to seven per week, alternating with pain-free intervals of days, weeks, or months.[83,87] Some 75% of patients suffer the associated features of ipsilateral conjunctival and ciliary injection and lacrimation.[83,87] Blurred vision, rhinorrhea, and dizziness are less common accompaniments. Neurologic examination is normal. In particular, hypesthesia in the territory of the trigeminal or cervical nerves is not present.

C2 neuralgia is distinguished from referred pain from the neck by its neurogenic quality, its periodicity, and its association with lacrimation and ciliary injection. The latter association has attracted the appellation of "cluster-like" headache.[85] The cardinal diagnostic feature is complete relief of pain following local anesthetic blockade of the suspected nerve root, typically the C2 spinal nerve, but occasionally the C3 nerve. These blocks are performed under radiologic control and employ discrete amounts (0.6–0.8 ml) of long-acting local anesthetic to block the target nerve selectively.[83]

There is no evidence that C2 neuralgia responds to pharmacotherapy.[87] Surgery appears to be the only definitive means of treatment. Nerves entrapped by scar may be liberated[84]; meningiomas may be excised.[85] With respect to venous anomalies, resection of the vascular abnormality alone does not reliably relieve the pain; resection or thermocoagulation of the nerve appears to be necessary to guarantee relief of pain.[87] This calls into question whether the vascular anomaly is really the responsible lesion, particularly in view of the fact that in 50% of cadavers the C2 roots are surrounded by a dense venous network.[89]

Third Occipital Headache

A number of studies have implicated the C2–3 zygapophyseal joint in the causation of headache. Trevor-Jones[50] first drew attention to this region when he reported three patients with headache in whom surgical exploration revealed entrapment of the third occipital nerve by osteophytes of the C2–3 zygapophyseal joint. Release of the nerve relieved the headache. Poletti[53] reported one patient who suffered from occipital headache and who had posttraumatic arthritis of the C2–3 zygapophyseal joint. Her pain was relieved by resection of the joint. Maigne[90,91] claimed that headaches arising from the C2–3 zygapophyseal joint could be diagnosed and treated by injections of local anesthetic and manual therapy.

Bogduk and Marsland[92,93] pursued Maigne's claims but used fluoroscopically controlled blocks instead of office procedures. They described a small number of patients whose headache could be relieved by anesthetizing either the C2–3 zygapophyseal joint or the third occipital nerve, which innervates that joint.

Although heralded by some,[94] third occipital headache has been disputed by others.[95,96] A recent study, however, using controlled diagnostic blocks of the third occipital nerve, has shown that third occipital headache is common among victims of whiplash injury, accounting for 58% of patients whose major complaint after whiplash is headache.[97]

Third occipital headaches exhibit no characteristic clinical features that distinguish them from other forms of headache,[92,93,97] but careful manual examination can elicit pathognomonic features of a symptomatic zygapophyseal joint at C2–3.[98] However, the mainstay of diagnosis is the use of controlled blocks of the third occipital nerve.[97]

There is no proven treatment for third occipital headache. Intra-articular corticosteroids do not offer reliable relief.[99] Percutaneous thermocoagulation of the third occipital nerve has been tried, but the results are unreliable. Dramatic and lasting relief can be achieved in some patients, but in others difficulties arise in adequately coagulating the target nerve.[100]

Atlantoaxial Joints

The lateral atlantoaxial joints can be anesthetized with periarticular[52] or intra-articular[101] injections of local anesthetic. Applying such blocks relieves headaches in some patients. Ehni and Benner[52] reported relief of headache in seven patients who showed noticeable osteoarthritis of the lateral atlantoaxial joint on roentgenography but who otherwise (clinically) would have been diagnosed as suffering from occipital neuralgia. They advocated treatment with repeated blocks, or with intradural C2 rhizotomy if blocks failed to achieve relief. Others have reported success with fusion of the C1–2 segment.[102]

Although these studies demonstrate in principle that the lateral atlantoaxial joint can be a source of headache, the prevalence of this etiology has not been established.

Occipital Neuralgia

The International Association for the Study of Pain (IASP) defines occipital neuralgia as "pain, usually deep and aching, in the distribution of the second cervical dorsal root."[103] The International Headache Society (IHS) defines it as "paroxysmal jabbing pain in the distribution of the greater or lesser occipital nerves, accompanied by diminished sensation or dysaesthesiae in the affected area."[4] However, although the IHS stipulates sensory abnormalities in its definition, they are not listed among the diagnostic criteria.

The two definitions differ in one critical respect: The IHS stipulates that the pain must be paroxysmal and jabbing pain, whereas the IASP describes it as deep and aching pain, and only sometimes stabbing in nature. The IASP states that "nerve block may give relief," but the IHS insists that temporary relief by anesthetic block is a diagnostic criterion. This inconsistency and contradiction are characteristic of the literature on occipital neuralgia. There is no consensus on definition or diagnostic criteria, and the rubric is used loosely if not arbitrarily to refer to any pain felt in the occipital region.

The term *neuralgia* explicitly means pain stemming from a nerve and should be reserved for such conditions. Paroxysmal lancinating pain is the hallmark of neuralgia and should be an essential diagnostic criterion for occipital neuralgia, if that term is to be used. In this respect the definition of the IASP is in error. Deep, aching pain in the occiput can arise from a variety of sources and causes, not the least of which are diseases of the posterior cranial fossa and base of skull[53] and the upper cervical joints.[52,92,93,97,101] Indeed, the IHS comments that occipital neuralgia must be distinguished from occipital referral of pain from the atlantoaxial or upper zygapophyseal joints.[4]

The IASP definition would include these latter conditions even though they do not involve irritation or compression of the greater occipital nerve or even the C2 spinal nerve. Deep, aching pain in the occiput is no more than deep, aching pain in the occiput, for which a specific cause should be found. The habit of ascribing such pain to irritation of the greater occipital nerve stems from an era when neurologists and neurosurgeons were oblivious to somatic referred pain and had to ascribe any and every pain to a nerve.

There is no compelling evidence that occipital pain is due to irritation of the greater occipital nerve. Lancinating occipital neuralgia has been recorded as a feature of temporal arteritis,[104] in which inflammation of the occipital artery could affect the companion nerve. However, in the majority of cases of so-called occipital neuralgia, no such pathology is evident.

No one has produced compelling evidence of entrapment of the greater occipital nerve. The response to liberation of the nerve where it pierces the trapezius relieves headache in some 80% of cases, but the relief has a median duration of only some 3–6 months.[105] Excision of the greater occipital nerve provides relief in some 70% of patients, but this has a median duration of only 244 days.[106]

The cardinal diagnostic criterion seems to be response to blocks of the greater occipital nerve; but these blocks are not target specific when they involve volumes such as 5[105] or 10 ml[107,108]; thus, they do not selectively implicate the greater occipital nerve (or the lesser occipital nerve if that is the target).

Of concern is the clinical similarity between lancinating occipital neuralgia and what has been described previously as C2 neuralgia. In the latter condition, Jansen and colleagues[83,87,88] portray the C2 ganglion as the site of irritation. Their evidence that vascular lesions are the cause is not convincing, but their histologic evidence of neuropathy at this site is. It may well be that in all cases of lancinating occipital neuralgia, clinicians should investigate for lesions proximal to the greater occipital nerve instead of fixing on a traditional site that has borne no therapeutic fruit. Meanwhile, deep and aching occipital pain should invite investigation of the upper cervical joints and the posterior cranial fossa.

There are mixed reports about the treatment of intractable, idiopathic occipital neuralgia. Dorsal rhizotomy at C1–3 or C1–4 has provided some patients with complete relief for 1–4 years, but some nevertheless suffer recurrences.[109] Partial posterior rhizotomy at C1–3 appears to provide good relief while preserving touch sensation, but not all patients respond adequately.[110] Unfortunately, these procedures are so radical that they provide us with little insight into the mechanisms of occipital neuralgia, save to warn that even complete deafferentation of the affected region does not guarantee pain relief.

DISCUSSION

Cervical headache is not a distinctive clinical entity like migraine. It is an expression of referred pain from the upper segments of the neck. There is no single cause of cervical headache; any of the muscles, joints, nerves, or other components of the upper cervical spine could be the source of pain. However, the source of pain in a given case cannot be identified by clinical examination, nor can it be inferred from the clinical features of the pain and its associated features.

Contemporary investigators have probably been addressing variants of the same phenomenon. Where they differ is only with respect to what they presume to be the source of pain or the degree to which they have pursued that source. Thus, proponents of cervicogenic headache[1,70] are not fundamentally at odds with those who espouse an arthropathic model.[52,92,93,97] The difference lies only in the strength of the evidence that implicates a particular source of pain.

The use of diagnostic blocks has emerged as the cardinal and critical tool in the modern study of cervical headaches. When imaging studies fail or are unable to reveal lesions of the neck that might reasonably be the cause of headache, diagnostic blocks are the only feasible means of pursuing a cervical source of pain. Diagnostic blocks have been used to implicate the C2 spinal nerve in C2 neuralgia,[83] the C2–3 zygapophyseal joint in third occipital headache,[92,93,97] and the lateral atlantoaxial joint in occipital neuralgia.[52] Blocks of the greater occipital nerve have been implemented in the pursuit of the source of cervicogenic headache.[70,74,77] They also have continued to be applied in the investigation and treatment of headache without regard to the nosologic status of the headache.[107,108]

Diagnostic blocks, however, are fraught with pitfalls and limitations. Although the use of large volumes may be justified on humanitarian grounds in that it secures relief (albeit temporary) for patients, it provides no useful scientific data. Volumes such as 5 or 10 ml spread extensively throughout the posterior muscles of the neck, and no specific target is selectively anesthetized. This nonspecificity prevents any scientific conclusions about cervical headache, even if the patients appear to respond.

Most critical is the need for controls. Without controls an observer cannot distinguish between the pharmacologic effects of the injection and nonspecific effects such as the charisma of the physician, the setting of the procedure, expectation, and conditioning; nor can they determine that the apparent therapeutic effect was not due simply to the hydraulic distension of the tissues injected. For these reasons, case series that report success with injections no longer constitute compelling evidence in any argument about the causes of headaches.

Injections of normal saline constitute the most rigorous control, but ethical considerations restrict their application. A single-blind injection of normal saline without informed consent could be construed as assault in some legal jurisdictions. Single-blind injections are also not immune to operator bias. Double-blind injections ensure that an operator tries just as hard with the active agent as with the dummy agent. No studies of cervical headache have yet employed the rigorous technique of double-blind, placebo-controlled diagnostic blocks.

A compromise is available, however. Saline controls can be circumvented without loss of scientific rigor by using comparative blocks. These require that the blocks be repeated on separate occasions but using different local anesthetic agents under double-blind conditions. A positive response is accepted only if the patient obtains complete relief of pain on both occasions but reports short-lasting relief when a short-acting agent is used, and long-lasting relief when a long-acting agent is used. This paradigm has been formally evaluated and vindicated.[111] Moreover, it has now been shown that positive diagnostic decisions based on this paradigm are robust against challenge with placebo.[112] Comparative blocks are able to rule in true positive responders. Failure to satisfy the diagnostic criteria does not prove that the patient *does not* have pain, but if a patient *does* satisfy the diagnostic criteria, he or she is almost certainly a true positive responder.

Comparative blocks have been used to date only in the study of third occipital headache.[97] Therefore, only that entity has survived and satisfied scientific criteria. Conclusions drawn from other studies remain to be corroborated by controlled studies.

Still of concern is the lack of any pathologic anchor for cervical headache. Blocks may indicate the nerves that mediate symptoms, but they do not reveal lesions. Even in patients who respond positively to controlled blocks, no evidence has been found of the actual cause of pain.

Those authors who have pursued an arthropathic model argue that, circumstantially, patients who have posttraumatic headache are likely to have injured joints in their neck, and they use diagnostic blocks to identify which joint is the source of pain. Studies have yet to appear that correlate morphologic evidence of joint damage to response to blocks. The same kind of correlation should be required of those who claim muscle injury or ligament damage to the neck. Neither controlled blocks nor pathologic data have been brought to bear on this argument, let alone a correlation between blocks and morphology.

Most vexatious is the persisting view that blocking the greater occipital nerve relieves headache. This nerve supplies only the skin of the scalp, and no lesions affect this skin that might reasonably be a source of chronic pain. If response to greater occipital nerve blocks can be shown to be a genuine phenomenon, a conceptual nightmare would arise. It would be evident that blocks in the cervical region do not exert a specific, peripheral antinociceptive effect, but somehow instead exert a modulatory effect on the trigeminocervical nucleus.

Indeed, this concept of modulatory effect has already been raised in critiques of cervical headache.[95] However, there is no objective evidence for the phenomenon; it remains only a speculative concept. Were it to be proved, however, it would put cervical headache squarely back into the central nervous system along with its relatives, migraine and tension-type headache.

REFERENCES

1. Sjaastad O, Saunte C, Hovdahl H, Breivik H, et al. "Cervicogenic" headache: An hypothesis. Cephalalgia 1983;3:249.
2. Fredriksen TA, Hovdal H, Sjaastad O. "Cervicogenic headache": Clinical manifestation. Cephalalgia 1987;7:147.
3. Sjaastad O, Fredriksen TA, Pfaffenrath V. Cervicogenic headache: Diagnostic criteria. Headache 1990;30:725.
4. Headache Classification Committee of the International Headache Society. Classification and diagnostic criteria for headache disorders, cranial neuralgias, and facial pain. Cephalalgia 1988;8(Suppl 7):1
5. Humphrey T. The spinal tract of the trigeminal nerve in human embryos between 7½ and 8½ weeks of menstrual age and its relation to early fetal behaviour. J Comp Neurol 1952;97:143.
6. Torvik A. Afferent connections to the sensory trigeminal nuclei, the nucleus of the solitary tract, and adjacent structures. J Comp Neurol 1956;106:51.
7. Kerr FWL. Structural relation of the trigeminal spinal tract to upper cervical roots and the solitary nucleus in the cat. Exp Neurol 1961;4:134.
8. Taren JA, Kahn EA. Anatomic pathways related to pain in face and neck. J Neurosurg 1962;19:116.

9. Kerr FWL. A mechanism to account for frontal headache in cases of posterior fossa tumors. J Neurosurg 1962;18:605.
10. Cyriax J. Rheumatic headache. BMJ 1938;2:1367.
11. Campbell DG, Parsons CM. Referred head pain and its concomitants. J Nerv Ment Dis 1944;99:544.
12. Feinstein B, Langton JBK, Jameson RM, Schiller F. Experiments on referred pain from deep somatic tissues. J Bone Joint Surg Am 1954;36A:981.
13. Wolff HG. Headache and Other Head Pain (2nd ed). New York: Oxford University Press, 1963;582.
14. Dwyer A, Aprill C, Bogduk N. Cervical zygapophyseal joint pain patterns. I: A study in normal volunteers. Spine 1990;15:453.
15. Dreyfuss P, Michaelsen M, Fletcher D. Atlanto-occipital and lateral atlanto-axial joint pain patterns. Spine 1994;19:1125.
16. Kimmel DL. Innervation of the spinal dura mater and dura mater of the posterior cranial fossa. Neurology 1960;10:800.
17. Lazorthes G, Gaubert J. L'innervation des articulations interapophysaire vertebrales. Comptes Rendues de l'Association des Anatomistes 1956;488.
18. Bogduk N. Local anaesthetic blocks of the second cervical ganglion: A technique with application in occipital headache. Cephalalgia 1981;1:41.
19. Bogduk N. The clinical anatomy of the cervical dorsal rami. Spine 1982;7:319.
20. PL Williams, R Warwick, M Dyson, LH Bannister (eds). Gray's Anatomy (37th ed). Edinburgh: Churchill Livingstone, 1989.
21. Hovelacque A. Anatomie des Nerfs Craniens et Rachidiens et du Systeme Grand Sympathique. Paris: Doin, 1927.
22. Bogduk N, Lambert G, Duckworth JW. The anatomy and physiology of the vertebral nerve in relation to cervical migraine. Cephalalgia 1981;1:1.
23. Kimmel DL. The cervical sympathetic rami and the vertebral plexus in the human foetus. J Comp Neurol 1959;112:141.
24. Bogduk N, Windsor M, Inglis A. The innervation of the cervical intervertebral discs. Spine 1989;13:2.
25. Mendel T, Wink CS, Zimny ML. Neural elements in human cervical intervertebral discs. Spine 1992;17:132.
26. Holmes G. Headaches of organic origin. Practitioner 1913;1:968.
27. Patrick HT. Indurative or rheumatic headache. JAMA 1913;71:82.
28. Luff AP. The various forms of fibrositis and their treatment. BMJ 1913;1:756.
29. Kelly M. Headaches, traumatic and rheumatic: The cervical somatic lesion. Med J Aust 1942;2:479.
30. Travell J. Mechanical headache. Headache 1962;7:23.
31. Travell J, Rinzler SH. The myofascial genesis of pain. Postgrad Med 1952;11:425.
32. Hackett GS, Huang TC, Raftery A. Prolotherapy for headache. Headache 1962;2:20.
33. Kayfetz DO, Blumenthal LS, Hackett GS, Hemwall GA, et al. Whiplash injury and other ligamentous headache: Its management with prolotherapy. Headache 1963;3:24.
34. Perelson HN. Occipital nerve tenderness: A sign of headache. South Med J 1947;40:653.
35. Olesen J. Some clinical features of the acute migraine attack: An analysis of 750 patients. Headache 1978;18:268.
36. Lous I, Olesen J. Evaluation of pericranial tenderness and oral function in patients with common migraine, muscle contraction headache, and combination headache. Pain 1982;12:385.
37. Langemark M, Olesen J. Pericranial tenderness in tension headache. Cephalalgia 1987;7:249.
38. Wolfe F, Simons DG, Fricton J, et al. The fibromyalgia and myofascial pain syndromes: A preliminary study of tender points and trigger points in persons with fibromyalgia, myofascial pain, and no disease. J Rheumatol 1992;19:944.
39. Hunter CR, Mayfield FH. Role of the upper cervical roots in the production of pain in the head. Am J Surg 1949;78:743.
40. Mayfield FH. Symposium on cervical trauma: Neurosurgical aspects. Clin Neurosurg 1955;2:83.
41. Chambers WR. Posterior rhizotomy of the second and third cervical nerves for occipital pain. JAMA 1954;155:431.
42. Cusson D, King A. Cervical rhizotomy in the management of some cases of occipital neuralgia. Bulletin of the Guthrie Clinic 1960;29:198.
43. Knight G. Post-traumatic occipital headache. Lancet 1963;1:6.
44. Hammond SR, Danta G. Occipital neuralgia. Clin Exp Neurol 1978;15:258.
45. Murphy JP. Occipital neurectomy in the treatment of headache. MD State Med J 1969;18:62.
46. Weinberger LM. Cervico-occipital pain and its surgical treatment. Am J Surg 1978;135:243.
47. Bogduk N. Greater Occipital Neuralgia. In DM Long (ed), Current Therapy in Neurological Surgery (2nd ed). Philadelphia: Decker, 1989;263.

48. Bogduk N. The anatomy of occipital neuralgia. Clin Exp Neurol 1980;17:167.
49. Dugan MC, Locke S, Gallagher JR. Occipital neuralgia in adolescents and young adults. N Engl J Med 1962;267:1166.
50. Trevor-Jones R. Osteoarthritis of the paravertebral joints of the second and third cervical vertebrae as a cause of occipital headache. S Afr Med J 1964;30:392.
51. Sigwald J, Jamet F. Occipital Neuralgia. In PJ Vinken, GW Bruyn (eds), Handbook of Clinical Neurology (Vol 5). New York: Elsevier, 1968;368.
52. Ehni G, Benner B. Occipital neuralgia and the C1-2 arthrosis syndrome. J Neurosurg 1984;61:961.
53. Poletti CE. Proposed operation for occipital neuralgia: C-2 and C-3 root decompression. Neurosurgery 1983;12:221.
54. Barré N. Sur un syndrome sympathique cervicale posterieure et sa cause frequente: L'arthrite cervicale. Rev Neurol (Paris) 1926;33:1246.
55. Gayral L, Neuwirth E. Oto-neuro-ophthalmologic manifestations of cervical origin: Posterior cervical sympathetic syndrome of Barré-Lieou. NY State J Med 1954;54:1920.
56. Neuwirth E. Neurologic complications of osteoarthritis of the cervical spine. NY State J Med 1954;54:2583.
57. Kovacs A. Subluxation and deformation of the cervical apophyseal joints. Acta Radiol 1955;43:1.
58. Stewart DY. Current concepts of "Barré syndrome" or the "posterior cervical sympathetic syndrome." Clin Orthop 1962;24:40.
59. Dutton CD, Riley LH. Cervical migraine: Not merely a pain in the neck. Am J Med 1969;47:141.
60. Pawl RP. Headache, cervical spondylosis, and anterior cervical fusion. Surg Annu 1977;9:391.
61. Bartschi-Rochaix W. Headaches of Cervical Origin. In PJ Vinken, GW Bruyn (eds), Handbook of Clinical Neurology (Vol 5). New York: Elsevier, 1968;192.
62. Lance JW. Mechanism and Management of Headache (4th ed). London: Butterworth, 1982.
63. Friedenberg ZB, Miller WT. Degenerative disk disease of the cervical spine. J Bone Joint Surg Am 1963;45A:1171.
64. Raney AA, Raney RB. Headache: A common symptom of cervical disc lesions. Arch Neurol Psychiatry 1948;59:603.
65. Schultz EC, Semmes RE. Head and neck pains of cervical disc origin. Laryngoscope 1950;60:338.
66. Peterson DI, Austin GM, Dayes LA. Headache associated with discogenic disease of the cervical spine. Bull Los Angeles Neurol Soci 1975;40:96.
67. Chirls M. Retrospective study of cervical spondylosis treated by anterior interbody fusion in 505 patients performed by the Cloward technique. Bull NY Hosp Joint Dis 1978;39:74.
68. Lord Brain. Some unsolved problems of cervical spondylosis. BMJ 1963;1:771.
69. Wilkinson M. Symptomatology. In M Wilkinson (ed), Cervical Spondylosis (2nd ed). London: Heinemann, 1971;59.
70. Pfaffenrath V, Dandekar R, Pollmann W. Cervicogenic headache: The clinical picture, radiologic findings, and hypotheses on its pathophysiology. Headache 1987;27:495.
71. Fredriksen TA. Cervicogenic headache: The forehead sweating pattern. Cephalalgia 1988;8:203.
72. Fredriksen TA, Wysocka-Bakowska MM, Bogucki A, Antonaci F. Cervicogenic headache: Pupillometric findings. Cephalalgia 1988;8:93.
73. Fredriksen TA, Fougner R, Tangerud A, Sjaastad O. Cervicogenic headache: Radiological investigations concerning head/neck. Cephalalgia 1989;9:139.
74. Sjaastad O. Cervicogenic headache: The controversial headache. Clin Neurol Neurosurg 1992;94:S147.
75. Bogduk N. Headache and the cervical spine. Cephalalgia 1984;4:167.
76. Sjaastad O, Fredriksen TA, Stolt-Nielsen A. Cervicogenic headache, C2 rhizopathy, and occipital neuralgia: A connection? Cephalalgia 1986;6:189.
77. Bovim G, Berg R, Dale LG. Cervicogenic headache: Anaesthetic blockades of cervical nerves (C2–C5) and facet joint (C2/C3). Pain 1992;49:315.
78. Lance JW, Anthony M. Neck tongue syndrome on sudden turning of the head. J Neurol Neurosurg Psychiatry 1980;43:97.
79. Bogduk N. An anatomical basis for neck tongue syndrome. J Neurol Neurosurg Psychiatry 1981;44:202.
80. Bertoft ES, Westerberg CE. Further observations on the neck-tongue syndrome. Cephalalgia 1985;5(Suppl 3):312.
81. Fortin CJ, Biller J. Neck tongue syndrome. Headache 1985;25:255.
82. Elisevich K, Stratford J, Bray G, Finlayson M. Neck tongue syndrome: Operative management. J Neurol Neurosurg Psychiatry 1984;47:407.
83. Jansen J, Markakis E, Rama B, Hildebrandt J. Hemicranial attacks or permanent hemicrania: A sequel of upper cervical root compression. Cephalalgia 1989;9:123.

84. Poletti CE, Sweet WH. Entrapment of the C2 root and ganglion by the atlanto-epistrophic ligament: Clinical syndrome and surgical anatomy. Neurosurgery 1990;27:288.
85. Kuritzky, A. Cluster headache–like pain caused by an upper cervical meningioma. Cephalalgia 1984;4:185.
86. Sharma RR, Parekh HC, Prabhu S, Gurusinghe NT, et al. Compression of the C2 root by a rare anomalous ectatic vertebral artery. J Neurosurg 1993;78:669.
87. Jansen J, Bardosi A, Hildebrandt J, Lucke A. Cervicogenic, hemicranial attacks associated with vascular irritation or compression of the cervical nerve root C2: Clinical manifestations and morphological findings. Pain 1989;39:203.
88. Hildebrandt J, Jansen J. Vascular compression of the C2 and C3 roots: Yet another cause of chronic intermittent hemicrania? Cephalalgia 1984;4:167.
89. Bovim G, Bonamico L, Fredriksen TA, Lindboe C, et al. Topographic variations in the peripheral course of the greater occipital nerve. Spine 1991;16:475.
90. Maigne R. Une signe evocateur et inattendu de cephalee cervicale: "La douleur au pince-roule du sourcil." Annales de Medicine Physique 1976;19:416.
91. Maigne R. Signes cliniques des cephalees cervicales: Leur traitement. Medecine et Hygiene 1981;39:1171.
92. Bogduk N, Marsland A. On the concept of third occipital headache. J Neurol Neurosurg Psychiatry 1986;49:775.
93. Bogduk N, Marsland A. The cervical zygapophyseal joints as a source of neck pain. Spine 1988;13:610.
94. Third-nerve headache [editorial]. Lancet 1986;2:374.
95. Edmeads J. The cervical spine and headache. Neurology 1988;38:1874.
96. Edmeads J, Soyka D. Headache Associated with Disorders of the Skull and Cervical Spine. In J Olesen, P Tfelt-Hansen, KMA Welch (eds), The Headaches. New York: Raven, 1993;741.
97. Lord S, Barnsley L, Wallis B, Bogduk N. Third occipital headache: A prevalence study. J Neurol Neurosurg Psychiatry 1994;57:1187.
98. Jull G, Bogduk N, Marsland A. The accuracy of manual diagnosis for cervical zygapophyseal joint pain syndromes. Med J Aust 1988;148:233.
99. Barnsley L, Lord SM, Wallis BJ, Bogduk N. Lack of effect of intraarticular corticosteroids for chronic pain in the cervical zygapophyseal joints. N Engl J Med 1994;330:1047.
100. Lord SM, Barnsley L, Bogduk N. Percutaneous radiofrequency neurotomy in the treatment of cervical zygapophyseal joint pain: A caution. Neurosurgery 1995;36:732.
101. McCormick CC. Arthrography of the atlanto-axial (C1-C2) joints: Technique and results. J Intervent Radiol 1987;2:9.
102. Joseph B, Kumar B. Gallie's fusion for atlantoaxial arthrosis with occipital neuralgia. Spine 1994;19:454.
103. Merskey H, Bogduk N (eds). Classification of Pain: Descriptions of Chronic Pain Syndromes and Definitions of Pain Terms (2nd ed). Seattle: International Association for the Study of Pain, 1994;64.
104. Jundt JW, Mock D. Temporal arteritis with normal erythrocyte sediment rates presenting as occipital neuralgia. Arthritis Rheum 1991;34:217.
105. Bovim G, Fredriksen TA, Stolt-Nielsen A, Sjaastad O. Neurolysis of the greater occipital nerve in cervicogenic headache: A follow-up study. Headache 1992;32:175.
106. Anthony M. Headache and the greater occipital nerve. Clin Neurol Neurosurg 1992;94:297.
107. Saadah HA, Taylor FB. Sustained headache syndrome associated with tender occipital nerve zones. Headache 1987;27:201.
108. Gawel MJ, Rothbart PJ. Occipital nerve block in the management of headache and cervical pain. Cephalalgia 1992;12:9.
109. Horowitz MB, Yonas H. Occipital neuralgia treated by intradural dorsal nerve root sectioning. Cephalalgia 1993;13:354.
110. Dubuisson D. Treatment of occipital neuralgia by partial posterior rhizotomy at C1-3. J Neurosurg 1995;82:581.
111. Barnsley L, Lord S, Bogduk N. Comparative anaesthetic blocks in the diagnosis of cervical zygapophyseal joint pain. Pain 1993;55:99.
112. Lord SM, Barnsley L, Bogduk N. The utility of comparative local anaesthetic blocks versus placebo-controlled blocks for the diagnosis of cervical zygapophyseal joint pain. Clin J Pain 1995;11:208.

23
Headache and the Temporomandibular Joint

Steven B. Graff-Radford

This chapter addresses the topic of temporomandibular disorders (TMD) and how they relate to headache, discussing the evidence for and against the relationship. Of particular interest is whether there is a relationship between headache and temporomandibular dysfunction (incoordination of intracapsular parts), and further, whether there is a relationship between the occlusion (how the teeth meet) and the temporomandibular joint. Another area of controversy to be discussed is the relationship of tension-type headache to the tender muscles seen with myofascial pain. Myofascial pain and tension-type headache are well-described clinical entities whose etiology is still unknown.

CLASSIFICATION AND ETIOLOGY

Tension-type headache has previously been called tension headache, muscle contraction headache, stress headache, essential headache, and psychogenic headache. Tension-type headache can be either episodic or chronic.[1] The International Headache Society[1] describes episodic tension-type headache as "recurrent episodes of headache lasting minutes to days." The pain is typically pressing or tightening in quality, of mild or moderate intensity, bilateral in location, and does not worsen with routine physical activity. Nausea is absent, but photophobia and phonophobia may be present. Chronic tension-type headache is present for at least 15 days per month during at least 6 months (see Chapters 11 and 12).

The relevance of pericranial tenderness is unknown. It resembles myofascial pain. Treatment of this type of head pain often involves a physical medicine approach accompanied by cognitive behavioral techniques. Additional treatments include pharmacotherapy, occlusal therapy, and surgery.

Temporomandibular disorders is a collective term embracing a number of clinical problems that involve the masticatory musculature, the temporomandibular joint, and associated structures. Numerous other terms have been used to describe this problem, including *oromandibular disorders.*[2] The most common symptom is pain, usually localized in the muscles of mastication, the preauricular area, or the temporomandibular joint. The pain is characteristically aggravated by jaw function. Additional characteristics are limited or asymmetric jaw movements as well as joint noise on movement, or locking on opening. The relationship of TMD to headache is still not certain; it may be causal, coincidental, or only an aggregating factor.

Epidemiologic studies of TMD have shown that approximately 75% of people have at least one sign of TMD, and about 33% have at least one symptom (e.g., pain, joint sounds, limited jaw range of motion).[3–5] It is estimated, however, that only 5% need treatment.[3,4,6] TMD seems to be a self-limiting condition that fluctuates over time, but rarely is seen in patients older than 40. Signs and symptoms of TMD do not increase in prevalence with age. Knowledge regarding the natural history of TMD is limited, and further investigation is required to determine which patients develop chronic problems.

Temporomandibular disorders are often separated into muscle disorders and disorders of the temporomandibular joints. In practice these problems usually coexist, but they may occur independently. The most common muscle disorder is myofascial pain, which is associated with pericranial tenderness (trigger points) with characteristic pain referral patterns.[7] The muscle pain and tenderness are thought to be secondary to muscle hyperactivity. Bruxism and parafunctional habits have been suggested as perpetuating factors. There is, however, at this time, little scientific evidence to support either claim. If muscle hyperactivity is present, one should at least be able to show some electrical or neurologic changes in the muscles. The International Headache Society classification makes clear that in tension-type headache, electromyelography is normal. Simons has hypothesized, based on findings of spontaneous electrical activity and spike potentials produced by compression or increased acetylcholine release, that there may be extrafusal motor end-plate changes in trigger points.[8] The initiation of this spontaneous electrical activity has not been determined. Only in myospasm or voluntary splinting are there obvious electromyelography changes. Additionally, clenching and grinding (bruxism) are almost universal,[9–13] and there does not appear to be a statistically significant association between these disorders and muscle pain.[14,15]

It is, therefore, possible that muscle tenderness is secondary to activation in a CNS pathway that drives the pain. The CNS change may be secondary to alteration in descending neural inhibition or activation of central On-cells. The CNS change may also help in explaining why anesthesia of the peripheral tender areas decreases pain. It may be postulated that the anesthesia decreases peripheral feedback, which in turn decreases CNS sensitivity.

The relationship found between frequent headache and muscle hyperactivity has also been explored. Tenderness on palpation in the jaw muscles and muscle fatigue suggest that the masticatory muscle disturbances may be the underlying cause of headache pain.[14–17] Muscle tenderness could be referred hyperalgesia, thus the etiologic factor may not be in the muscle.[18,19]

The common painful disorders of the temporomandibular joint are internal derangements associated with inflammation. Internal derangement implies an anatomic disturbance of the disk–condyle relationship with consequent changes in the mechanics of the joint such as clicking, popping, locking, or momentary catching.[2] When inflammation is present with internal derangement, the patient experiences pain.

Other hypotheses for the etiology of TMD have included trauma, emotional stress, and occlusal disharmony; but, as is the case with the muscle hyperactivity hypothesis, none has been scientifically validated. The role of functional occlusal relationships in temporomandibular disorders has been reviewed by Seligman and Pullinger.[14,15] Their reviews do not support the role of occlusion as a principal causative factor in TMD. Seligman and Pullinger point out that controlled studies fail to demonstrate an association between occlusal interferences and TMD signs and symptoms in symptomatic nonpatients or in TMD patients. The frequency of occlusal interferences in the presence of TMD or when TMD does not exist is no different. Therefore, the finding of an occlusal problem does not indicate its involvement in TMD. There is speculation that a significant movement (> 2 mm) of the condyle from an intercuspal (teeth locked) position to a retruded condyle position is a cause of joint pathology. Seligman and Pullinger concluded that osteoarthrosis may cause the slides (from intercuspal position to retruded condyle position), rather than the slide causing the degeneration. There was insufficient evidence associating TMD with slides (movement from the intercuspal position to a retruded position). These findings are controversial, and other studies need to be done to prove or disprove the claims. Currently, there is a lack of evidence that the composition of an idealized occlusion through complex occlusal therapy is necessary for TMD management.[13–15] There is agreement that multiple factors influence the evolution of TMD and their interrelationship is yet to be determined.

The evaluation of the patient with TMD should include a history and physical examination, complemented by joint imaging in selective cases and psychological evaluation in cases that display chronic pain characteristics. The physical examination should cover range of motion, joint and muscle tenderness assessment through palpation, evaluation of joint sounds, and the effect of manipulation and functional (bite pressure) forces on the pain. Evaluation of the occlusion is thought to be important by some and not by others.[2] It is the present author's opinion that the occlusion is not a prominent factor in TMD. The use of mandibular movement recordings, electromyography, and Doppler auscultations are all considered experimental and at this time offer little if any information of use in diagnosis of TMD.[20,21]

TREATMENT

There are several treatment approaches to TMD, with little difference in outcome demonstrated. Caution should be taken against assuming that if a treatment is effective, it points to the etiology. Ideally, in treating TMD we would like to eliminate the cause, but too often the cause is unknown and we are left with only the option of managing the symptoms. In general, simple and reversible treatments are preferred to complicated and irreversible procedures. Patient education and home care constitute the mainstay of treatment for TMD.[2,8] The home program includes instruction on what can be chewed, muscle exercise with the aid of cold vapocoolant sprays, and behavioral modification addressing postural and oral habits, as well as controlling operant (behavioral) factors. Emotional stressors may be addressed through a number of stress management and relaxation techniques including biofeedback.

Appliance therapy is a physical medicine technique used routinely in management of TMD. It has been proposed that the effects seen with this technique are due to alteration of occlusal disharmony through an indirect effect on the muscles, or are related to an effect on bruxism. Clinical evidence suggests that appliance treatment is effective, but the reason it works is unknown.[2,22] Pharmacologic intervention for TMD is also useful. Tricyclic antidepressants decrease symptoms,[23] and anti-inflammatory drugs, the most commonly used medications, help manage the symptoms of inflammation.[2]

ASSOCIATION BETWEEN HEADACHE AND TEMPOROMANDIBULAR DISORDERS

Berlin et al.[24] were the first to draw attention to the association between TMD and headache. They noted in their study of bruxism and headache that treatments directed toward functional disturbances in the masticatory system has a positive effect on headache. Although several studies support a positive association between chronic oral parafunctional habits and TMD, these studies are based on patient reports of parafunction. Electromyographic research and dental attrition studies, which more accurately reflect the incidence of parafunctional habits, suggest that they are almost universal.[6,25–27] There is also increasing evidence that bruxism is not provoked by long-standing, naturally occurring occlusal variations. Despite the fact that men show greater occlusal wear, women more commonly are the TMD and headache patients. Some clinicians suggest that symptoms are caused by bruxism where the trauma exceeds the tolerance of muscles and joints, and that this breakdown is more common in women.[7]

In a headache population in whom bruxism was identified, an intraoral stabilization appliance markedly decreased the headache but did not alter the bruxism.[28] Further investigation is required to understand the role of bruxism and pain, but at this time the causal relationship is based on clinical speculation.

Reik described patients with headaches that were unilateral and continuous and did not fulfill criteria identified by the Ad Hoc Committee on Classification of Headache for temporomandibular joint pain dysfunction syndrome.[29] He identified these patients as a unique headache population. They responded to treatment with exercise and antidepressants as well as soft diet and salicylates. This description offers little evidence to clarify the relationship between TMD signs and antidepressant therapies.

About 70% of patients diagnosed with TMD are reported to suffer from headache.[30,31] Correlations between headaches and signs and symptoms of TMD have been found in children, adolescents,[32,33] and adults.[14,34,35] Further study is required to determine the causal relationship, especially considering the 70% incidence of signs in a nonpatient population. Is TMD the cause of headache or do the two simply coexist? Schiffman et al.[36] evaluated 27 tension headache patients and 28 migraine sufferers, in addition to 63 TMD (internal derangement) and 62 myofascial pain patients. There were significant differences in the specific signs of jaw dysfunction between the latter two groups. The TMD internal derangement group could be differentiated from the headache cohort using the presence of clicking and pain with maximal mouth opening, and pain with joint palpation. These two criteria had 92% sensitivity and 91% specificity. The myofascial pain group could be differentiated from the headache group using pain with maximum mouth opening, palpation of the joint, and lateral jaw movement. These criteria had a sensitivity of 77% and specificity of 85%. Because of the study's cross-sectional design, Schiffman et al. make no implication as to the relationship of TMD to headache.

The association between headache and TMD has been underscored by investigations showing improvement in recurrent headache from TMD treatment. This purported cause-and-effect relationship should be carefully evaluated in the context of each study. It is only when controlled populations are appropriately evaluated that these treatments prove no more effective than placebo. The following paragraphs review some studies that demonstrate the inadequacy of noncontrolled investigations, comparing them with the few available controlled studies.

Magnusson treated headache patients who had ill-fitting dentures with new dentures and reported a reduction in head pain. Little description is provided as to the headache type or the mechanism associated with success.[37] It is implied that the vertical dimension change that resulted from inserting the new dentures was the reason for headache reduction. The possible role of looking better or of eating better in pain reduction was not commented on. In an uncontrolled study, 33 TMD patients were treated by occlusal splint therapy.[30] Following 4 weeks of therapy, 64% of patients reported a decrease in the number of weekly headaches, and 30% showed a complete remission of headaches. Patients with high headache frequencies (four or more per week) responded more favorably to occlusal splint therapy. The placebo response was not controlled for, nor was there a clear definition of the type of headache. Treatment with splints is probably effective. The reasons and relationship to etiology are still unknown.

In another uncontrolled study of TMD patients, changes in headache were evaluated 1 year after the start of TMD treatment.[38] The treatment consisted of occlusal splints, therapeutic exercise for the lower jaw, occlusal adjustment, or, most often, combinations of these measures. Seventy percent of the patients reported less frequent headache than 1 year earlier. Forty-two percent reported less severe head pain. None of the treatments or combinations of treatments was significantly better in resolving headache frequency or severity than any other. This study suggests an important factor rarely controlled for in headache treatment: feelings of self-control. The treatment may have helped patients to better deal with their pain (with self-help techniques), even though the severity of pain was changed in only 42%. If we do anything for our patients, and give them an adequate explanation for their problems, many will improve. In an uncontrolled study by Graff-Radford et al. on 25 myofascial headache pain patients (without internal derangements), 90% had pain reduction at the end of treatment and at 12 months posttreatment. This study suggested that altering perpetuating factors such as posture, body mechanics, and stress was the reason for relief. The role of reduction of symptomatic medications or the relationship between the treatment and possible central nervous system headache was not considered.[39]

Recurrent headache patients, referred for neurologic examination, were invited for a functional examination of their stomatognathic system.[40] Among them,

55 patients had pain caused by TMD. In 51 patients the pain was myogenic, and in four it was arthrogenic. The 55 patients were divided at random into two groups.[41] One group was treated by the neurologist, according to conventional headache treatment regimens, and the other group was treated with stabilization splints for 6 weeks, supplemented in some cases by physical therapy. Two patients with arthrogenic pain received infrared laser treatment. In the TMD treatment group, headache frequency decreased in 56%, compared with 32% in the neurologic treatment group. The two groups also reported taking significantly different amounts of symptomatic medication to control headache. However, the TMD group had much greater exposure to the treating clinician, which could in part account for the difference. Additionally, the reduction in medication itself could have been an important factor in the reduction of pain (see discussions of drug-dependent headache in Chapters 8 and 12).

The study described previously did not use a control group. Forssell et al., in 1985, conducted a double-blind trial on 56 patients from a neurology clinic diagnosed with tension-type headache.[42] Treatments included an occlusal equilibration (adjustment) or a placebo equilibration. Patients were randomly assigned to active and placebo groups, and after a 4- to 8-month follow-up period a neurologist evaluated the treatment outcome. In the active group, headache frequency was reduced in 80% of patients and its intensity in 47%; in the placebo group, frequency and intensity were reduced in 50% and 16%, respectively. Forssell treated some of the patients from the placebo group and reported a significant reduction in headache frequency.[43] Except for the possible confound that the same clinician did both treatments (active and placebo) unblinded, this study again supports TMD treatment for headache associated with TMD signs and symptoms.

In a more recent study, Tsolka et al. studied 51 patients with TMD and divided them into two groups: One group received a mock occlusal adjustment, the other received adjustments to remove significant slides and nonworking slide interferences. Both groups received identical counseling. There was no significant difference in outcome between the two groups.[44] Although headache was not the primary description of pain, Goodman et al. used mock equilibration as a treatment in 25 myofascial pain patients. After the treatment 14 (64%) reported total or nearly total remission of their symptoms. This study emphasizes the power of placebo in this population group.[45]

The influence of the doctor–patient relationship was explored by Laskin[46] in myofascial pain dysfunction patients. A placebo drug, "Myolax" was presented to 50 patients with pain. A placebo effect was reported in 52% of the subjects.

Because TMD is believed to have a multifactorial etiology, it is usually assumed that the best results are achieved by using several different treatment methods to eliminate as many predisposing or perpetuating factors as possible. Most studies that look at treatment outcome use numerous treatment modalities and cannot describe the contribution of each. Wennenberg attempted to determine the effect of occlusal adjustment alone versus a combination therapy with occlusal splint, exercises, and in selected cases, minor occlusal adjustment. Significantly greater improvement occurred in the combination group compared with the equilibration group. In a well-controlled study, TMD patients receiving different treatments were compared.[47] Each group had 15 subjects; group O received occlusal equilibration, and group S received an intraoral appliance and home exercises.[1]

Although the exposure to the clinician was more than twice that of the S group, the O group achieved a poorer outcome.[2] This study again cautions the clinician against the overuse of occlusal equilibration. It was noted that headache symptoms were also reduced significantly more in the S group than in the O group.

Although it seems evident that TMD treatment is effective in headache management, it is still unclear which factors in treatment are responsible. In the case of arthrogenous pains, there appears to be an important relationship between function and pain. If functional manipulation in the presence of joint tenderness or internal derangement aggravates the pain, there is likely to be an association between joint pathology and the pain. Forssell et al.[48] showed that patients who had pain while chewing responded more favorably to TMD therapy in terms of headache reduction.

In a contrasting study, 100 headache patients were studied by Reik,[29] of whom 20 had previously received dental therapies without success. It was determined by the author that four of the 20 fit criteria for temporomandibular joint pain dysfunction syndrome and 16 fit criteria for other headache disorders. Care should be taken to clearly classify the pain using positive inclusion criteria, rather than to infer that if there is pain in the head, a dental therapy is likely to be effective.

In perhaps the best-controlled longitudinal study (3 years) of the association between occlusal interference and craniomandibular disorders (TMD), no association could be found when the effect of reduction in occlusal interferences was compared with that of mock equilibration.[49]

Temporomandibular joint surgery is considered to be useful treatment for certain TMDs. There are few temporomandibular surgery studies where headache symptoms are an outcome variable. Vallerand and Hall[50] reported on 50 patients diagnosed with temporomandibular joint internal derangement, myalgia, and headaches who had not responded to nonsurgical management. The surgical procedures the patients received included disk repositioning, repair of disk perforation, disk recontouring, lysis of adhesions, diskectomy, or a combination of those procedures. In the retrospective evaluation, most patients reported decreases in headache in addition to decreases in joint pain and noise. Headache frequency decreased from 80% pretreatment to 13% postsurgery, and severe headaches from 87–27%. The surgeons offer the explanation that the change in head pain is a secondary result of decreasing joint pain, which allowed the patients to cope better with other pains. In another study, Montgomery et al.[51] reported significant changes in temporomandibular joint, ear, neck, and shoulder pains, whereas headaches were less consistently changed following arthroscopy.

CONCLUSION

The treatment of TMD has a lot to offer the headache patient. There is significant evidence that the pain may be greatly helped through nonpharmacologic means. There is a need for an acceptable and tested classification system for TMD, which would facilitate determination of the mechanism by which treatments aimed at the joint, muscles, or teeth work. Could chronic pain arising from TMD activate central centers, causing migraine and tension-type headache? Could central nervous system events that initiate migraine produce peripheral nociception, so that mechanical problems become painful? It is essential to look beyond the joint, muscles, and teeth. What is the role of the central nervous system and the trigeminal system? Caution should be taken not to oversimplify the etiologic factors causing headache or to assume that if a treatment is effective, then the cause necessarily lies where the treatment is aimed.

REFERENCES

1. Headache Classification Committee of the International Headache Society (Olesen J, et al.). Classification and diagnostic criteria for headache disorders, cranial neuralgias, and facial pain. Cephalalgia 1988;8(Suppl 7):1.
2. McNeill C (ed). Craniomandibular Disorders: Guidelines for Evaluation, Diagnosis, and Management (2nd ed). Chicago: Quintessence, 1992.
3. Dworkin SF, LeResche LR, Von Korff, Howard J, et al. Epidemiology of signs and symptoms in temporomandibular disorders. I: Clinical signs in cases and controls. J Am Dent Assoc 1990;120:273.
4. Rugh JD, Solberg WK. Oral health status in the United States: Temporomandibular disorders. J Dent Educ 1985;49:393.
5. Schiffman E, Fricton JR. Epidemiology of TMJ and Craniofacial Pain. In JR Fricton, RJ Kroening, KM Hathaway (eds), TMJ and Craniofacial Pain: Diagnosis and Management. St. Louis: Ishiyaku EuroAmerica, 1988;1.
6. Schiffman E, Fricton JR, Haley D, Shapiro BL. The prevalence and treatment needs of subjects with temporomandibular disorders. J Am Dent Assoc 1989;120:295.
7. Travell JG, Simons D. Myofascial Pain and Dysfunction: The Trigger Point Manual. Baltimore: Williams & Wilkins, 1988.
8. Simons DG. Clinical and etiological update of myofascial pain from trigger points. J Musculoskel Pain 1996;4:93.
9. Attanasio R. Nocturnal bruxism and its clinical management. Dent Clin North Am 1991;35:245.
10. Faulkner KDB. Bruxism: A review of the literature, Part I. Aust Dent J 1990;35:266.
11. Faulkner KDB. Bruxism: A review of the literature, Part II. Aust Dent J 1990;35:355.
12. Ingerall B, Mohlin B, Thailander B. Prevalence of symptoms of functional disturbances of the masticatory system in Swedish men. J Oral Rehabil 1980;7:185.
13. Seligman DA, Pullinger AG, Solberg WK. The prevalence of dental attrition and its association with factors of age, gender, occlusion, and TMD symptomatology. J Dent Res 1988;67:1323.
14. Seligman DA, Pullinger AG. The role of functional occlusal relationships in temporomandibular disorders. J Craniomandib Disord Facial Oral Pain 1991;5:96.
15. Seligman DA, Pullinger AG. The role of intercuspal occlusal relationships in temporomandibular disorders: A review. J Craniomandib Disord Facial Oral Pain 1991;5:96.
16. Isacsson G, Linde C, Isberg A. Subjective symptoms in patients with temporomandibular joint disk displacement versus patients with myogenic craniomandibular disorders. J Prosthet Dent 1989;61:70.
17. Lous I, Olesen J. Evaluation of pericranial tenderness and oral function in patients with common migraine, muscle contraction headache, and combination headache. Pain 1982;12:385.
18. Mense S. Considerations concerning the neurobiological basis of muscle pain. Can J Physiol Pharmacol 1991;69:610.
19. Fricton JR, Dall'Arancio D, Schiffman E. Stretching exercises for myofascial pain: A randomized clinical trial. Pain 1997, in press.
20. Mohl ND, McCall WO, Lund JP, Plesh O. Devices for the diagnosis and treatment of temporomandibular disorders. Part I: Introducing scientific evidence and jaw tracking. J Prosthet Dent 1990;63:198.
21. Mohl ND, Lund JP, Widmer CG, McCall WO. Devices for the diagnosis and treatment of temporomandibular disorder. Part II: Electromyography, sonography. J Prosthet Dent 1990;63:332.
22. Lamay PJ, Barcley SC. Clinical effectiveness of occlusal splint therapy in patients with classic migraine. Scott Med J 1987;32:11.
23. Sharar Y, Singer E, Schmidt E, Dionne RA, et al. The analgesic effect of amitriptyline on severe facial pain. Pain 1987;31:199.
24. Berlin R, Dessner L. Bruxism and chronic headache. Lancet 1960;9:289.

25. Chun DS, Koskienen-Moffett L. Distress jaw habits and connective tissue laxity as predisposing factors to TMJ sounds in adolescents. J Craniomandib Disord Facial Oral Pain 1990;4:165.
26. Clark GT, Jow RW, Lee JJ. Jaw pain and stiffness levels after repeated maximum voluntary clenching. J Dent Res 1989;68:69.
27. Sherman RA. Relationship between jaw pain and jaw muscle contraction level: Underlying factors and treatment effectiveness. J Prosthet Dent 1985;54:114.
28. Holmgren K, Sheilcholeslam A, Rise C. Effect of a full-arch maxillary occlusal splint on parafunctional activity during sleep in patients with nocturnal bruxism and signs and symptoms of craniomandibular disorders. J Prosthet Dent 1993;9:293.
29. Reik L, Hale M. The temporomandibular joint pain and dysfunction syndrome: A frequent cause of headache. Headache 1981;21:151.
30. Kemper JT, Okeson JP. Craniomandibular disorders and headaches. J Prosthet Dent 1983;49:702.
31. Magnusson T, Carlsson GE. Comparison between two groups of patients in respect of headache and mandibular dysfunction. Swed Dent J 1978;2:85.
32. Egermark-Eriksson I. Mandibular dysfunction in children and individuals with dual bite. Swed Dent J 1982;6(Suppl 10):230.
33. Wanman A, Agerberg G. Headache and dysfunction of the masticatory system in adolescents. Cephalalgia 1986;6:247.
34. Forssell H, Kangasniemi P. Mandibular dysfunction in patients with migraine. Proc Finn Dent Soc 1984;80:211.
35. Magnusson T, Carlsson GE. Recurrent headaches in relation to temporomandibular joint pain dysfunction. Acta Odontol Scand 1978;36:333.
36. Schiffman E, Heley D, Baker C, Lindgren B. Diagnostic criteria for screening headache patients for temporomandibular disorders. Headache 1995;35:121.
37. Magnusson T. Changes in chronic headache and mandibular dysfunction after treatment with new complete dentures. J Oral Rehabil 1982;9:95.
38. Magnusson T, Carlsson GE. Changes in recurrent headache and mandibular dysfunction after various types of dental treatment. Acta Odontol Scand 1980;38:311.
39. Graff-Radford SB, Reeves JL, Jaeger B. Management of head and neck pain: The effectiveness of altering perpetuating factors in myofascial pain. Headache 1987;27:186.
40. Schokker RP, Hansson TL, Ansink BJJ. The results of treatment of the masticatory system of chronic headache patients. J Craniomandib Disord Facial Oral Pain 1990;4:126.
41. Schokker RP, Hansson TL, Ansink BJJ. Craniomandibular disorders in headache patients. J Craniomandib Disord Facial Oral Pain 1989;3:71.
42. Forssell H, Kirveskari P, Kangasniemi P. Changes in headache after treatment of mandibular dysfunction. Cephalalgia 1985;5:229.
43. Forssell H, Kirveskari P, Kangasniemi P. Response to occlusal treatment in headache patients previously treated by mock occlusal adjustment. Acta Odontol Scand 1987;45:77.
44. Tsolka P, Morris RW, Preiskel HW. Occlusal adjustment therapy for craniomandibular disorders: A clinical assessment by a double-blind method. J Prosthet Dent 1992;68:957.
45. Goodman P, Greene CS, Laskin DM. Response of patients with myofascial pain dysfunction syndrome to mock equilibration. J Am Dent Assoc 1976;92:755.
46. Laskin DM, Greene CS. Influence of the doctor-patient relationship on placebo therapy for patients with myofascial pain dysfunction (MPD) syndrome. J Am Dent Assoc 1972;85:892.
47. Wennenberg B, Nystrom T, Carlsson G. Occlusal equilibration and other stomatognathic treatment in patients with mandibular dysfunction and headache. J Prosthet Dent 1988;59:478.
48. Forssell H, Kirveskari P, Kangasniemi P. Distinguishing between headaches responsive and irresponsive to treatment of mandibular dysfunction. Proc Finn Dent Soc 1986;82:219.
49. Kirveskari P, Alarin P, Jamsa T. Association between craniomandibular disorders and occlusal interferences. J Prosthet Dent 1989;61:66.
50. Vallerand WP, Hall MB. Improvement in myofascial pain and headaches following TMJ surgery. J Craniomandib Disord Facial Oral Pain 1991;5:197.
51. Montgomery MT, Van Sickels JE, Harms SE, Thrash WJ. Arthroscopic TMJ surgery: Effects on signs, symptoms, and disk position. J Oral Maxillofac Surg 1989;47:1263.

Index

In this index, page numbers in italic indicate figures, and t indicates a table.